W0050693

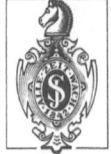

A. Uchida · K. Ono (Eds.)

Recent Advances in Musculoskeletal Oncology

With 97 Illustrations

Springer Japan KK

Associate Professor ATSUMASA UCHIDA, M.D.
Professor KEIRO ONO, M.D.
Department of Orthopedic Surgery, Osaka University Medical School, Fukushima, 1-1-50, Osaka, 553 Japan

ISBN 978-4-431-68366-7   ISBN 978-4-431-68364-3 (eBook)
DOI 10.1007/978-4-431-68364-3

© Springer Japan 1992

Originally published by Springer-Verlag Tokyo Berlin Heidelberg New York in 1992
Softcover reprint of the hardcover 1st edition 1992

This work is subject to copyright. All rights are reserved, whether the whole or part of the material is concerned, specifically the rights of translation, reprinting, reuse of illustrations, recitation, broadcasting, reproduction on microfilms or in other ways, and storage in data banks.
The use of registered names, trademarks, etc. in this publication does not imply, even in the absence of a specific statement, that such names are exempt from the relevant protective laws and regulations and therefore free for general use.
Product liability: The publisher can give no guarantee for information about drug dosage and application thereof contained in this book. In every individual case the respective user must check its accuracy by consulting other pharmaceutical literature.

Typesetting: Best-set Typesetter Ltd., Hong Kong

Preface

Je le pensay, et Dieu le guarist

Ambroise Paré

This was not fully validated in malignant tumors, whichever systems or organs they may have originated in. Amputation immediately after diagnosis was not rewarding for patients with musculoskeletal malignancy until the development in the last 20 years of adjuvant chemotherapy and oncologic surgical techniques based on the appropriate staging system.

Ever since the advent of effective systemic chemotherapy, further improvements in its regimen have been made, based on various theories concerning cell-cycle-dependent drug sensitivity, drug combinations to minimize tumor resistance, and dose intensity to enhance the fractional kill of tumor cells. Histologic subtype, aggressiveness, and particularly the anatomic setting of the lesions were found to be the determinants of surgical results in the treatment of musculoskeletal malignancy and hence integrated as a surgical staging system by Ennecking.

It is essentially important for all orthopedic surgeons, oncologists, radiologists, nurses, and co-medical staff to dedicate their whole-hearted devotion to the cause of a modern oncology regimen to combat the patients' suffering before God's mercy is bestowed on them. Fortunately expenditure for the treatment of these malignant diseases is covered by the national medical insurance scheme in Japan. Yet the physical, psychological, educational, and occupational costs for the patients accompanying the management of the oncology should not be ignored. Less than 70% survivorship for osteogenic sarcoma seems to be less than rewarding for all these events related to the whole process of treatment.

What will the next breakthrough be in musculoskeletal oncology? The answer to this question should focus on achieving earlier detection of the lesions, inhibiting and suppressing spread, and improving systematized treatment by medical, surgical, and physical modalities, in other words, the rational method, including enhancement of a patient's self-cure potential, as Paré prayed for his patients. This was enthusiastically discussed at the 23rd Annual Meeting of the Musculoskeletal Oncology Society of the Japanese Orthopedic

Association, 1990, in Osaka. Plenary lectures, selected papers at the Meeting, and further invited papers have been collected and organized here in this book, with the aim of introducing recent advances in musculoskeletal oncology in Japan and the world. As a potential breakthrough, emphases are placed on the following subjects: new image technology, new assessment modalities of tumor aggressiveness, development and refinement of chemotherapy and heavy particle irradiation, limb saving surgery and newly developed tumor prostheses, progress in assessment and surgical management of metastatic bone disease, comprehensive supportive care for patients, and rehabilitation programs.

Even the children, knowing fully well the grave situation in which they are placed by these malignant tumors, make efforts with nausea and fatigue to reconcile themselves to their lot, hiding the tragedy of the mental agony of loneliness within themselves. We should never forget that any progress in oncology could not be accomplished without the patient's positive collaboration. This book is dedicated to all our undefeated patients.

KEIRO ONO
ATSUMASA UCHIDA

Contents

Part 4 Surgical Treatment

Part 5   Prognostic Factors

Part 6   Total Care

List of Contributors

Part 1
Diagnosis

Section I
Diagnostic Technology

Imaging Diagnosis in Orthopedics: A Basic Introduction to the Interpretation of MRI

Hitoshi Katayama[1]

Introduction

Although interpretation of simple X-ray films is an excellent first step in imaging diagnosis in orthopedics, the recent advance of magnetic resonance imaging (MRI) has had a great impact on this field. MRI is often compared with X-ray computerized tomography (CT) due to the similarity of their images. The principles of X-ray absorption governing the reading of conventional X-ray film can be directly applied to the interpretation of X-ray CT. However, MRI is produced by the principle of magnetic resonance, a technique fundamentally different from that of roentgenography. Thus, it is essential for clinicians to understand the basic principle of MR in order to correctly interpret the information provided by MRI.

MRI: Fundamental Principles

The understanding of fundamental MRI principles are essential to the interpretation of the findings. MRI can be performed after a human body becomes a macroscopic bar magnet (M_0) by placing the body in a strong magnetic field (B_0). This bar magnet (M_0) maintains a certain angle to the direction (Z axis) of a magnetic field (B_0), and precesses around the Z axis (in a motion resembling the movement of a top aligned with the earth's gravitational field) at a certain speed called the "resonance frequency," which is determined by various nuclei and the strength of the static magnetic field (B_0) (Fig. 1).

Next, a magnetic field (B_1), rotating at a certain speed and at a right angle to the static magnetic field (B_0), is applied from outside. This second magnetic field (B_1) has a frequency equal to the resonance frequency (ω_0) of the bar magnet (M_0).

[1] Department of Radiology, Juntendo University, School of Medicine, Bunkyo-ku, Tokyo, 113 Japan

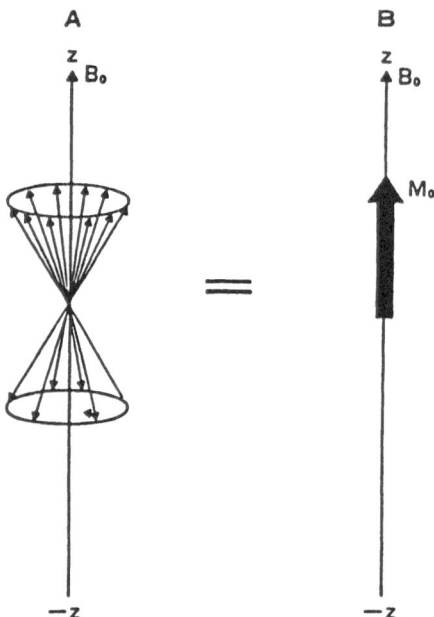

Fig. 1. A In a strong static magnet (B_0), proton magnets array at the same angle to the Z-axis, pointing either towards Z or $-Z$. **B** The macroscopic bar-magnet (M_0) winds up in the Z-direction because of the predominance of Z-direction proton magnets. (From [19] with permission)

The second magnetic field (B_1) is actually provided in the form of high frequency waves (radiowaves). Thus, a macroscopic bar magnet (M_0) can be laid down to the plane crossing the Z axis at a right angle (X-Y plane), when energy is applied as radiowaves for a certain duration. This high frequency pulse is called a "90 degree pulse" (Fig. 2).

In this manner, M_0 rotates around the axis of the B_1 direction by a pulse of 90 degrees. Because B_1 also rotates at the resonance frequency ω_0, M_0 has, therefore, a complicated movement: M_0 rotates around the axis of the B_1 direction by a pulse of 90 degrees while rotating around the Z axis at ω_0. When the 90 degree pulse is turned off at a certain point in time, M_0 continues to rotate around the Z axis at the resonance frequency ω_0 because B_0 is the only external magnetic field. As M_0 moves back to the B_0 direction, an AC current is induced. This is an MR signal. The various MR signals provide MR images through Fourier transformation (Fig. 3). There are various pulse sequences of MRI, but the spin echo (SE) is predominantly used for routine MRI of the musculoskeletal system.

How to Read MRI

We should have some understanding of different MR signal intensities in order to read MRI properly. The signal intensity of MRI depends on internal factors being endogenically present in objects (tissues or lesions) and also on external factors which can be determined by the operator. The internal factors include (1) proton density (P), (2) longitudinal relaxation time (T1), and (3) transverse

Fig. 2. A macroscopic bar magnet (M_0) is laid down at an angle of 90 degrees to the X-Y plane with a charge of a magnetic field (B_1), which directs it to the X-Y plane and rotates it at a resonance frequency (ω_0). (From [19] with permission)

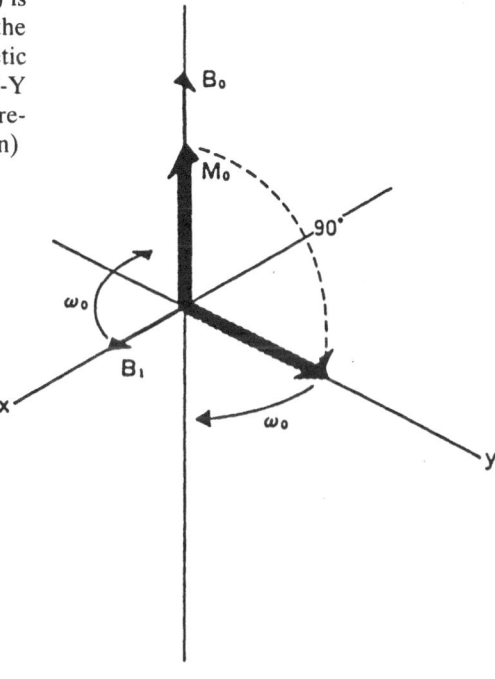

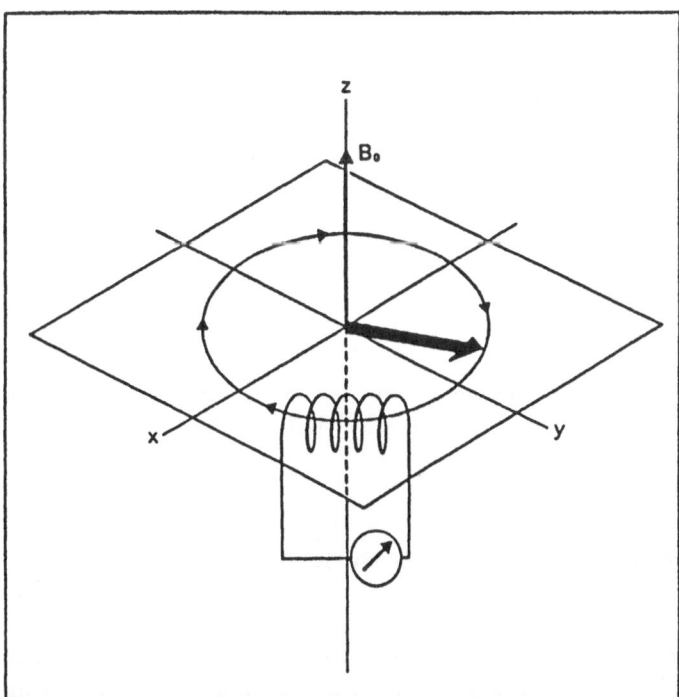

Fig. 3. An induction current is obtained on the X-Y plane by a rotating magnetic field. This is a magnetic resonance signal. *Large arrow*, macroscopic bar magnet at 90 degrees to the X-Y plane; *small arrow*, direction of static magnet. (From [19] with permission)

relaxation time (T2). The external factors include repetition time (TR) and echo time (TE).

Spin echo (SE) is a universal technique in MRI of bones and joints, and understanding of the significance of these parameters and their reciprocal correlation is essential for MRI interpretation.

TR (repetition time) indicates the duration between a 90 degree pulse and the next 90 degree pulse, applied to create a spin echo signal. When a short TR is selected, images weighting the effect of T1 relaxation time are obtained.

TE (echo time) indicates the duration between a 90 degree pulse and an echo signal peak. When a long TE is selected, the images' weighting effect of T2 relaxation time are obtained.

A spin is laid down by a 90 degree pulse in the direction at a right angle to the magnetic field, and the spin starts to return to the original position when the 90 degree pulse is switched off. The speed of returning to the original position (direction of the magnetic field) differs among tissues and lesions. There are two relaxation times. They are T1 (longitudinal relaxation time) and T2 (transverse relaxation time), which act as vector components. Since these parameters (T1 and T2) differ according to the state of an individual tissue and lesion, they have different signal intensities and different contrasts on MRI.

Images mainly reflecting a difference in parameters T1 and T2 are called T1- and T2-weighted images, respectively. There is a third image mainly reflecting proton density, the proton-weighted image. MRI, having different contrasts even in the same site, can be easily obtained with a different selection of the parameters. In other words, a contrast on MRI can be reversed technically. Such a conversion never occurs on X-ray CT. Before reading an MRI, it is mandatory to determine the sequence of the MRI by checking the parameters (TR, TE) (Fig. 4). The relation of TR and TE to T1-, T2-, and proton-weighted images is shown in Table 1. The above is only a cursory background for MRI interpretation, and further study of the physics of MRI is necessary for effective clinical use of this information.

Normal and Abnormal MRI of Bone and Soft Tissue

The cortical bone creates almost no signals because of its very low proton density, and is observed as a black band on ordinary MRI. The tendon, ligament, joint capsule, and fibrous cartilage also have a low signal intensity. The hyaline cartilage shows an intermediate signal intensity. The fatty tissue of the bone marrow and of other sites shows markedly short T1 and appears white, indicating an area of high signal intensity, especially on the T1-weighted image.

Bone tumors are usually observed as an area of low signal intensity on T1-weighted images, showing apparent contrast to bone marrow fat. Bone tumors invading into soft tissue are observed as an area of high signal intensity on T2-weighted images, giving useful information of their relation to soft part components such as neurovascular bundles (Fig. 5) [1]. We occasionally

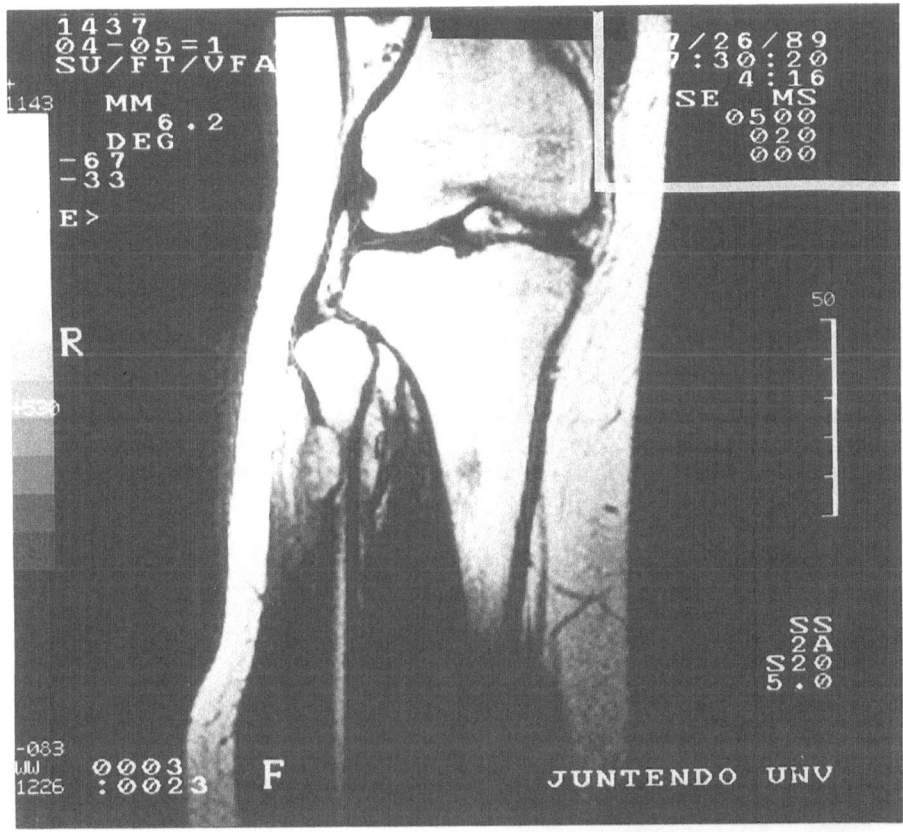

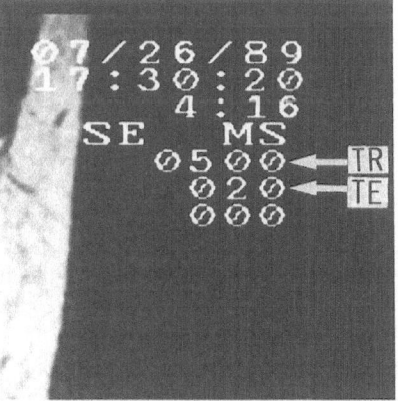

Fig. 4. A T1-weighted image of the knee joint (Toshiba MRT-200). The pulse sequence (TR, TE) is indicated in the *right upper corner*. This is an image of spin echo (SE) with TR 500 ms/TE 20 ms. A close-up view is shown *below*

see fluid levels in bone cyst, aneurysmal bone cyst, giant cell tumor, and teleangiectatic osteosarcoma (Fig. 6). Normal muscle shows low signal intensity. It should be borne in mind that an area of abnormal signal intensity does not always correspond to the extent of the tumor because surrounding reactive changes, such as edema and congestion, also show a similar abnormal signal

Table 1. Relation of TR, TE, and MRI (T1, T2, and proton images)

TR	TE	SE Image
Short (<500 ms)	Short (<20 ms)	T1-Weighted image
Long (>2,000 ms)	Long (>70 ms)	T2-Weighted image
Long (>5,000 ms?)	Short (<10 ms?)	Proton-weighted image

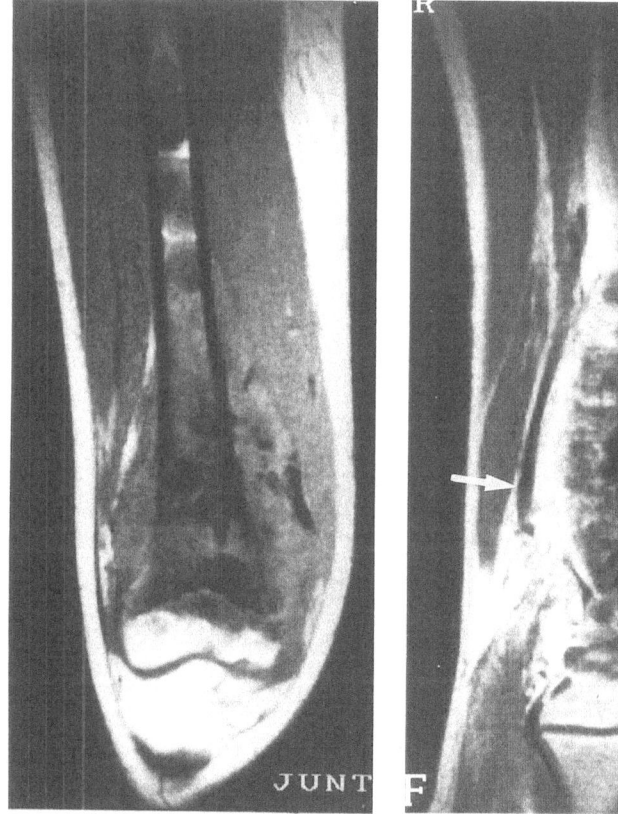
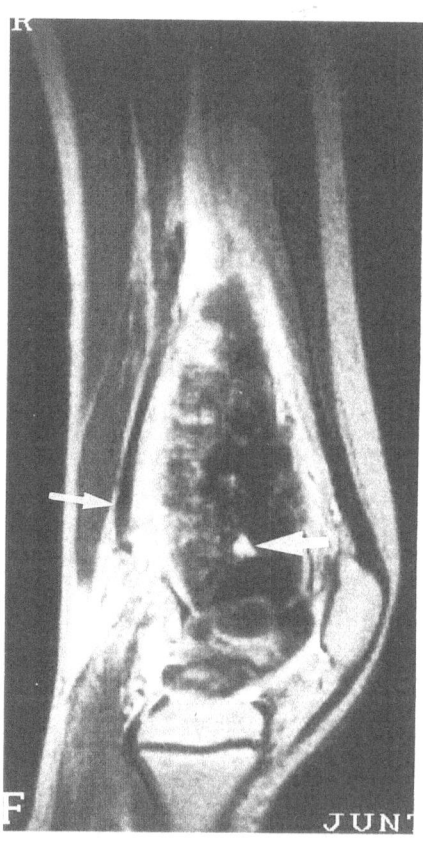

Fig. 5a,b. An osteosarcoma of the right femur in a 9-year-old female. **a** T1-weighted image (SE 500/20). Intraosseous extension of the tumor is shown as an area of low signal intensity (*dark area*). **b** A T2-weighted image (SE 2000/80). A soft part involvement is shown as an area of high signal intensity (*white*). The popliteal artery is probably involved (*arrow*). *Arrow* indicates hemorrhage

intensity. MR contrast media would help to differentiate in such circumstances [2]. A marginal sclerotic rim on the roentgenogram, indicating a benign process, appears as a dark rim on T1-weighted images (Fig. 7). Periosteal reactions can be demonstrated on MRI (Fig. 8). There is much controversy about

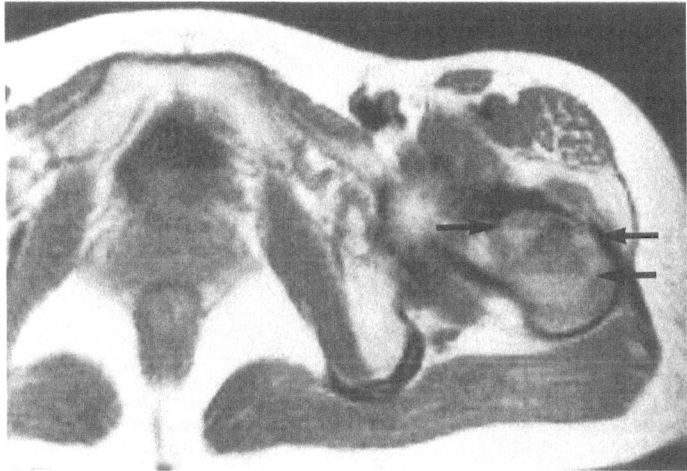

Fig. 6. A giant cell tumor of the left femur in a 37-year-old female. The T1-weighted image (TR 460/TE 35) shows multiple fluid levels (*arrows*)

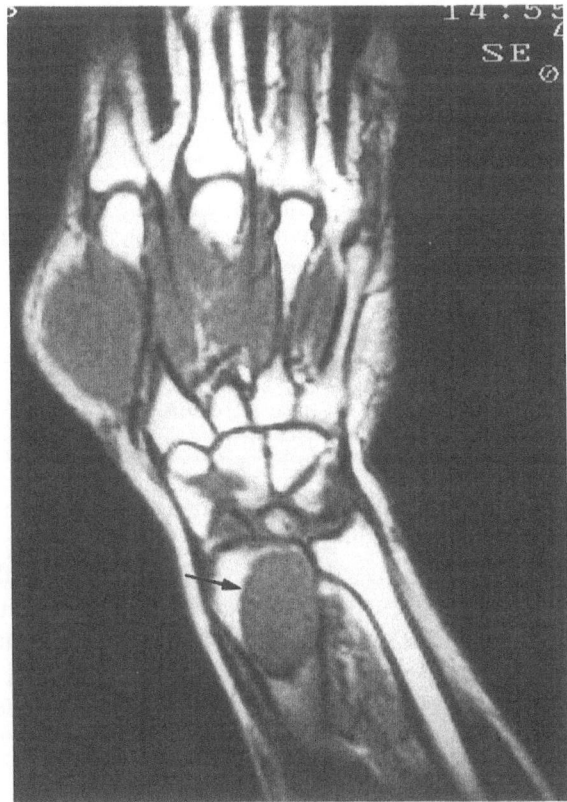

Fig. 7. A bone cyst of the right radius in a 50-year-old female. A dark rim is seen (*arrow*) in the T1-weighted image (TR 500/TE 20)

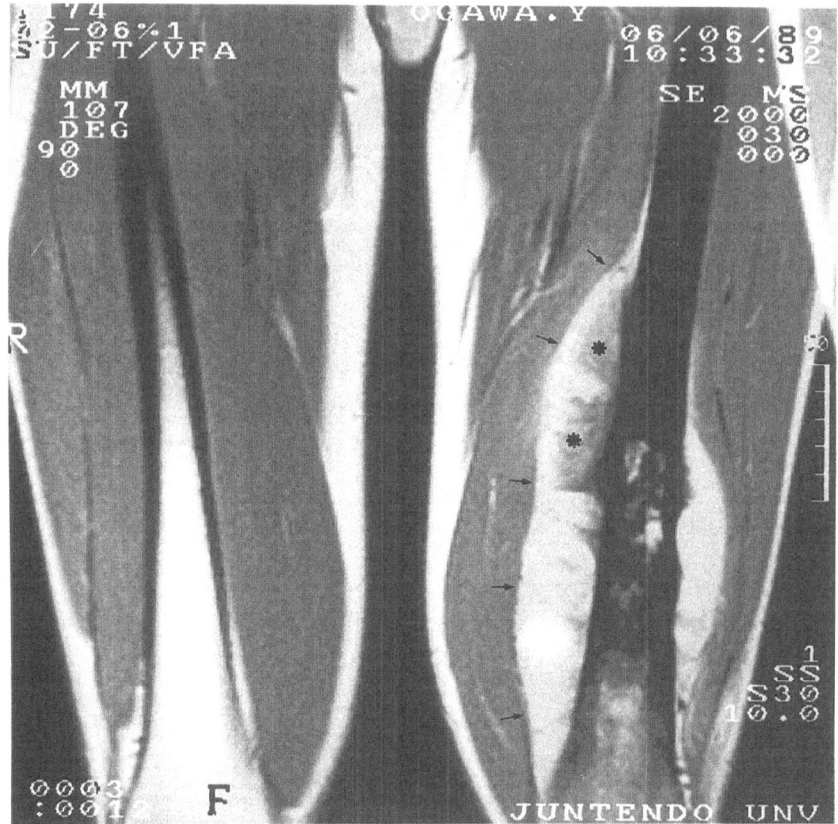

Fig. 8. Osteosarcoma of the left femur in a 12-year-old male. In the T2-weighted image (TR 2000/TE 80) a soft tissue extension appears clearly as an area of high signal intensity (*arrows*). Periosteal reaction is well defined (*asterisks*)

the ability to differentiate between benignancy and malignancy on MRI [3–6]. This is also true with regard to pre- and post-chemotherapeutic changes of the tumors [7].

Hematomas should be identified with special care because their signal intensities alter according to the stage of the process. T1 is shortened and signal intensity is increased on T1-weighted images as the amount of methemoglobin increases. Hemorrhage shows high signal intensity both on T1 and T2 images. Table 2 shows signal intensity and MRI of various tissues and lesions [8].

Imaging diagnosis of tumors of the bone and soft tissue has been dramatically changed since MRI was introduced. The usefulness of MRI includes (1) early detection of the tumor, (2) better evaluation of the extent of the tumor, (3) selection of an operative procedure [9], and (4) evaluation of chemotherapy [10, 11].

Table 2. Signal intensity and MRI on T1- and T2-weighted images (spin echo) (From [8] with permission)

T1-Weighted image

T1 \ T2	Low	Slightly low	Intermediate	Slightly high	High
High	◇ Methemoglobin (intra-erythrocyte) ◇ Melanin pigment — melanoma ◇ Coagulation necrosis (varied by stage)		◇ Fat (low*) ◇ Yellow marrow (low*) ◇ Elastic cartilage	◇ Hemorrhage (methemoglobin, extra-erythrocyte) ◇ Hemorrhagic necrosis ◇ Protein-rich fluid — ganglion	
Slightly high			White matter Liver Pancreas		
Slightly low		◇ Muscle (intermediate ~ slightly high*)	◇ Gray matter ◇ Thyroid	◇ Hyaline cartilage (incl. joint cartilage) ◇ Mucous membrane ◇ Spleen ◇ Kidneys	
Low	◇ Fibrous tissue — fibrous dysplasia ◇ Calcification, ossification, sclerotic foci, osteoid. ◇ Tendon, ligament ◇ Hemosiderin ◇ Rapid flow ◇ Air		◇ Red marrow (intermediate ~ low*) ◇ Nerves (intermediate ~ low*)	◇ Tumor ◇ Inflammation ◇ Coagulation necrosis (varied by stage) ◇ Lymph nodes ◇ Urine ◇ CSF	◇ Hemangioma ◇ Free fluid ◇ Cyst ◇ Liquefying necrosis ◇ Edema

T2-Weighted image
(* indicates signal intensity on STIR)

STIR, short inversion time inversion recovery

In delineating the extent of the tumor, MRI is useful for the determination of not only its parameters in bone marrow, but its distance from the epiphyseal plate or joint as well. Skip lesions are also readily detected.

Other Benefits of MRI

In addition to the usefulness of MRI in the diagnosis of tumorous conditions, MRI has a great potential in the field of orthopedics. The advantages of MRI have already been established in vertebral body and spinal cord abnormalities [12], and early detection of bone necrosis is well known [13, 14]. Abnormalities of joints are also well visualized on MRI, especially in larger joints like the shoulder [15], hip, and knee. For example, arthrography has almost been replaced by MRI. Menisci, crucial ligaments, and other articular structures are well visualized on MRI without the aid of contrast media [16–18]. MRS (magnetic resonance spectroscopy) is another possible technique for evaluating muscular disease. Finally, surgical intervention of meniscal injuries can be performed without prior knee arthrography.

References

1. Tehranzadeh J, Mnaymneh W, Ghavam C, Morillo G, Murphy BJ (1989) Comparison of CT and MR imaging in musculoskeletal neoplasms. J Comput Assist Tomogr 13(3):466–472
2. Elemann R, Reiser MF, Peters PE, Vasallo P, Nommensen B, Kusnierz-Glaz CR, Ritter J, Roessner A (1989) Musculoskeletal neoplasms: Static and dynamic Gd-DTPA-enhanced MR imaging. Radiology 171(3):767–773
3. Nurenberg P, Harms SE (1988) Magnetic resonance imaging of musculoskeletal tumors. Crit Lev Diagn Imaging 28(4):331–366
4. Kattapuram SV, Khurana JS, Rosenthal DI, Ehara S (1989) Musculoskeletal application of MRI. Radiat Med 7(2):47–54
5. Sundaram M, McDonald DJ (1989) The solitary tumor or tumor like lesion of bone. Top Magn Reson Imag 1(4):17–29
6. Sartoris DJ, Resnick D (1987) MR imaging of the musculoskeletal system: Current and future status. AJR 149(3):457–467
7. Hanna SL, Fletcher BD, Fairclongh DL, Jenkins JH 3d, Le AH (1991) Magnetic resonance imaging of disseminated bone marrow disease in patients treated for malignancy. Skel Radiol 20(2):79–84
8. Otake H, Nishimura H, Uchida M (1990) Skeletal MR diagnosis (in Japanese). Clin Imagiol (Jpn) 6(5):48–59
9. Sandaram M, McGuire MH, Herbold DR, Wolverson MK, Heiberg E (1986) Magnetic resonance imaging in planning limb-salvage surgery for primary malignant tumors of bone. J Bone Joint Surg [Am] 68(6):809–819
10. Holscher HC, Bloem JL, Nooy MA, Taminiau AH, Eulderink F, Hermans J (1990) The value of MR imaging in monitoring the effect of chemotherapy on bone sarcomas. AJR 154(4):763–769
11. Pan G, Raymond AK, Carrasco CH, Wallace S, Kim EE, Shirkhoba A, Jaffe N, Murray JA, Benjamin RS (1990) Osteosarcoma: MR imaging after preoperative chemotherapy. Radiology 174(2):517–526

12. Sugimura K, Yamasaki K, Kitagaki H, Tanaka Y, Kono M (1987) Bone marrow diseases of the spine: Differentiation with T1 and T2 relaxation times in MR imaging. Radiology 165(2):541–544

13. Shuman WP, Castagno AA, Baron RL, Richardson ML (1988) MR imaging of avascular necrosis of the femoral head: Value of small field-of-view sagittal surface-coil images. AJR 150(5):1073–1078

14. Mitchell DG, Rao VM, Dalinka MK, Spritzer CE, Alavi A, Steinberg ME, Fallon M, Kressel HY (1987) Femoral head avascular necrosis: Correlation of MR imaging, radiographic staging, radionuclide imaging, and clinical findings. Radiology 162(3):709–715

15. Holt RG, Helms CA, Steinback L, Neumann C, Munk PL, Genant HK (1990) Magnetic resonance imaging of the shoulder: Rationale and current applications. Skel Radiol 19(1):5–14

16. Crues JV 3d, Mink J, Levy TL, Lotysch M, Stoller DW (1987) Meniscal tears of the knee: Accuracy of MR imaging. Radiology 164(2):445–448

17. Stoller DW, Martin C, Crues JV 3d, Kaplan L, Mink JH (1987) Meniscal tears: Pathologic correlation with MR imaging. Radiology 163(3):731–735

18. Lee JK, Yao L, Phelps CT, Wirth CR, Czajka J, Lozman J (1988) Anterior cruciate ligament tears: MR imaging compared with arthoscopy and clinical tests. Radiology 166(3):861–864

19. Araki T (1989) Magnetic resonance signal intensity: For the beginner in MRI. J Med Imaging Suppl 6:10–11, Figs. 3–5

MR Imaging of Bone and Soft Tissue Sarcoma: Significance of MRI in Planning Surgical Margins and Check Points in Clinical Evaluation

MITSURU TAKAHASHI[1], KEIJI SATO, KEISUKE NAKANISHI, NAOKI FUKAYA, and TAKAYUKI MIURA[2]

Introduction

Limb salvage surgery has had almost as many successful results as amputation surgery for bone and soft tissue sarcoma. This is attributable to the standardization of procedure for wide resection based on the theory of the "barrier" which has an ability to prevent tumor penetration [1–3]. A critical area for concern is ensuring that resection is performed using the smallest surgical margin consistent with safety, to preserve good function of the affected extremity. However, in many cases, the lesion may have already extended beyond the adjacent region (extra-compartment lesion), i.e., stage IIB of Enneking's criteria [2]. For the lesion adjacent to a major neurovascular bundle, it may be impossible to secure a "curative margin" corresponding to the criteria of the Evaluation Method of Surgical Margin for Musculoskeletal Sarcoma of the Japanese Orthopaedic Association Musculoskeletal Tumor Committee (JOA criteria) [1]. This type of case requires some kind of reliable method of preoperative imaging in order to determine the margin of tumor extension referred to by the sub-type of histology as well as to measure the effectiveness of adjuvant therapy at the planning stage of a limb salvage operation.

Since 1985, we have utilized magnetic resonance imaging (MRI) as the main preoperative imaging examination method for musculoskeletal sarcomas, and have tried to clarify the barrier as well as the tumor-surrounding "tumor-reactive zone". In the present study, we examine the safety of planning the surgical margin based on an assessment of peritumoral findings by MRI, and compare the results with the post-operative evaluation of the surgical margin according to JOA criteria.

[1] Division of Orthopaedic Surgery, Nagoya Memorial Hospital, Nagoya, Japan
[2] Department of Orthopaedic Surgery, Nagoya University School of Medicine, Nagoya, Japan

Materials and Methods

Cases

Our study included 33 cases whose MRI assessment was comparable with the postoperative evaluation based on JOA criteria, out of a total of 45 patients with musculoskeletal sarcomas surgically treated in our clinic from 1985 to 1989.

All 10 cases with osteosarcoma had primary lesions and all had been treated with preoperative adjuvant therapy; 4 received only systemic chemotherapy and 6 were administered local chemotherapy with either intra-arterial (IA) infusion or radiation, or both. In the cases of soft tissue tumors, 8 patients had malignant fibrous histiocytomas (MFH), 5 of whom were initially operated cases, and 3 were recurrent cases: 5 patients were treated preoperatively with hyperthermia and/or chemotherapy by local IA infusion, while the other 3 received no preoperative therapy. Other diagnoses include 3 rhabdomyosarcomas, 2 chondrosarcomas, 3 synovial sarcomas, 2 liposarcomas, 1 Ewing's sarcoma, 1 neurosarcoma, 1 MFH of bone, and 1 leiomyosarcoma of bone.

MRI Imaging Method

MRI was performed for the patients who had undergone preoperative therapy before the onset of therapy and again at one week before surgery. MRI was carried out 2 weeks before surgery for the patients who had not received preoperative therapy. Images were always obtained in two orthogonal planes; axial plane images were necessary in all cases, while either coronal plane or sagittal plane images or both were obtained on a case-by-case basis.

Evaluation of Tumor Involvement in MRI

We detected areas which showed moderately higher signal intensity than that of tumor and normal muscles on T1-weighted images, and the same or moderately lower signal intensity than the tumor images on T2-weighted images. We regarded such an area as a tumor-reacting zone in MRI, and named it the reactive edematous zone (REZ). We paid special attention to the black line frequently detected in the outer margin of tumors and in the intermuscular space (low signal intensity line; low SI line). The detection of a low SI line was made by a comparison of T1- and T2-weighted images; in addition, the data from proton density images was included in some cases.

Since we discovered some cases which showed different appearances of REZ in various parts of the affected area, we counted each finding as an individual case, resulting in a total of 51 cases.

Macroscopic Evaluation of the Surgical Margin

Resected surgical specimens were fixed in 10% formalin according to the method described in the JOA criteria [1], and segments equivalent to the slices studied in MRI were prepared. The outer margin of the tumor was evaluated using the following points:

1. Findings in the *tumor capsule*.
   a) Was the tumor sufficiently covered with a thick capsule?
   b) Was the capsule of a continuously unchanging color and was it even in thickness?
2. Findings and width of the *tumor-reactive zone* adjacent to the tumor (the area surrounding tumor). The microvascular new-growths and hemorrhage which were directly related to the tumor extension, and the edema or color change of the soft tissue adjacent to the tumor which occurred following preoperative adjuvant therapy or the mass-effect of the tumor existence (as opposed to the tumor itself), were recorded according to the JOA criteria.
3. The relationship of the tumor-reactive zone to fascia or periosteum, that was designated as the *barrier* by the JOA criteria. Special attention was given to whether or not the tumor-reactive zone was retained inside the barrier.

Histopathological Investigation

Histological findings of REZ in MRI were classified into the following groups: (1) tumor cell permeation, (2) secondary bleeding, microvascular new-growth and peritumoral scar formation which were regarded as the sign of tumor cell invasion (tumor-reactive zone), and (3) edema or inflammation caused by the mass-effect or by local therapy.

Reliability of the low SI line as a safety barrier was studied by the histological findings of the line and adjacent tissues.

Results

REZ Recognition in MRI

We were able to recognize an area showing high signal intensity (REZ) around the tumor images in 43 cases, but not in the remaining 8 cases. In 28 of the 43 cases, REZs were observed outside the tumor images with a low SI line on both T1- and T2-weighted images (strong low SI line). In the other 15 cases, although the REZ had a faintly differing signal intensity from the tumor images, it was not bounded by a strong low SI line but by a variable SI line with a differing pulse sequence (faint low SI line). A REZ was found both in 24 cases out of 28 who had received local therapy and in 19 cases out of 23 without local therapy, showing no significant difference.

Histological Findings of REZ

Based on the difference in relation of the REZ to tumor images, we classified the cases into 2 groups.

REZ separated from tumor image with strong low SI line (28 cases). REZs involving tumor-reactive zones were seen in 16 cases (57%), and in edematous

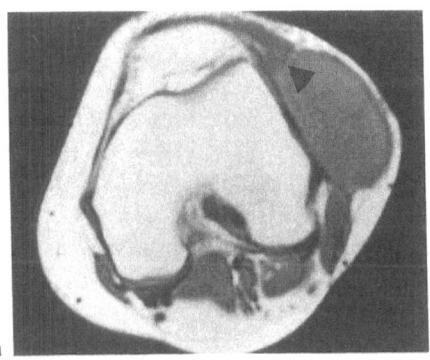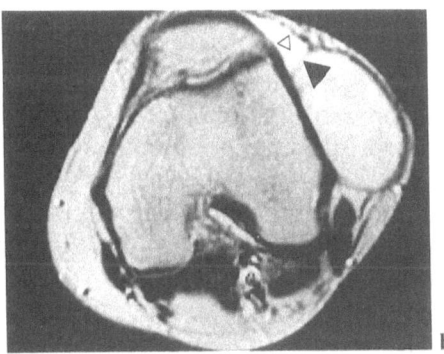

a   b

Fig. 1a,b. Malignant fibrous histiocytoma of the left knee (axial image; GE: SIGNA). **a** T1-weighted image (TR500, TE20). **b** T2-weighted image (TR2000, TE80). The REZ was recognized in the anterior of the tumor image. It had the same signal intensity as the surrounding muscle in the T1-weighted image and a higher intensity than the tumor image in the T2-weighted image (*open triangle*). There was only a faint low SI line in the border of the tumor image (*solid triangle*). In this case, tumor cell invasion of the REZ was observed by histopathological investigation

tissue in 12 cases (43%) as seen by macroscopic investigation of the surgical margin. In the 13 cases not receiving local therapy, 9 cases (69%) involved tumor-reactive zones and 4 cases (31%) involved edematous tissue. On the other hand, 7 cases (47%) involved tumor-reactive zones and 8 (53%) involved edematous tissue among the 15 cases who had received local therapy. Thus cases without local therapy had a higher REZ frequency of tumor-reactive zones and those with local therapy had a higher REZ frequency of edematous tissue.

Microscopically, the REZ was seen to involve microvascular new-growth and secondary hemorrhage in 9 out of 13 cases without local therapy, which was the same finding as that from the macroscopic investigation. On the contrary, in 15 cases with preoperative local therapy, only 4 cases (27%) involved tumor-reactive zones, and the other 9 cases had edema, inflammation, or muscle degeneration related to preoperative local therapy. Two cases showed almost normal tissue. No tumor cells were found in the REZ of this group with/without local therapy.

REZ without a strong low SI line in border of tumor image (15 cases). Macroscopically, the REZ of all 6 cases without local therapy were evaluated as a reactive zone, while in 9 cases with local therapy, 6 involved tumor-reactive zones in REZ, but 3 proved to have only edematous tissue by macroscopic investigation. In addition, by microscopic investigation, four (67%) out of 6 cases without local therapy and 3 (33%) out of 9 cases with local therapy were shown to have been infiltrated by tumor cells in the area which corresponded to the REZ (Fig. 1).

Histopathology of Low SI Line

Cases with strong low SI lines. This line was identified in 18 cases of bone tumors and 10 cases of soft tissue sarcoma. In 7 cases of bone tumors with local therapy, the line corresponded to the fascia beyond the REZ in 4 cases (57%), while a thick periosteum, a thick ligamentous capsule, and clear thin fascia adjacent to the tumor mass were observed in each of the other cases. On the other hand, the line was formed most frequently by tumor capsules (7 cases, 64%), and by periosteum (3 cases, 27%) for 11 bone tumors without local therapy. The line was indicative of fascia beyond the tumor-reactive zone in only 1 case (9%).

The line corresponded to the fascia existing at the border between normal tissue and an edematous lesion outside the tumor-reactive zone (3 cases, 50%) among 6 cases of soft tissue sarcomas. In addition a thin membrane covering the tumor mass formed the line in 2 cases (33%). In 4 of the locally untreated cases, the line was made by a thin tumor capsule in 3 cases (75%) and the fascia corresponded to the line in only 1 case (25%).

Tumor cell invasion into tissue corresponding to a low SI line was observed in a ligamentous capsule of a bone tumor without local therapy and in fascia and the tumor capsule of each case of locally treated soft tissue sarcoma.

Causes of disappearance of strong low SI line (23 cases). A strong low SI line was not observed in 12 locally treated cases. Histopathological findings on the line included degeneration of fascia and periosteum in 3 cases (25%), an edematous scar, which was not separable from a tumor in MRI, in 3 cases (25%) (1 case also involved tumor cells), and a thin incomplete tumor capsule in 5 cases (42%) (2 cases with infiltration of tumor cells). Destruction of the barrier by a tumor also caused disappearance of the line (1 case, 8%). The 3 cases with tumor infiltration and tumor destruction were the previously mentioned cases with tumor cells evidenced in REZ.

In 11 locally untreated cases, 1 case (9%) had degenerated periosteum with tumor infiltration, 2 cases (18%) edematous scar (1 case with tumor cells), 3 cases (27%) thin tumor capsules without tumor infiltration, and 1 case (9%) a clear tumor capsule. Four cases (36%) had destruction of the barrier and corresponded to cases with tumor cells in REZ (Fig. 2).

Discussion

Sundaram and colleagues have reported that MRI is more efficient than other image examination methods to delineate tumor extension in soft tissue as well as in bone marrow, even when a normal-conductive imaging method is used [4, 5]. Since super-conductive imaging methods became available with their excellent sensitivity and especially clear images, many studies have appeared reporting on the use of such images in the differential diagnosis of tumors and the evaluation of the effects of chemotherapy [6, 7]. However, in our previous study [9], as well as in a report by Aisen et al. [10], current MRI techniques

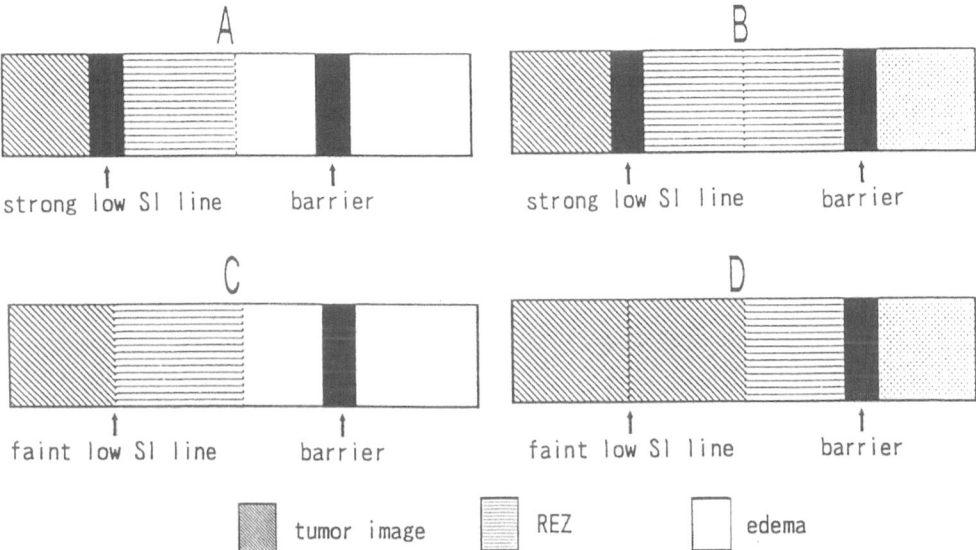

Fig. 2A–D. Detection of the REZ and the low SI line. **A** Cases not receiving local therapy. The REZ was separated from the tumor image by a strong low SI line and did not reach the barrier outside it. The REZ had a high percentage of tumor-reactive zone (69%), but no tumor cells were found. **B** Cases receiving local therapy. The REZ was separated from the tumor image by a strong low SI line and reached the barrier outside it. The REZ had a high percentage of edematous tissue (53%), and no tumor cells were found. **C** Cases not receiving local therapy. The REZ was separated from the tumor image by a faint low SI line not a strong low SI line, and did not reach the barrier outside it. In this case, the REZ had a high percentage of tumor-reactive zone (67%), and tumor cell infiltration was found in 4 of 6 cases. **D** Cases receiving local therapy. The REZ was not separated from the tumor image and reached the barrier outside it because of inflammation and muscle degeneration caused by the local therapy. This area was regarded as the tumor image, and the higher intensity area outside the barrier (edematous change followed by the local therapy) was regarded as the REZ

were not shown to have suitable specificity for the assessment of tumor characteristics. Although Mizuta attempted the differential diagnosis of various tumors and the estimation of their viability by measuring T1 and T2 values in NMR studies, he did not succeed since the T1 and T2 values were widely scattering in each tumor [11]. Nidecker et al. tried to estimate the viability of tumor cells with MR spectroscopy (MRS) [12]. However, their setting in the region of interest was not accurate for examining the spectral change between pre- and post-chemotherapy images, and complete measuring of viability in tumors was impossible, suggesting that using MRS for routine evaluation would be difficult. These considerations indicate that the primary function of current MR imaging remains the anatomical detection of tumor location.

With regard to surgical approaches for osteosarcoma extending into soft tissue, Enneking et al. and Kawaguchi et al. have reported on resection techniques based on evaluations of the surgical margin [2, 13]. The work was based on the concept of the barrier originated by the "compartment" theory, which provided the anatomical location of tumor extension. Although these reports are based on a relationship between a reactive zone at the tumor's outer margin and the barrier, routine examination methods did not permit the zone to be converted into clear images. Therefore, a comparison of MRI findings in a tumor's outer margin with histological results of resected tissue is essential for making a guide line in preoperative MRI assessment of the surgical margin of musculoskeletal sarcoma. Beltran et al. examined the histopathological findings in 7 cases that showed an increased signal intensity in the muscles surrounding a tumor [14]. However, they did not elaborate on either the existence of tumor cells or their relation to the findings of the affected region in MRI. We were able to find only 2 case reports describing a change around the tumor margin related to the effect of treatment and surgical intervention [15, 16].

It has been reported that the area around a tumor's outer margin has a higher signal intensity than normal muscle: this is termed peritumoral edema. However, in our experience, the high signal intensity area around a tumor includes not only edematous tissues caused by the mass-effect, degeneration, and scar formation induced by preoperative therapy, but also includes other pathology such as tumor infiltration, hemosiderin deposits, and microvascular growth following secondary hemorrhage due to rapid tumor extension, which correspond to the tumor-reactive zone in an evaluation of the surgical margin [8, 9]. Therefore, expressing the MRI finding of all of these areas in one all-inclusive word, edema, is thought to lead to a confusion in semantics when conducting pre- and post-operative assessments of the surgical margin. In discussing the safety of a tumor's outer margin, we propose the use of the term reactive edematous zone (REZ) which includes the above-mentioned tumor-reactive zone and the degenerated surrounding tissue caused by both the mass-effect and edema. This zone is distinguishable from a tumor image due to the different signal intensity and was detected in 43 out of 51 (84%) of our examined cases. We examined the histology of areas with a low SI line and a REZ observed by MRI and assessed their security in the surgical margin.

Relation Between REZ and Histology in Cases with a Strong Low SI Line

When classifying the cases with a strong low SI line (28 cases) into locally treated and untreated groups, the untreated cases showed a 69% tumor-reactive zone involvement, while the treated cases showed 47%. This result led us the following considerations:

Locally untreated cases. When the line is regarded as a surgical margin with the intent of preserving important organs, it is possible to ensure the safety of the procedure (comparable to wide procedure in JOA criteria) due to its function as a barrier, even though the line is considered a marginal margin according to the assessment criteria of JOA.

Locally treated cases. Inflammation is induced within and outside of the tumor capsule, and the signal difference among the tumor and the reactive zone is likely to disappear. As a result, the tumor images are over-evaluated and the recognizable REZ is moved outwardly. Thus, it often reflects secondary edema outside the tumor-reactive zone. In addition, a low SI line is likely to reflect fascia or periosterum, which can be evaluated as a normal barrier outside the tumor reactive zone. Therefore, in the assessment of a surgical margin, a low SI line is, at least, a reliable indicator of a wide margin. Contrarily, in cases of surgery combined with preoperative local therapy to preserve important organs, the tumor image may be enlarged on MRI, thus requiring a comparison with the pre-treated image.

Cases without a strong low SI line in the REZ at a border of the tumor image. If resection crossing this REZ is performed in this group, an evaluation of the surgical margins obtained might be less than a marginal margin in 100% of locally untreated cases and in 60% of locally treated cases. In order to establish a surgical margin within the wider margin where no tumor cells exist, it is essential to include an operation field extending beyond REZ. It is impossible to obtain such a secure outer margin, however, since the REZ width can change with different equipment as well as with varying pulse sequences or choice of window. Resection must therefore be carried beyond the normal fascia or joint capsule identified as a low SI line outside the REZ. In such cases, careful planning of the curative procedure is mandatory.

References

1. The JOA Musculoskeletal Tumor Committee (1989) Evaluation method of surgical margin for musculo-skeletal sarcoma (in Japanese). Kanehara, Tokyo
2. Enneking WF, Spanier SS, Goodman MA (1980) A system of surgical staging of musculoskeletal sarcoma. Clin Orthop 153:106–120
3. Sterner B (1978) The management of soft tissue tumors. Int Orthop 1:289–298
4. Sundaram M, McGuire MH, Herbold DR (1987) Magnetic resonance imaging of osteosarcoma. Skeletal Radiol 16:23–29
5. Sundaram M, McGuire MH, Herbold DR (1986) Magnetic resonance imaging in planning limb-salvage surgery for primary malignant tumors of bone. J Bone Joint Surg [Am] 68:809–819
6. Vanel D, Lacombe MJ, Couanet D, Klifa C, Spielmann M, Genin J (1987) Musculoskeletal tumors: Follow-up with MR imaging after treatment with surgery and radiation therapy. Radiology 164:243–245
7. Bohndorf K, Reiser M, Lochner B, Feaux de Lacroux W, Steinbrich W (1986) Magnetic resonance imaging of primary tumors and tumor like lesions of bone. Skeletal Radiol 15:511–517
8. Gomeri JM, Grossman RI, Goldberg HI, Zimmerman RA, Bilaniuk LT (1985) Intracranial hematomas: Imaging by high field MRI. Radiology 157:87–93

9. Takahashi M, Sato K, Nakanishi K, Fukaya N (1990) MRI diagnosis of bone and soft tissue tumors: Reference to the resected specimens (in Japanese). Orthopedics 41:349–355

10. Aisen AM, Martel W, Braunstein EM, McMillin KI, Phillips WA, Kling TF (1986) MRI and CT evaluation of primary bone and soft tissue tumors. AJR 146:749–756

11. Mizuta H (1984) Nuclear magnetic resonance studies on human bone and soft tissue tumors. J Jpn Orthop Assoc 58:97–106

12. Nidecker AC, Müller S, Aue WP, Seelig J, Fridrich R, Hartweg H, Benz UF (1985) Extremity bone tumors: Evaluation by P-31 MR spectroscopy. Radiology 157:167–174

13. Kawaguchi T, Amino K, Matsumoto S, Manabe J, Huruya K, Isobe Y (1986) Limb salvage operation for osteosarcoma (in Japanese). Orthop Surg Traumatr 29:863–874

14. Beltran J, Simon DC, Katz W, Weis LD (1987) Increased MR signal intensity in skeletal muscle adjacent to malignant tumors. Radiology 162:251–255

15. Pan G, Raymond AK, Carrasco CH, Wallace S, Kim EE, Shirkhoda A, Jaffe N, Murray JA, Benjamin RS (1990) Osteosarcoma:MR imaging after preoperative chemotherapy. Radiology 174:517–526

16. Sanchez RB, Quinn SF, Walling A, Estrada J, Greenberg H (1990) Musculoskeletal neoplasms after intraarterial chemotherapy: Correlation of MR images with pathologic specimens. Radiology 174:237–240

1.3

Determination of Surgical Margins by Intraoperative Ultrasonography in Malignant Soft Tissue Tumors

SHINJI HIRABAYASHI, ATSUMASA UCHIDA, HIDEKI YOSHIKAWA, and KEIRO ONO[1]

Introduction

Diagnosis and treatment of malignant soft tissue tumors have advanced as the result of rapid progress in diagnostic imaging techniques, such as CT and MRI. The availability of accurate information preoperatively allows the surgery to be performed more easily and precisely.

Recently, ultrasonography for the examination of tumors has come into clinical use because of the following advantages: (1) the easier use of ultrasound compared to other diagnostic imaging methods to determine the size and location of a tumor, (2) the availabity of ultrasonography in real time, and the possibility of conducting examinations in any location as well as repeating examinations, and (3) the ultrasound technique is simple and harmless.

However, ultrasound does have some disadvantages. Ultrasonographic imaging can not determine with certainty whether a tumor is malignant or benign. Also, in malignant tumors, ultrasonography cannot detect the difference between normal tissues and the reactive zone surrounding the tumor edge.

Ultrasonography was mainly utilized for the screening examination or for guidance of percutaneous needle biopsy [1, 2]. In making wide surgical excisions of tumors, the location and shape of the lesion change markedly, and, therefore, an imaging apparatus can be used intraoperatively in order to detect tumors precisely. There have been some reports concerning the intraoperative application of ultrasound for the purpose of surgical guidance, especially in the orthopedic field [3, 4]. In this paper, we describe the feasibility and effectiveness of intraoperative ultrasonographic imaging for safe wide local resection of tumors.

---

[1] Department of Orthopedic Surgery, Osaka University Medical School, Fukushima, 1-1-50, Osaka, 553 Japan

Table 1. Histological diagnosis

	Extremity		Total
	Upper	Lower	
Liposarcoma	0	4	4
Malignant fibrous histiocytoma	1	2	3
Rhabdomyosarcoma	1	1	2
Malignant schwannoma	0	1	1
Synovial cell sarcoma	1	0	1
Mesenchymal chondrosarcoma	0	1	1
Infantile fibrosarcoma	0	1	1
Desmoid	0	2	2
Total	3	12	15

Materials and Methods

We reviewed 15 patients with malignant soft tissue tumors who underwent wide excision surgery with the assistance of intraoperative ultrasonography. These included primary lesions in 12 cases, a recurrent tumor in 1 case, and additional resections in 2 cases. There were 6 males and 9 females in this series, and their ages ranged from 7 months to 79 years (average age: 40.9 years). The histological diagnosis was liposarcoma (4), MFH (malignant fibrous histiocytoma) (3), rhabdomyosarcoma (2), malignant schwannoma (1), synovial cell sarcoma (1), mesenchymal chondrosarcoma (1), infantile fibrosarcoma (1), and desmoid (2) (Table 1).

There were 3 upper limb and 12 lower limb tumors. After the tumors were discovered by incisional biopsy to be malignant, preoperative chemotherapy was performed for 2 months in all cases. The preoperative surgical planning for wide excision was based on the information obtained with CT and MRI.

The intraoperative ultrasound studies were performed with linear scanners (Toshiba SSA-250, SAL-38B). Transducers were sterilized with etylene oxide gas and were used at frequencies between 5.0–7.5 MHz.

After the incision was made, the transducer was placed directly onto the fat or muscle fascia. Longitudinal and transverse scanning of the affected site was then performed. The location and size of the tumor were evaluated in the longitudinal scan, while the relations of the soft tissues adjacent to the tumor were assessed in the transverse scan. Surgical resection was performed away from the tumor border as identified by ultrasonography. The distance between the excisional edge and the tumor border was measured on the machine by using calipers. In the patients undergoing additional wide excisions without tumor, the excision was performed away from the scar tissue. The tumor borders detected by intraoperative ultrasonography were confirmed by scanning of the excised specimen postoperatively, and histological examination was then performed.

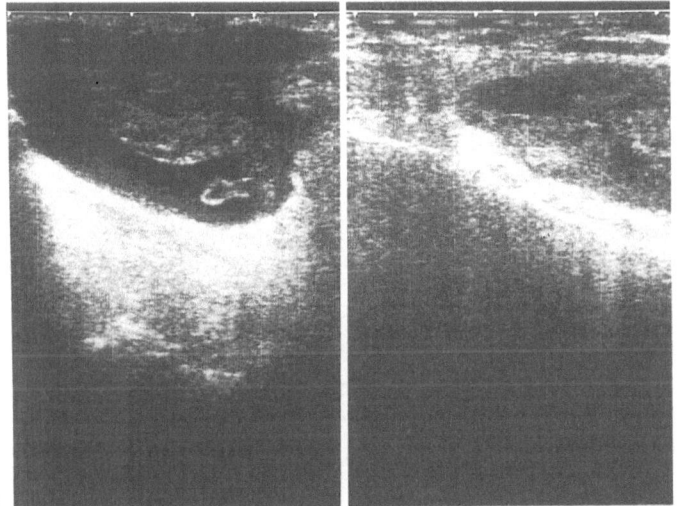

Fig. 1a,b. Liposarcoma (case 1). **a** In the transeverse scan, the internal tumor echoes were low and heterogeneous. **b** In the longitudinal scan, the boundary echo of the tumor was clear. The *scale* is in 1 cm units. The distance between the tumor border and the surgical excisional edge could be measured intraoperatively using callipers and this scale

All cases were followed by CT, MRI, and garium scintigraphy for 3–24 months (average follow-up period: 12 months) in order to assess local recurrence or distant metastasis.

Results

The surgical procedure provided a sufficient resectional margin macroscopically in all cases. Furthermore, the borders of the tumor that had been determined by intraoperative ultrasonography were shown to correspond to the actual tumor borders confirmed by histological examination. Distinctive characteristics were detected by ultrasonography in each case.

Case 1

The patient was a 47-year-old female with liposarcoma. In the longitudinal scan, the main ultrasonographic features were that the boundary echoes were clear, the internal echoes had low echogenicity, and the posterior echoes of the tumor were enhanced compared with the surrounding tissues. Utilizing the scale on the ultrasound units, the surgical procedure was performed 3 cm away from the tumor border delineated by the scanning (Fig. 1).

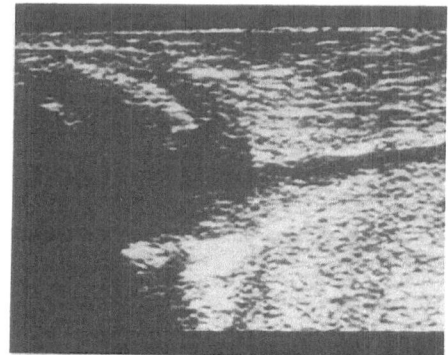

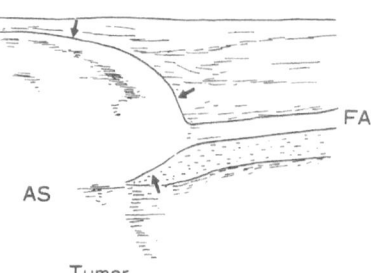

Tumor
FA : Femoral artery
AS : Acoustic shadow

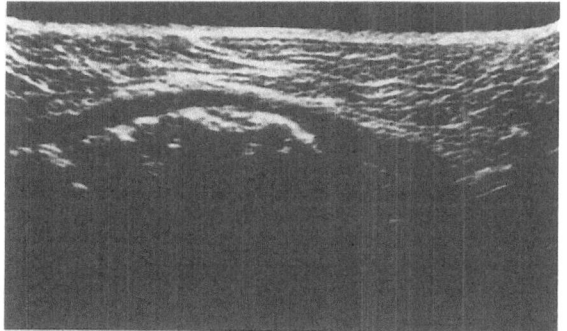

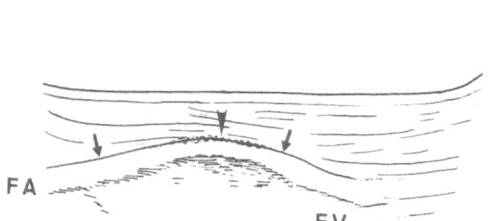

Tumor
AS : Acoustic shadow
FA : Femoral artery
FV : Femoral vein

Fig. 2a,b. Mesenchymal chondrosarcoma (case 2). Ultrasonography showed an acoustic shadow due to calcification in the tumor. The high echogenicity at the wall of the femoral artery was suspected to be due to tumor invasion (*arrows*). The echoes of the vessel wall were thick and irregular (*arrow head*), and no tumor emboli were seen in the artery

Case 2

The patient was a 33-year-old female with mesenchymal chondrosarcoma which was invading along the femoral artery. The images of a thick, irregular, and high echogenesity of the wall of the artery were suspected to indicate tumor invasions. No tumor emboli were seen in the artery both at surgery and during scanning (Fig. 2).

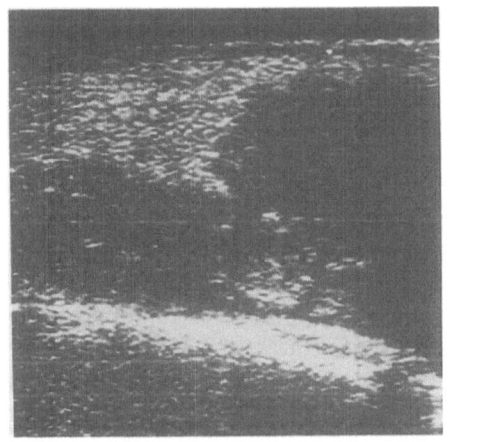
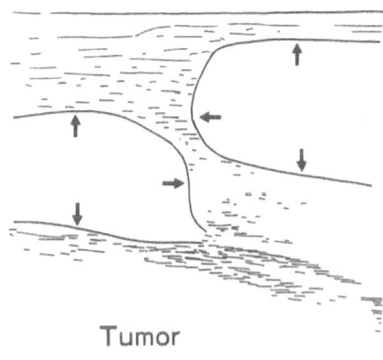

Tumor

Fig. 3. Desmoid tumor (case 3). Boundary echoes of the tumor were unclear and irregular (*arrows*). Internal echoes were homogeneous and of low echogenicity. The tumors were not connected in one plane

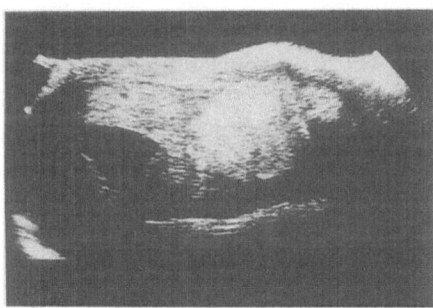
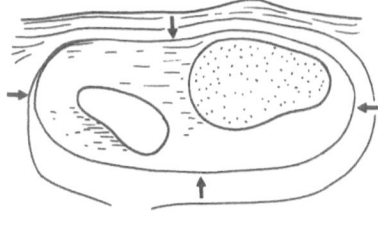

Tumor

Fig. 4. Rhabdomyosarcoma (case 4). The *arrows* represent the tumor border. Most parts of the tumor were necrotic due to chemotherapy. The internal echo was coarse. Areas of low echogenicity areas represented cysts, and areas of high echogenicity indicated bleeding

Case 3

The patient was a 29-year-old female with desmoid tumor. Tumor borders were not clearly discrete nor were they connected to each other (Fig. 3).

Case 4

The patient was a 16-year-old female with rhabdomyosarcoma. Cystic and necrotic changes in the tumor after chemotherapy were clearly detected. These changes were revealed both at ultrasonography and during histological examination (Fig. 4).

Discussion

We had found intraoperative ultrasonography to have many advantages. It can detect the location of the tumor in real time and at any surgical stage, such as skin incision, wide excision, and loosening of the resected border. The tumor can be resected safely since ultrasonography allows a regular interval from the tumor margin to be maintained. Ultrasonography facilitated the recognition of the relations between surrounding tissues such as bone, arteries, nerves and the tumor itself. Resection of the surrounding tissues was minimized, e.g., by virtue of knowing that muscle fascia was acting as a barrier to tumor invasion and guiding the line of resection outside of it. Furthermore, the presence of 3–5 mm skip lesions and tumor invasion was clearly detected. In malignant soft tissue tumors of over 5 cm, high frequency transducers (over 7.5 MHz, linear array) can find the total tumor image within a multidimensional scan because ultrasonography could be done directly into deep layers. In addition, scar tissues were differentiated from normal tissues.

Ultrasonography had some disadvantages, particularly in that the production of pictures is less clear than that of other imaging methods. Higher freqency transducers are needed in order to overcome this deficiency. However, such transducers can not propagate their waves into deep tissues due to attenuation. Furthermore, ultrasonography was useless in assessing bone involvement since bone has a high acoustic impedance which prevents ultrasound waves from spreading through it and reflect them completely at the surface. Ultrasonography could give some limited information about tumor invasion along the vessels and nerves.

Conclusions

Intraoperative ultrasonography during wide excision of malignant soft tissue tumors was performed in 15 patients. Ultrasonography gave useful information concerning the tumor and the surrounding tissues, enabling surgical procedures to be more easily and safely performed. None of the patients had recurrences during a mean follow-up period of 12 months. Intraoperative ultrasonography was shown to be very useful in the surgical treatment of malignant soft tissue tumors.

References

1. Lange TA, Austin CW, Seibert JJ, Angutuaco TL, Yandow DR (1987) Ultrasound imaging as a screening study for malignant soft tissue tumors. J Bone Joint Surg [Am] 69:100–105
2. Amino K, Kawaguchi T, Matumoto S, Manabe A, Furuya K, Wada N, Isobe Y, Tako M, Kitagawa T (1986) A clinicopathologic study of liposarcoma. J Jpn Orthop Assoc 60(9):S210–211

3. Hirabayashi S, Uchida A, Yoshikawa H, Ono K (1990) The utilization of ultrasonography during wide excision of malignant soft tissue tumors. J Jpn Orthop Assoc 64(6):S673–674
4. Machi J, Bernard S, Kurohiji T, Zaren HA, Joaquin S (1990) Operative ultrasound guidance for various surgical procedures. Ultrasound Med Biol 16:37–42

1.4

Gene Analysis for Bone and Soft Tissue Tumors

Nobuhito Araki, Atsumasa Uchida, Tomoatsu Kimura,
Hideki Yoshikawa, Yasuaki Aoki, Takafumi Ueda,
and Keiro Ono[1]

Introduction

It is generally accepted that malignant tumors arise from some genetic disorders which lead to abnormal proliferation and differentiation of the tumor cells. Moreover, some disorders may modulate the malignant properties, such as invasiveness or metastatic potential. Recent advances in molecular biology revealed these characteristic gene abnormalities in many cancers, and they have been classified as oncogenes, anti-oncogenes and modulator genes [1]. An oncogene usually codes some growth regulatory sequence, such as growth factor or its receptor, and controls tumor development positively. On the other hand, an anti-oncogene regulates the tumor cell negatively, normally suppressing tumorigenicity. Inactivation of the anti-oncogene will cause a tumor. Modulator genes are defined as the genes which can influence secondary malignant properties as, for example, in multidrug-resistant genes [2]. Analyses of these disordered genes in various tumors will offer a useful diagnostic tool to understand the characteristic behavior of the tumor and to decide upon appropriate therapy, because they reflect the essential properties of the disease. There is also a possibility that a new diagnostic classification can be made by adding the genetic information to the ordinary pathological classification. However, in bone and soft tissue, these analyses have just begun in only a few kinds of tumors. We report the involvement of c-*fos* gene expression as an oncogene and Rb (retinoblastoma) gene disorders as an anti-oncogene in some bone and soft tissue tumors.

The retinoblastoma gene is the first isolated anti-oncogene in which loss of activity of both normal alleles is thought to be associated with tumorigenesis of retinoblastoma [3]. An etiologic association between osteosarcoma and retinoblastoma has been suggested in the analysis of the Rb gene [4]. In

[1] Department of Orthopaedic Surgery, Osaka University Medical School, Fukushima, 1-1-50, Osaka, 553 Japan

order to clarify to what degree the Rb gene mutation is responsible for a tumorigenetic factor of the bone and soft tissue tumors, we have analyzed the Rb gene structure in 23 osteosarcomas and in 34 other bone and soft tissue sarcomas [5].

Oncogene *fos* was initially identified as v-*fos* from the FBJ murine osteosarcoma virus [6, 7]. Although there have been few reports on the correlation between the *fos* gene and human osteosarcoma, recent analysis in the transgenic mouse that carries c-*fos* gene suggests some involvement of this gene in bone and cartilage tumors [8]. Therefore, we examined the *fos* gene expression by RNA blot analysis in 16 musculoskeletal tumors.

Materials and Methods

Tumor Tissue Samples

Tumor tissue samples (0.5–2.0 g) were obtained from patients at either biopsy or wide resection. Retinoblastoma gene analyses were performed on 23 osteosarcomas and 34 cases of other bone and soft tissue tumors, such as malignant fibrous histiocytomas, synovial sarcomas, Ewing's sarcomas, giant cell tumors, and others. All diagnoses were confirmed by open biopsy. None of the patients had a history of retinoblastoma. C-*fos* gene expression was examined in 16 musculoskeletal tumors, including 11 osteosarcomas, 3 chondrosarcomas, 2 Ewing's sarcomas, 4 soft-tissue tumors, and others.

DNA Blot Analysis

High molecular weight DNA was extracted from tumor tissues and from white blood cells (WBC) according to a modified method described by Sambrook et al. [9]. DNA (15–20 µg) was digested with *Hind* III restriction enzyme, electrophoresed through 0.7% agarose gel, and transferred to nylon filters (Gene Screen Plus, New England Nuclear) with 20 × SSC (SSC is 0.15M NaCl, 0.015M trisodium citrate, pH 7.0).

RNA Blot Analysis

Total cellular RNA was isolated from some of the above patients using the Guanidinium/ScCl method as previously described [9]. Total RNA (20 µg) was electrophoresed in 0.8% agarose gel by the glyoxal method and transferred to a nylon filter with 20 × SSC.

Probes

The cDNA probes of the Rb gene, p0.9R and p3.8R, were generous gifts from Dr. S.H. Friend [3]. *Nco* I/*Stu* I fragments of the human pc-*fos* gene was used as a c-*fos* probe [7]. Probes were labeled with ^{32}P using the random primer procedure (Amersham, USA).

Hybridization

Nylon filters were hybridized with a ^{32}P-labeled p3.8R probe or a c-*fos* probe and then were rehybridized with ^{32}P-random primed β-actin probe by the procedure recommended by the manufacturers. Hybridization was performed for 16h at 65°C in a solution containing 1M NaCl, 1% SDS, 10% Dextran sulfate, and denatured salmon sperm DNA at 100 μg/ml. Filters were washed twice at room temperature in 2 × SSC and once at 65°C in 2 × SSC and 1% SDS. Autoradiography was done on Kodak X-AR film with an intensifying screen at −80°C.

Results

In the DNA blot analysis of the Rb gene, 8 out of 23 patients with osteosarcoma showed structural abnormalities in their DNA (Fig. 1). In case 1, the genomic DNA from tumor tissue represented only 6.2 and 2.05 kb bands, while DNA from WBC in the same patient showed the following normal six bands: 10.0, 7.5, 6.2, 5.3, 4.5, and 2.05 kb (Fig. 1, lane 1). This result indicates that the DNA from tumor tissue of this case lacks both of the 4.5, 7.5, 5.3, and 10.0 kb *Hind* III fragments of the Rb alleles (homozygous deletion). A schematic pattern of these deletions in this case is shown in Fig. 1, lower column. In case 3, the 4.5 and 7.5 kb *Hind* III fragments are missing (Fig. 1, lane 3). The intensities of the remaining Rb fragments imply the existence of only a single copy of the aberrant Rb locus (heterozygous deletion). Thus, cases 1–3 showed homozygous deletions at various sites of the Rb locus and cases 4–8 showed heterozygous deletions mainly in the 7.5 kb *Hind* III fragment of the Rb gene. There were no detectable abnormalities in the DNA blot analysis of the remaining 15 cases. In 34 cases of other bone and soft tissue sarcoma, there were only 2 cases of malignant fibrous histiocytoma which showed structural alterations and heterozygous deletion at the Rb locus in DNA blot analysis (data not shown).

By RNA blot analysis using total cellular RNA extracted from some osteosarcoma tissues, 7 of the 8 samples expressed no detectable Rb transcripts, and 1 case showed a truncated Rb transcript of the 3.5 kb band in addition to the normal-sized 4.7 kb band (Fig. 2). The absence of degradation of RNA was confirmed by the presence of mRNA hybridizable with a β-actin probe on the same nylon filter (Fig. 2, lower column). These results indicate that in many cases, Rb gene inactivation may be detectable only by using RNA blot analysis.

In order to investigate other genetic alterations specific to osteosarcoma, we studied c-*fos* gene expression by RNA blot analysis. Some of the results are shown in Fig. 3. *Fos* gene expression was detected by RNA blot analysis in all osteosarcoma cases and other malignant bone tumors but was not present in either soft tissue tumors or in normal tissues. Moreover, although the degree of *fos* gene expression varied with different cases, the levels were relatively higher level in osteosarcomas and chondrosarcomas when the band intensity was

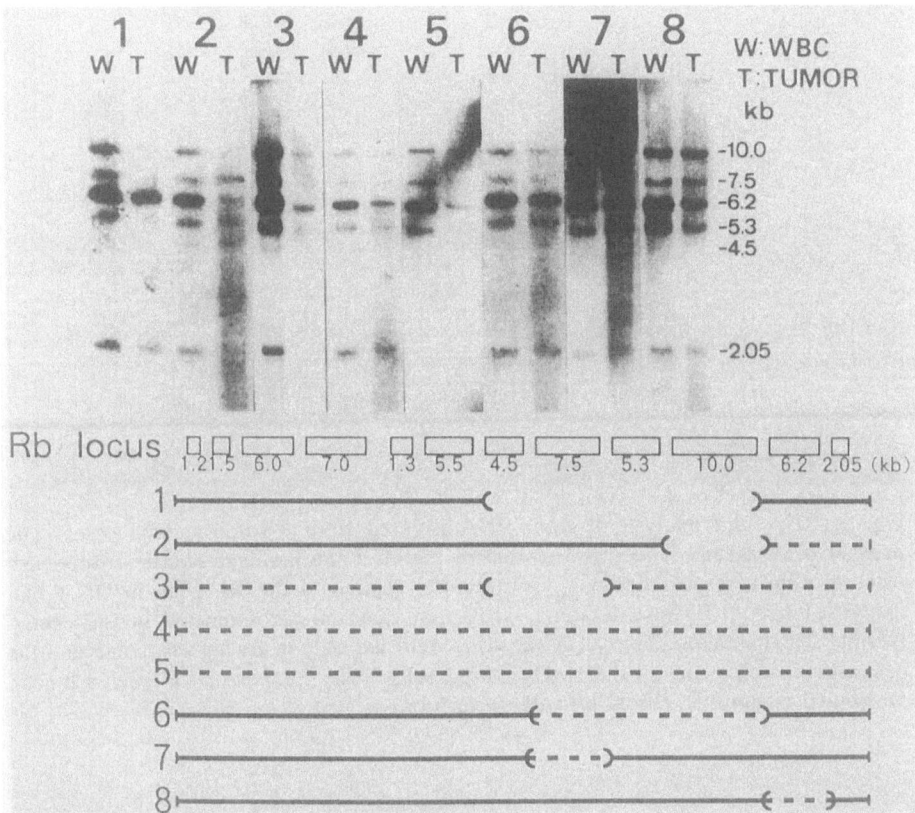

Fig. 1. DNA blot analysis of osteosarcomas (*upper*) and the schematic representation of their deletion patterns (*lower*) *Upper* DNA blot analysis of genomic DNA from white blood cell (*W*) and tumor tissue (*T*) of patients with osteosarcoma. The same amount of DNA was digested with *Hind* III restriction endonuclease and hybridized with a p3.8R probe. *OS 1–3*, homozygous deletion; *OS 4–8*, heterozygous deletion. Molecular weight markers are shown on the *right* side in kilobase pairs (kb). *Each band* shows a DNA fragment detected with the p3.8R probe: 10.0, 7.5, 6.2, 5.3, 4.5, and 2.05 kb DNA fragments in the Rb locus. Deletion patterns of the Rb loci in each tumor DNA are represented in the *lower* scheme. *Lower* Schematic ordering of deletions in the genomic DNA from each cases of osteosarcoma. Each of the boxes at the *top line* represents a discrete *Hind* III fragment detectable with p0.9R and p3.8R. The sizes of each fragment are indicated by the *number* under the boxes in kilobase. The number of each line is identical with the number of lanes in DNA blotting (*upper*). *Dotted lines* between brackets show heterozygous deletion, *open bracket*, homozygous deletion. (From [5] with permission)

measured by a densitometer (Fig. 4). Densitometric analysis of these *fos* band intensities revealed that some of the osteosarcoma cases showed very high *fos* expression in comparison with the β-actin expression. These results of *fos* gene expression were very useful as an indicator of malignant tumors with osteogenic or chondrogenic potential.

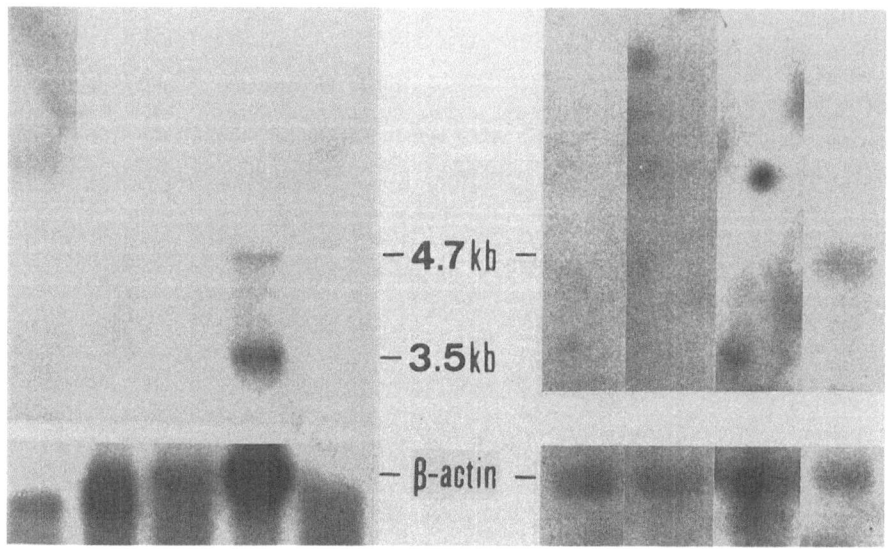

Fig. 2. RNA blot analysis of total RNA isolated from 8 osteosarcoma cases. The number of each lane is identical to that of Fig. 1. Lane numbers above 10 represent osteosarcoma cases without obvious structural change of the Rb gene in DNA blot analysis. *Lane C* Ewing's sarcoma. Molecular markers are indicated in the *center*. Normal Rb gene expressions of 4.7 kb were detected only in Ewing's sarcoma and the osteosarcoma case 23. On the *bottom panel*, rehybridized bands of ^{32}P-labeled β-actin are shown as controls. (From [5] with permission)

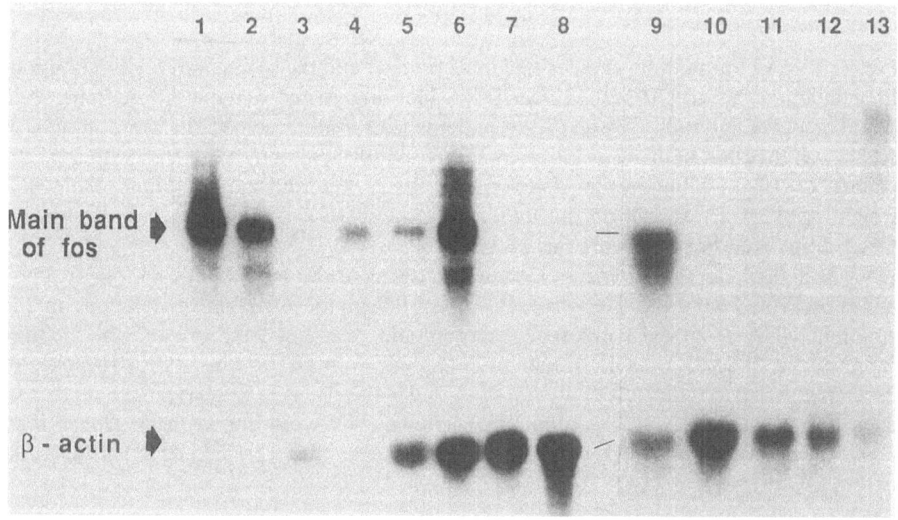

Fig. 3. C-*fos* gene expression of various bone and soft tissue tumors. Each *lane* represents the following tumors: osteosarcoma *1, 2, 3, 6* and *9*; chondrosarcoma *4, 5*; cultured osteosarcoma cell *7*; normal bone marrow *8*; malignant fibrous histiocytoma *10, 12*; malignant lymphoma *11*; synovial sarcoma *13*. *Bottom panel* shows a β-actin band of the same filter

Fig. 4. Densitometric analysis of c-*fos* gene expression. The highest intensity was assigned as 100%. Osteosarcoma and chondrosarcoma are represented by a relatively high intensity. The differences between malignant and benign tumors are apparent. *MFH*, Malignant fibrous histiocytoma

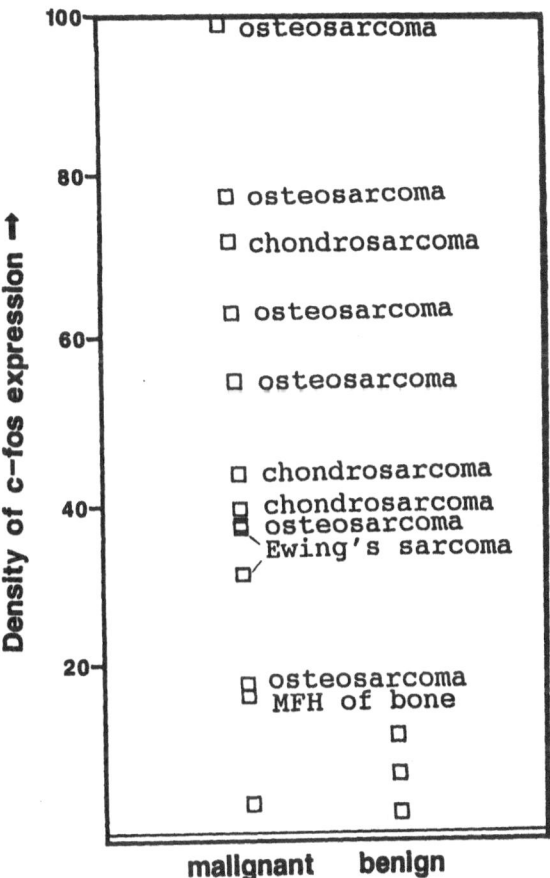

Discussion

With regard to the genetic abnormality responsible for the induction of bone and soft tissue tumors, no characteristic or specific disorder has been found for these mesenchymal cell-originated tumors. In this study, we showed that structural alterations of genomic DNA at the Rb locus were detected by DNA blot analysis in 35% of 23 osteosarcoma cases, and that Rb mRNA was undetectable or truncated in all 8 available tissue samples. These frequencies are consistent with the data on retinoblastoma in that approximately 40% of the patients with retinoblastoma showed apparent structural changes in DNA and most of the remaining patients showed either no expression or expression of a truncated transcription in RNA blot analysis [3, 10–12]. Therefore, our results suggest that abnormality in this anti-oncogene is strongly connected with osteosarcoma. Moreover, there is a report that introduction of a normal Rb gene into retinoblastoma cells suppresses their neoplastic phenotype, including tumorigenicity in nude mice [13]. These results prove that the Rb gene suppresses tumor cell progression and that the inactivation of this gene is intimately concerned with tumorigenesis of osteosarcoma.

In addition, we showed high expression of the c-*fos* gene which may be correlated with this tumor. The characteristic expression of this gene only in malignant bone tumors, especially in osteosarcoma and chondrosarcoma, suggests that c-*fos* might be correlated with bone or cartilage formation in these bone tumors. Densitometric analysis of the degree of this gene expression represents a useful diagnostic tool for osteosarcoma. However, analysis in a greater number of patients is necessary.

Conclusions

We found that abnormalities in these two genes are not specific but are so common to osteosarcoma that we should be able to use these data for an additional diagnostic tool. Although there is not yet enough data, investigation of the clinical association of these involvements of genes will be able to offer a new grading or staging system in addition to the ordinary classifications presently in clinical use. There are also many other important genes on which analyses are being undertaken, such as *mdr* [14] and p53 [15]. The final purpose of these analyses is not only to understand the etiologic factor of these tumors but also to use the result as a definitive characteristic of each tumor. In order to establish this information as a clinical marker, we must accumulate more data from gene analyses in bone and soft tissue tumors.

Acknowledgments. The authors would like to thank Dr. S.H. Friend for kindly providing the cDNA probe of the Rb gene and Ms. D. Robinson for helpful comments during preparation of the manuscript.

References

1. Klein G (1987) The approaching era of the tumor suppressor genes. Science 238:1539–1545
2. Fojo AT, Ueda K, Slamon DJ, Poplack DG, Gottesman MM, Pastan I (1987) Expression of a multidrug-resistant gene in human tumors and tissues. Proc Natl Acad Sci USA 84:265–269
3. Friend SH, Bernards R, Rogeli S, Weinberg RA, Rapaport JM, Albert DM, Drija TP (1986) A human DNA segment with properties of the gene that predisposes to retinoblastoma and osteosarcoma. Nature 323:643–646
4. Abramson DH, Ellsworth RM, Kitchin FD, Tung G (1984) Second nonocular tumors in retinoblastoma survivors. Ophthalmology 91:1351–1355
5. Araki N, Uchida A, Kimura T, Yoshikawa H, Aoki Y, Ueda T, Takai S, Miki T, Ono K (1991) Involvement of the retinoblastoma gene in primary osteosarcoma and other bone and soft-tissue tumors. Clin Orthop 270:271–277
6. Finkel MP, Biskis BO, Jinkins PB (1966) Virus induction of osteosarcoma in mice. Science 151:698–701

7. Curran T, Macconnell WP, Straaten FV, Verma IM (1983) Structure of the FBJ murine osteosarcoma virus genome: Molecular cloning of its associated helper virus and the cellular homolog of the v-*fos* gene from mouse and human cells. Mol Cell Biol 3:914–921
8. Rüther U, Garber C, Komitowski D, Muller R, Wagner EF (1987) Deregulated c-*fos* expression interferes with normal bone development in transgenic mice. Nature 325:412–416
9. Sambrook J, Fritsch EF, Maniatis T (1989) Molecular cloning: A laboratory manual, 2nd edn. Cold Spring Harbor Laboratory, New York
10. Fung YKT, Murphree AL, T'Ang A, Qian J, Hinrichs SH, Benedict WF (1987) Structural evidence for the authenticity of the human retinoblastoma gene. Science 236:1657–1661
11. Lee WH, Bookstein R, Hong F, Young LJ, Lee EYHP (1987) Human retinoblastoma susceptibility gene: Cloning, identification, and sequence. Science 235:1394–1399
12. Toguchida T, Ishizaki K, Sasaki MS, Ikenaga M, Sugimoto M, Kotoura Y, Yamamuro T (1988) Chromosomal reorganization for the expression of recessive mutation of retinoblastoma susceptibility gene in the development of osteosarcoma. Cancer Res 48:3939–3943
13. Huang HJS, Yee JK, Shew JY, Chen PL, Bookstein R, Friedmann T, Lee EYHP, Lee WH (1988) Suppression of the neoplastic phenotype by replacement of the Rb gene in human cancer cells. Science 242:1563–1566
14. Wunder J, Bell RS, Czitrom A, Andrulis I (1991) MDR1 expression and clinical outcome in osteosarcoma: A pilot study. ORS Transaction, 37th 16:264
15. Miller CW, Aslo A, Tsay C, Slamon D, Ishizaki K, Toguchida J, Yamamuro T, Lampkin B, Koeffler P (1990) Frequency and structure of p53 rearrangements in human osteosarcoma. Cancer Res 50:7950–7954

Section II
Histological Diagnosis

1.5

Histopathological Diagnosis of Soft Tissue and Bone Tumors by Cytological, Architectural, and Matrical Characteristics

HIDEO NAMIKI[1]

Introduction

Pathological diagnosis of tumors generally depends upon the clinical information, gross appearance, and microscopic features of the tissue specimen. The microscopic features include the cytological characteristics of the tumor cells, their arrangement, the interrelationship between the tumor cells and the supportive tissue, and the results of special studies.

Microscopic diagnosis of epithelial tumors is usually simpler than that of non-epithelial tumors. Epithelial tumors are composed of compact groups of cells, referred to as "nests", which are supported by a non-neoplastic supportive stroma. Depending upon the type of differentiation, epithelial tumors are classified into a relatively small number of groups: gland-forming tumors, tumors with squamous differentiation, neuroendocrinic tumors closely resembling their native tissue (such as tumors of most endocrine glands and tumors of hepatocellular origin), and undifferentiated carcinomas.

In contrast, microscopic diagnosis of non-epithelial tumors can be a difficult task due to their heterogenous origins. There are many non-epithelial tumors, mostly benign, which are associated with clinical and pathological presentations so characteristic that the diagnosis can easily be established by routine hematoxylin and eosin preparations. However, there are also a number of benign and malignant non-epithelial tumors with microscopic features resembling those of other tissue origins.

Pathologists with little experience with tumors of non-epithelial tissues are easily bewildered when they face the complexity of the histopathology of these tumors. There should be a way to overcome this problem. A classification of soft tissue tumors by their cytological, and architectural characteristics, which I

[1] Department of Pathology, The Queen's Medical Center, PO Box 861, Honolulu, Hawaii, 96808 USA

prepared, was found to be useful and practical. By categorizing the tumor under investigation according to this scheme, the number of types of tumor to be differentiated is relatively limited. The examiner, then, establishes the final pathological diagnosis based upon clinical information, gross characteristics of the submitted specimen, and the detailed microscopic features of the tumor, including those of special stains.

Assessment of the histogenesis of soft tissue tumors has been difficult even for experienced pathologists. Recent advances in immunohistochemistry have contributed greatly to the histogenetically differential diagnosis of these tumors. Currently, immunohistochemical studies have become an integral part in the diagnosis of soft tissue tumors; conversely, conventional special stains and electron microscopy play a relatively limited role because of difficulty in the interpretation of the results inherent to the former study, and the time-consuming procedures and high cost of the latter.

It is believed that a combination of subtyping of soft tissue tumors by their cytological, architectural, and matrical characteristics, a careful observation of microscopic features as seen in routine and common histochemical stains, and application of proper immunohistochemical stains provides a simple and accurate approach to the diagnosis of soft tissue tumors. According to the proposed classification, one tumor may have features fitting 2 or more categories. For example, a so-called monophasic synovial sarcoma may fit the categories of "spindle cell tumors," "tumors with prominent lobulation," and, partly, "biphasic tumors."

A comparable classification of bone tumors has been also prepared and found to be quite useful in the histopathological diagnosis of bone tumors.

Histopathological Diagnosis of Soft Tissue Tumors by Cytological, Architectural, and Matrical Characteristics

Spindle Cell Tumors

1. *Tumors and tumor-like lesions of fibrous tissue*: fibromatoses, nodular fasciitis, proliferative fasciitis, fibrous granulation tissue, scar and keloid, elastofibroma, fibroma of tendon sheath, fibrous hamartoma of infancy, calcifying aponeurotic fibroma, infantile digital fibroma, infantile myofibromatosis, nasopharyngeal angiofibroma, cranial fasciitis of childhood, fibroosseous pseudotumor of the digit, fibrosarcoma
2. *Tumors and tumor-like lesions of peripheral nerves*: traumatic neuroma, nerve sheath myxoma, neuromuscular hamartoma, schwannoma, solitary neurofibroma, neurofibromatosis, epithelioid neurofibroma, ganglioneuroma, malignant schwannoma
3. *Tumors of smooth muscle*: leiomyoma, angioleiomyoma, "epithelioid smooth muscle tumors" (stromal tumors of the gastrointestinal tract), leiomyosarcoma

4. *Tumors of skeletal muscle*: rhabdomyoma (infantile and genital), rhabdomyosarcoma
5. *Fibrohistiocytic tumors*: fibrous histiocytoma (dermatofibroma), dermato-fibrosarcoma protuberans, giant cell fibroblastoma [1], malignant fibrous histiocytoma
6. *Tumors of adipose tissue*: spindle cell lipoma, angiolipoma, sclerosing type of well-differentiated liposarcoma
7. *Tumors of blood vessels*: spindle cell hemangioendothelioma, spindle cell dominant angiosarcoma, Kaposi's sarcoma
8. *Tumors of the serous membrane*: localized fibrous tumor of serous membrane, diffuse sarcomatoid mesothelioma
9. *Synovial sarcoma*
10. *Hemangiopericytoma*
11. *Melanocytic tumors*: Spitz nevus (spindle cell type), cellular blue nevus, melanoma
12. *Bone tumors*: fibrous dysplasia, periosteal desmoid, fibroma, fibro-sarcoma, osteosarcoma
13. *Sarcomatoid variant of carcinomas*: squamous cell carcinoma, renal cell carcinoma
14. *Tumors of the central nervous system*: fibrous meningioma, pilocytic astrocytoma

Small-Cell Tumors (Little Blue Cell Tumors)

These are neoplasms with small cells, less than 20 microns in diameter, with hyperchromatic nuclei and scanty cytoplasm.

1. *Embryonal rhabdomyosarcoma*
2. *Extraskeletal Ewing's sarcoma*
3. *Peripheral neuroepithelioma/neuroblastoma*
4. *Lymphoma/leukemia*
5. *Small cell undifferentiated carcinoma*
6. *Neuroendocrinic tumors*
7. *Merkel cell carcinoma*
8. *Hemangiopericytoma*
9. *Mesenchymal chondrosarcoma*
10. *Nephroblastoma metastatic to soft tissue*
11. *"Epithelioid smooth muscle tumor, small cell variant"*
12. *Plasmacytoma*
13. *Mastocytosis*
14. *Intra-abdominal desmoplastic small round-cell tumor [2]*

Pleomorphic Cell Tumors with Giant Cells

1. *Malignant fibrous histiocytoma*
2. *Atypical fibroxanthoma of the skin*
3. *Fibrous histiocytoma (dermatofibroma)*

4. *Pleomorphic rhabdomyosarcoma*
5. *Pleomorphic liposarcoma and lipoma*
6. *Malignant schwannoma and ancient schwannoma*
7. *Leiomyosarcoma*
8. *Atypical (symplastic; bizarre) leiomyoma of the uterus*
9. *"Epithelioid smooth muscle tumors"*
10. *Malignant melanoma and Spitz nevus (epithelioid cell type)*
11. *Malignant lymphoma (diffuse, large-cell, polymorphous type)*
12. *Large (giant) cell undifferentiated carcinoma*
13. *Osteosarcoma* extending/metastatic to soft tissue
14. *Giant cell tumor of the tendon sheath, localized/diffuse/malignant*
15. *Giant cell fibroblastoma*

Large Round/Polygonal-Cell Tumors

1. *Mesothelioma*
2. *Synovial sarcoma*
3. *Epithelioid sarcoma*
4. *Clear cell sarcoma*
5. *Malignant fibrous histiocytoma*
6. *Alveolar soft part sarcoma*
7. *Malignant rhabdoid tumor*
8. *Hibernoma*
9. *Granular cell tumor*
10. *Proliferative fasciitis and myositis*
11. *"Epithelioid smooth muscle tumors"*
12. *Epithelioid hemangioma and angiosarcoma*
13. *Epithelioid neurofibroma, epithelioid malignant schwannoma, ganglioneuroma*
14. *Nevi and malignant melanoma*
15. *Malignant lymphoma*
16. *Benign and malignant epithelial tumors*
17. *Meningioma*

Biphasic Tumors

1. *Synovial sarcoma*
2. *Diffuse mesothelioma*
3. *Malignant mixed Müllerian (mesodermal) tumor* (a highly malignant tumor arising from the endometrial stroma; common sarcomatous components include embryonal rhabdomyosarcoma, stromal sarcoma, leiomyosarcoma, chondrosarcoma, and osteosarcoma, in order of frequency)
4. *Tumors of the sweat gland (nodular hidradenoma), breast (fibroadenoma and phyllode tumor), and salivary and related glands (pleomorphic adenoma)*

5. *Poorly differentiated carcinoma with foci of osseous and/or cartilaginous metaplasia (e.g., metaplastic carcinoma of the breast)*
6. *Malignant melanoma with foci of osseous and/or cartilaginous metaplasia*
7. *Poorly differentiated squamous cell carcinoma with spindle cell foci ("carcinosarcoma")*
8. *Ovarian carcinoma with sarcoma-like stromal proliferation, particularly clear cell carcinoma*

Tumors with a Pericytomatous Vascular Pattern

1. *Hemangiopericytoma*
2. *Mesenchymal chondrosarcoma*
3. *Synovial sarcoma*
4. *Malignant fibrous histiocytoma*
5. *Osteosarcoma* extending/metastatic to soft tissue
6. *Many other sarcomas* (the pericytomatous vascular pattern being usually limited to focal areas)
7. *Localized fibrous tumor of the serous membrane, cellular variant*
8. *Thymoma, particularly spindle cell type*
9. *Stromal sarcoma of the uterus*
10. *Glomangioma*

Highly Vascularized Tumors

1. *Tumors and tumor-like lesions of the blood and lymph vessels:* hemangioma, lymphangioma, vascular malformations, telangiectasis, angiosarcoma
2. *Pyogenic granuloma*
3. *Masson's "vegetant intravascular hemangioendothelioma"*
4. *Kaposi's sarcoma*
5. *Angiolipoma and myxoid liposarcoma*
6. *Glomangioma*
7. *Alveolar soft part sarcoma*
8. *Paraganglioma*
9. *Osteosarcoma* extending/metastatic to soft tissue
10. *Highly vascularized carcinomas* (e.g., hepatoma and renal cell carcinoma)
11. *Endocrinic tumors*
12. *Giant cell fibroblastoma*
13. *Bacillary angiomatosis [3]*

Tumors with Prominent Myxoid Matrices

1. *Ganglia and related lesions*
2. *"Myxomas"*
3. *Nodular fasciitis*

4. *Schwann cell tumors, benign and malignant*
5. *Lipogenic tumors*: spindle cell lipoma, myxolipoma, benign lipoblastoma and lipoblastomatosis, myxoid liposarcoma
6. *Myxoid variant of dermatofibrosarcoma protuberans*
7. *Myxoid variant of malignant fibrous histiocytoma*
8. *Extraskeletal chondroid tumors*: extraskeletal chondroma, extra skeletal myxoid chondrosarcoma
9. *Chordoma* extending/metastatic to soft tissue
10. *Ossifying fibromyxoid tumor of soft parts [4]*
11. *Most spindle cell malignancies not listed above*
12. *Mucin-secreting carcinoma* metastatic to soft tissue

Tumors with Chondroid/Chondroid-Like Matrices

1. *Extraskeletal chondroma and chondrosarcoma*
2. *Extraskeletal myxoid chondrosarcoma*
3. *Chordoma* extending/metestatic to soft tissue
4. *Juvenile aponeurotic fibroma*
5. *Apocrine and eccrine mixed tumor*
6. *Pleomorphic adenoma of salivary gland and related tumors*
7. *Synovial chondromatosis and chondrometaplasia*
8. *Chondroid metaplasia in benign and malignant tumors*

Tumors with an Osteoid/Osseous Matrix

1. *Myositis ossificans*
2. *Fibrodysplasia (myositis) ossificans progressiva*
3. *Extraskeletal osteosarcoma*
4. *Ossifying fibromyxoid tumor of soft parts*
5. *Fracture callus*
6. *Osseous metaplasia in non-osseous tumor*
7. *Osseous metaplasia in foci of dystrophic calcification*

Tumors with Melanin Production

1. *Nevi and malignant melanoma*
2. *Melanotic Schwann cell tumors*: melanotic neurofibroma, melanotic schwannoma, malignant melanocytic schwannoma
3. *Pigmented neuroectodermal tumor of infancy*
4. *Bednar tumor (pigmented dermatofibrosarcoma protuberans)*
5. *Clear cell sarcoma*

Tumors with Marked Hemorrhaging and Hemosiderin Formation

1. *Tenosynovial giant cell tumor, localized and diffuse types*
2. *Pigmented villonodular synovitis*

3. *Synovial hemangioma*
4. *Angiomatoid "malignant fibrous histiocytoma" [5, 6]*
5. *Schwannoma*

Superficially Located Tumors

Common benign dermal tumors are omitted from this category. Those included in this category arise in the subcutaneous tissue, tenosynovial tissue, fascia, and other superficially located tissues.

1. *Dermatofibrosarcoma protuberans and giant cell fibroblastoma*
2. *Malignant fibrous histiocytoma*
3. *Angiomatoid "Malignant fibrous histiocytoma"*
4. *Leiomyosarcoma (in which superficially located leiomyosarcomas commonly pursue less aggressive courses than those located deep in the soft tissue)*
5. *Malignant schwannoma complicating neurofibromatosis*
6. *Epithelioid sarcoma*
7. *Clear cell sarcoma*
8. *Synovial sarcoma*
9. *Extraskeletal chondroma*
10. *Nodular and proliferative fasciitis*

Histopathological Diagnosis of Bone Tumors by Cytological, Architectural, and Matrical Characteristics

Osteoid/Bone-Forming Tumors and Tumor-Like Lesions

1. *Osteoma*
2. *Enostosis (medullary osteoma)*
3. *Osteochondroma (osteocartilaginous exostosis)*
4. *Callus*
5. *Traumatic periostisis*
6. *Osteoid osteoma*
7. *Osteoblastoma*
8. *Fibrous dysplasia*
9. *Osteofibrous dysplasia*
10. *Hamartoma (mesenchymoma) of chest wall*
11. *"Reactive" bone to other benign lesions*
12. *Osteosarcoma, intramedullary type*
13. *Parosteal (juxtacortical) osteosarcoma*
14. *Periosteal osteosarcoma*
15. *Telangiectatic osteosarcoma*
16. *High-grade surface osteosarcoma*
17. *Low-grade central osteosarcoma*
18. *Small cell osteosarcoma [7]*

19. *"Reactive" bone to other malignancies*
20. *Fibro-osseous lesions of jawbones*: fibrous dysplasia, ossifying fibroma, cemento-ossifying fibroma

Intraosseous Cartilage- and Chondroid-Forming Tumors/Lesions

 1. *Osteochondroma*
 2. *Multiple osteochondromas (osteochondromatosis)*
 3. *Subungual exostoses*
 4. *Extraskeletal chondroma*
 5. *Enchondroma (chondroma)*
 6. *Periosteal (juxtacortical) chondroma*
 7. *Multiple chondromas (multiple enchondromatosis; Ollier's disease)*
 8. *Chondroblastoma*
 9. *Chondromyxoid fibroma*
10. *Fibrous dysplasia*
11. *Cartilaginous callus*
12. *Chordoma*
13. *Chondrosarcoma* (classified as primary or secondary, central or peripheral, and typed as conventional, dedifferentiated, clear-cell, mesenchymal, or myxoid)
14. *Osteosarcoma, chondroblastic variant*
15. *Periosteal osteosarcoma*

Intraosseous and Juxtaosseous Spindle Cell Tumors/Lesions

 1. *Fibrous dysplasia*
 2. *Periosteal desmoid (avulsive cortical irregularity; fibrous cortical defect)*
 3. *Fibroma (metaphyseal fibrous defect; non-ossifying fibroma)*
 4. *Schwannoma (neurilemoma)*
 5. *Benign reactive fibrosis and fibrous scar*
 6. *Chondromyxoid fibroma*
 7. *Fibrosarcoma*
 8. *Malignant fibrous histiocytoma*
 9. *Osteosarcoma, fibroblastic variant*
10. *Dedifferentiated chondrosarcoma*
11. *"Monophasic" synovial sarcoma in the parosteal region*
12. *Adamantinoma*
13. *Metastatic sarcomatoid variant of carcinomas and melanomas*

Intraosseous Tumors/Lesions with Giant Cells

 1. *Giant cell tumor*
 2. *Giant cell reparative granuloma*
 3. *Non-ossifying fibroma*
 4. *Aneurysmal bone cyst*

5. *Brown tumor of hyperparathyroidism*
6. *Unicameral bone cyst*
7. *Chondroblastoma*
8. *Fibrous dysplasia*
9. *Osteosarcoma*
10. *Chondromyxoid fibroma*
11. *Osteoblastoma and osteoid osteoma*
12. *High-grade chondrosarcoma*
13. *Malignant fibrous histiocytoma*
14. *Metastatic carcinoma/melanoma*

Intraosseous and Parosteal Small-Cell Tumors

1. *Ewing's sarcoma*
2. *Malignant lymphoma of bone*
3. *Metastatic neuroblastoma/neuroepithelioma*
4. *Small cell osteosarcoma*
5. *Metastatic small cell undifferentiated carcinoma*
7. *Mastocytosis (mast cell disease)*

Intraosseous Round-Cell/Polygonal-Cell Tumors/Lesions

These tumors/lesions are composed of relatively large, round/polygonal cells with a fair amount of cytoplasm often producing an appearance like that of carcinomas.

1. *Histiocytosis X (eosinophilic granuloma/Hand-Schüller-Christian disease/ Letterer-Siwe disease; Langerhans' cell granulomatosis)*
2. *Gaucher's disease*
3. *Adamantinoma*
4. *Epithelioid variant of hemangioma and angiosarcoma*
5. *Chordoma, myxoid chondrosarcoma, and clear cell chondrosarcoma*
6. *Synovial sarcoma invading the bone*
7. *Metastatic carcinoma, melanoma, and sarcomas having an epithelioid appearance*

Intraosseous Highly Vascularized Tumors/Lesions

1. *Hemangioma and vascular malformations*
2. *Massive osteolysis (disappearing bone; phantom bone; Gorham's disease)*
3. *Lymphangioma*
5. *Angioblastic meningioma invading the skull bone*
6. *Angiosarcoma*
7. *Hemangiopericytoma*
8. *Aneurysmal bone cyst*
9. *Osteosarcoma and malignant fibrous histiocytoma*
10. *Metastatic carcinoma with high vascularity*

Intraosseous and Parosteal Epithelioid Tumors/Lesions

1. *Epidermal inclusion cyst*
2. *Adamantinoma of long bone*
3. *Synovial sarcoma* metastatic to or invading bone
4. *Metastatic carcinoma/melanoma*

Intraosseous Myxoid Tumors/Lesions

1. *Myxoma (fibromyxoma) of bone*
2. *Chondromyxoid fibroma*
3. *Benign chondroid tumors with myxoid change (enchondroma, osteo-chondroma, and callus)*
4. *Fibrous dysplasia with myxoid change*
5. *Malignant chondroid tumors (chondrosarcoma and chordoma)*
6. *Other malignant tumors with myxoid change (fibrosarcoma, malignant fibrous histiocytoma, etc.).*

Intraosseous Cystic Tumors/Lesions

1. *Intraosseous ganglion*
2. *Cystic lesions in inflammatory (rheumatoid arthritis) or degenerative (osteoarthritis) joint diseases*
3. *Solitary (unicameral; simple) bone cyst*
4. *Aneurysmal bone cyst*
5. *Telangiectatic osteosarcoma*
6. *Fracture callus with superimposed recent hemorrhages (hematomas)*
7. *Fibrous dysplasia*

References

1. Shmookler BM, Enzinger FM, Weiss SW (1989) Giant cell fibroblastoma: A juvenile form of dermatofibrosarcoma protuberans. Cancer 64:2154–2161
2. Gerald WL, Miller HK, Battifora H, et al. (1991) Intra-abdominal desmoplastic small round-cell tumor: Report of 19 cases of a distinctive type of high-grade polyphenotypic malignancy affecting young individuals. Am J Surg Pathol 15: 499–513
3. Relman DA, Loutit JS, Schmidt TM, et al. (1990) The agent of bacillary angiomatosis: An approach to the identification of uncultured pathogens. N Engl J Med 323:1573–1580
4. Enzinger FM, Weiss SW, Liang CY (1989) Ossifying fibromyxoid tumor of soft parts: A clinicopathological analysis of 59 cases. Am J Surg Pathol 13:817–827
5. Costa MJ, Weiss SW (1990) Angiomatoid malignant fibrous histiocytoma: A follow-up study of 108 cases with evaluation of possible histologic predictors of outcome. Am J Surg Pathol 14:1126–1132

6. Fletcher CD (1991) Angiomatoid "malignant fibrous histiocytoma": An immuno-histochemical study indicative of myoid differentiation. Hum Pathol 22:563–568
7. Ayala AG, Ro JY, Raymond AK, et al. (1989) Small cell osteosarcoma: A clinicopathologic study of 27 cases. Cancer 64:2162–2173

1.6

Preliminary Histomorphometric Study on Pathological Grading of Giant Cell Tumors of Bone

RUI-ZONG LEE, SHUN-LU YU, and ZHAO-HAN BIAN[1]

Introduction

Since Jaffe and his associates [1, 2], emphasized the importance of histological grading of giant cell tumor (GCT) of bone and classified them into three grades, benign or low aggressive, more aggressive or malignant, and frankly malignant, most of the orthopedists, radiologists, and pathologists in China adopted this grading system [3–6]. Pathological grading of GCT of bone is a complicated process and different opinions may exist among individual pathologists for the same specimen. However, histopathological observation of GCT of bone is benificial for predicting prognosis, and we attempted to determine the pathological grading of GCT of bone using histomorphometry.

Materials and Methods

A retrospective analysis was carried on 24 cases of GCT of bone encountered between 1980–1984. All the diagnoses were confirmed pathologically. The male to female ratio was 2:1 and the peak incidence occurred in the age range of 21–40 years. In 10 cases the lesions were located in the femur, 8 in the tibia, 4 in the radius, and 1 each in the fibula and rib. With the conventional method of pathological grading, there were 4 cases of grade I (Fig. 1), 17 of grade II (Fig. 2), and 3 of grade III (Fig. 3). For the histomorphometric study, the paraffin-embedded specimens were made into sections of 3–5 μ in thickness and stained with hematoxylin and eosin. The slides were first examined and photographed under a high power light microscope ($\times$400) and 5 fields were taken for each specimen producing a total of 120 pictures. The pictures were scanned with a Houston Instrument 8042 linked to an IBM AT Auto program. The data

[1]Department of Pathology, Orthopedic Institute, Tianjin Hospital, Tianjin, 300211 China

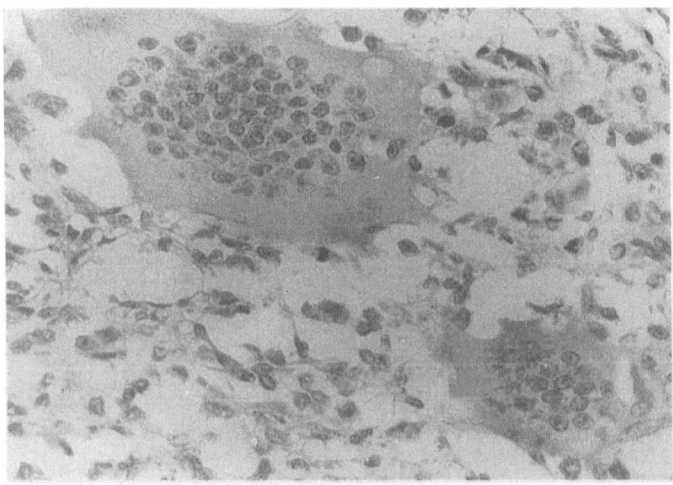

Fig. 1. Pathological appearance of giant cell tumor (GCT) of bone. Grade I, ×400

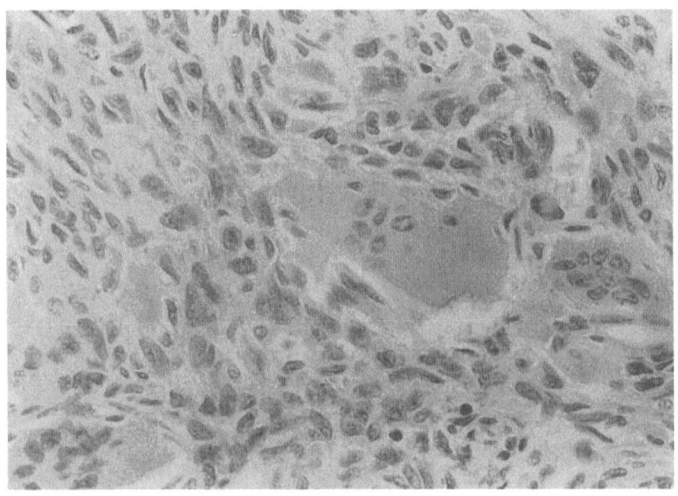

Fig. 2. Pathological appearance of grade II giant cell tumor (GCT) of bone, ×400

were obtained with calculations done by the IBM program and evaluated statistically.

The value of volume occupied by the giant cells (Vol. GC), volume of the space of giant cells (GC) between stroma cells (Vol. Space GC), and volume of maximal GC (Max. Vol. GC) were measured. A linear intercept method was used to determine the number of GC (No. GC), the number of stroma cells (No. SC), and the maximal number of nuclei of GC (Max. No. N. GC). The calculations were done for the volume of SC (*Vol. SC*, total volume − volume of GC − space of GC), volume index of GC and SC (*Vol. Ind. GC. SC*,

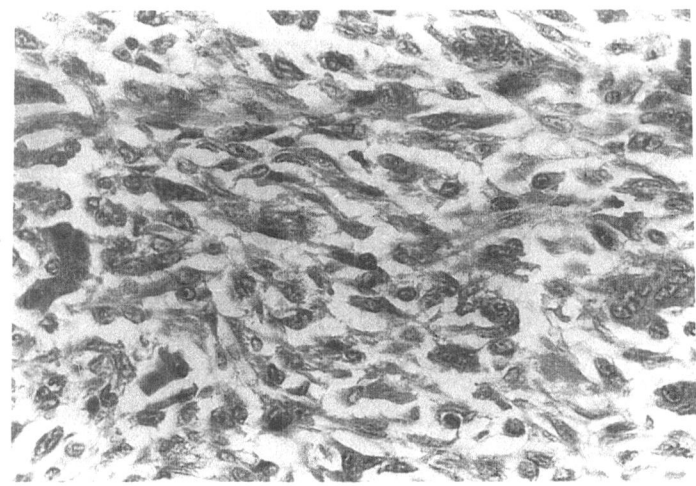

Fig. 3. Pathological appearance of giant cell tumor (GCT) of bone. Grade III, ×400

volume of GC:volume of SC), morphologic index of GC (*Morph. Ind. GC*, volume of GC:perimeter of GC), size index of GC (*Size Ind. GC*, No. GC:Vol. GC), and quantity index of GC and SC (*Quant. Ind. GC. SC*, number of SC). The result revealed statistical differences in the individual determinations as shown in Tables 1–4. (In each table, *S.S.* indicated statistical significance, * significance, and ** remarkable significance.)

Results

A remarkable statistical significance was seen in the data of the volume of GC and SC between grades I–III, I–II, and II–III tumors. The volume of space of GC showed a similar significance to the volume of GC, SC, while no significant difference was seen in grades II–III lesions. The volume index of GC and SC revealed significant differences in grades I–III tumors, followed by grades II–III and I–III lesions (Table 1). The number of GCs showed remarkable differences between grades I–III and I–II tumors, while no significance was evident in the II and III lesions. No statistical significance was observed in the number of SCs between the specimens of different grades. The quantity index of GC and SC showed marked significance in grades I–III and II–III tumors, while the difference was slight between the I and II lesions (Table 2). The statistical significance of the size index and morphological index of GC followed in a decreasing order from I–III, I–II, and II–III (Table 3). Table 4 shows the statistical differences of the maximal number of nuclei of GC and maximal volume of GC and the data followed in a decreasing order from I–II, II–III, and I–III.

Table 1. Volume of giant cells (GC) and stroma cells (SC), volume index of GC and SC, volume space of GC

	Grade	$\bar{X}$	A–B	$\bar{X}a-\bar{X}b$	a	q	$P = 0.05$	$P = 0.01$	S.S.
GC Vol.	I	23.6700	1–3	17.5008	3	23.9130	3.40	4.28	**
	II	12.3185	1–2	11.3515	2	15.5251	2.83	3.76	**
	III	6.1692	2–3	6.1493	2	8.3880	2.83	3.76	**
SC Vol.	III	87.4367	3–1	25.7943	3	21.0873	3.40	4.28	**
	II	78.8028	3–2	8.6339	2	6.8933	2.83	3.76	**
	I	61.6424	2–1	17.1604	2	14.1941	2.83	3.76	**
Vol. Ind. GC. SC.	III	14.1731	3–1	11.5689	3	10.2135	3.40	4.28	**
	II	6.3971	3–2	7.7760	2	6.3787	2.83	3.76	**
	I	2.6042	2–1	3.7929	2	2.9348	2.83	3.76	*
Vol. GC. Space	I	14.6631	1–3	7.9691	3	10.1486	3.40	4.28	**
	II	8.8787	1 3	5.7011	2	7.3663	2.03	3.76	! !
	III	6.6940	2–3	2.1847	2	2.1847	2.83	3.76	

Abbreviations: see text

Table 2. Number of giant cells (GC) and stroma cells (SC), quantity index of GC and SC

	Grade	$\bar{X}$	A–B	$\bar{X}a-\bar{X}b$	a	q	$P = 0.05$	$P = 0.01$	S.S.
No. SC	II	171.9667	2–1	19.3000	3	2.9816	3.40	4.28	
	III	162.7000	2–3	9.2667	2	1.4316	2.83	3.76	
	I	152.6667	3–1	10.0333	2	1.5500	2.83	3.76	
No. GC	I	6.6667	1–3	2.1000	3	5.9797	3.40	4.28	**
	II	6.0667	1–2	0.6000	2	1.7084	2.83	3.76	
	III	4.5667	2–3	1.5000	2	4.2712	2.83	3.76	**
Quant. Ind. GC. SC.	III	35.6274	3–1	12.7276	3	6.0518	3.40	4.28	**
	II	28.3460	3–2	7.2814	2	3.9894	2.83	3.76	**
	I	22.8998	2–1	5.4462	2	2.1624	2.83	3.76	

Abbreviations: see text

Table 3. Size index and morphologic index of giant cells (GC)

	Grade	$\bar{X}$	A–B	$\bar{X}a-\bar{X}b$	a	q	$P = 0.05$	$P = 0.01$	S.S.
Size Ind. of GC.	I	3.5504	1–3	2.1995	3	11.4445	3.40	4.28	**
	II	2.0305	1–2	1.5199	2	7.2024	2.83	3.76	**
	III	1.3509	2–3	0.6796	2	3.1321	2.83	3.76	*
Morph. Ind. of GC.	I	0.3852	1–3	0.1818	3	15.3957	3.40	4.28	**
	II	0.2720	1–2	0.1132	2	9.5841	2.83	3.76	**
	III	0.2034	2–3	0.0686	2	5.8116	2.83	3.76	**

Abbreviations: see text

Discussion

Giant cell tumor of bone is one of the most common neoplastic bony lesions seen in China, with an incidence of 26.4%, following that of osteosarcoma (34.2%) and osteochondroma (31.6%) [7]. The determination of the prognosis

Table 4. Maximal number of nuclei of giant cells (GC), maximal volume of GC

	Grade	X̄	A–B	X̄a–X̄b	a	q	P = 0.05	P = 0.01	S.S.
Max. No. N. of GC.	I	25.5000	1–3	15.1334	3	7.5300	3.40	4.28	**
	II	13.4333	1–2	12.0667	2	6.0041	2.83	3.76	**
	III	10.3666	2–3	3.0667	2	1.5259	2.83	3.76	
Max. Vol. of GC.	I	6.8213	1–3	4.9796	3	11.5868	3.40	4.28	**
	II	2.7707	1–2	4.0506	2	9.4251	2.83	3.76	**
	III	1.8417	2–3	0.9290	2	2.1616	2.83	3.76	

Abbreviations: see text

of GCT of bone is a complicated process. Besides pathological differentiation, the anatomical location, surgical staging system, and methods of treatment must all be taken into account for making any judgment [8]. Histomorphometry was generally used for the analysis of metabolic disturbance of bone and its treatment, but was used only rarely in lesions of the gastrointestinal tract for the study of tumor pathology [9, 10]. The presence of a great number of huge-sized multinucleated giant cells corresponding to many times the mononucleated stroma cells in GCT of bone provided with us the possibility to pursue further research with histomorphometry for the criteria of pathological grading of these lesions. Bone quantification can be done with simple eye-piece graticules, semiautomatic instruments, as well as fully automatic computer-linked image analysis equipment. In this study, semiautomatic instruments were used for measurement and calculation of individual determinations.

The above results revealed statistical significance between the different histopathological differentiation and the pathological grading of GCT of bone. The measured values tended to be higher in the comparatively well-differentiated lesions. This was seen in the data of the volume, space of volume, maximal volume, size index, and morphologic index of GC. A corresponding significance was noticed between grades I–III, and I–II, and declined between grades II and III. However, the volume of SC, volume index of GC and SC and quantity index of GC and SC were smaller in the well-differentiated lesions. A significant difference was seen between the grades I and II lesions, followed by grades I and III, and then grades II and III tumors. Generally, the statistical difference was much more significant between grades I and II, and I and III lesions, and mild between grades II and III specimens.

References

1. Jaffe HL, Lichtenstein L, Portis RB (1940) Giant cell tumor of bone. Arch Pathol 30:993–1031
2. Lichtenstein L (1972) Bone tumors, 4th edn. C.V. Mosby, Saint Louis
3. Lee RZ (1965) Giant cell tumor of bone. Chin J Pathol (Suppl):416–420
4. Guo BF, Cai TD, Chang HS, Shen CW, Chang PT, Liu CM (1981) Giant cell tumor of bone. Chin J Orthop 1:8–14

5. Lee RZ, Yu SL (1983) A pathological observation of giant cell tumor of bone. Chin J Orthop 3:121–123
6. Ma JK, Yan SY, Han XC (1984) Giant cell tumor of bone. Chin J Orthop 4:82–85
7. Liu ZJ, Lee RZ, Liu CM, Chang RY, Han Xun, Yang SY, Liang ZK, He TQ, Wang LT (1986) Pathological survey and analysis of tumors and tumor-like lesions of bone. Chin J Orthop 6:162–169
8. Lee RZ (1984) Correct comprehension of correlation between pathologic grading and prognosis of giant cell tumor of bone. Chin J Orthop 4:82–85
9. Reveall PA (1983) Histomorphometry of bone. J Clin Pathol 36:1323–1331
10. Riddle RH, Goldman H, Ransonglio CM (1982) Dysplasia in inflammatory bowel disease. Hum Pathol 14:931–966

Part 2
Chemotherapy

Principles of Adjuvant Chemotherapy for Bone and Soft Tissue Tumors

SHUICHI FUJIMOTO[1]

Introduction

The recent progress in the success of therapeutic effects on osteogenic sarcoma has been extraordinary and greatly enhanced by the contribution of adjuvant chemotherapy [1]. The number of treatment courses in adjuvant chemotherapy that will be adequate to eradicate all tumor cells has become a matter of concern. The principles involved in this matter and a tentative conclusion are presented by an analysis of the therapeutic results of 48 patients with osteogenic sarcoma.

Macroscopic and Microscopic Diseases

In order to obtain a cure, the accomplishment of total tumor cell kill is essential. The number of tumor cells in macroscopic diseases is in the range of 10^9 (approximately 1 g in weight and 1 cm in diameter) to 10^{12}. On the other hand, microscopic diseases have less than 10^9 of tumor cells. Thus, following the log cell kill theory [2], "3-times" more tumor cells exist in a microscopic disease than in a macroscopic disease.

Microscopic diseases consist of 9 populations from a 10^8-10^0 order of tumor cells. In patients with osteogenic sarcoma who had received no adjuvant chemotherapy, there were about 20% of continuous disease-free survivals (CDFS) [3], and who were probably cured of the disease with no residual tumor cells. Therefore, the remaining 80% of patients would theoretically be distributed equally over these 9 populations, indicating that the CDFS rate increases by 9% following each log kill of tumor cells and, thus, 100% of CDFS could be attained by 9 log kills.

A patient in the CDFS category (Fig. 1) in the present study received adjuvant chemotherapy with standard regimens according to Rosen's T-12

[1] Division of Chemotherapy, Chiba Cancer Center Research Institute, Chiba, Japan

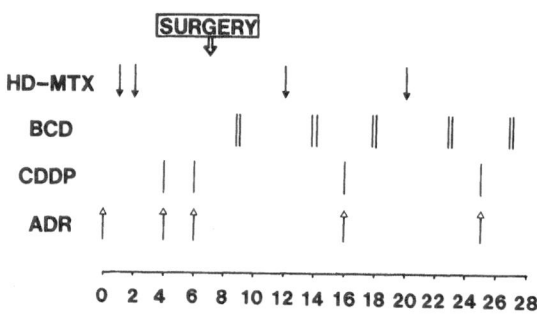

Fig. 1. Adjuvant chemotherapy given to a CDFS case (N.M.)

Table 1. Estimation of log kill potentials of various regimens used in the present study

Regimen	L[a]	Regimen	L
ADR (×2) + CDDP	1.66	ADR (×1) + CDDP	1.25
BCD (×2)	0.92	BCD (×1)	0.46
High dose MTX	0.87		
ADR (×2)	0.83	ADR (×1)	0.42
CDDP	0.83		
CPM (×2)	0.34	CPM (×1)	0.17

[a] Log tumor cell kill/course

pilot chemotherapy protocol [3]. This consisted of high-dose methotrexate with leucovorin rescue (HD-MTX), the combination of bleomycin, cyclophosphamide, and dactinomycin (BCD), and cisplatinum (CDDP) and Adriamycin (ADR) either alone or in combination. Using this regimen, it is clearly impossible to be certain how many numbers of log tumor cell kills could be performed after therapy, and, as a result, it becomes necessary to know the cell kill potential per course of each regimen.

Cell Kill Potential of Adjuvant Chemotherapy

Frei et al. [4] estimated the log kill potential per course of HD-MTX from the cytokinetic aspects of adjuvant chemotherapy of osteogenic sarcoma and deduced it to have a potential of 0.90 log tumor cell kill per course. After using their estimation method as well as a more detailed calculation method, we arrived at the log kill potentials of regimens used in the present study. (Table 1). For example, a HD-MTX regimen was recalculated as follows:

$$(100 - 16) \div 9 = 9.3\%/\log$$
$$(60 - 16) \div 9.3 = 4.7 \log s$$

If the CDFS rate of patients with surgery alone is 16%, the 84% rate of patients with microscopic deposits of the disease should be distributed over the

9 steps of the populations. Therefore, the CDFS rate increases by 9.3% following each log kill of tumor cells. By applying HD-MTX therapy, the CDFS rate reached 60%, 44% of which being attributable to adjuvant chemotherapy. It follows that by dividing 44% by 9.3%, the maximal log tumor cell kill of a HD-MTX regimen was calculated to be 4.7 logs. With this substitution in the kinetic formula of adjuvant chemotherapy [4], the log tumor cell kill per course of HD-MTX was estimated to be 0.87.

The log kill potential of the combination chemotherapy of ADR ($\times2$) and CDDP was similarly calculated from Rosen's T-12 pilot chemotherapy protocol [3]. In the grades I–II histological changes of primary tumor, preoperative adjuvant chemotherapy is considered to be ineffective not only for primary tumor but also for metastatic disease [1] and so postoperative adjuvant chemotherapy, the combination of ADR ($\times2$) and CDDP, induced 84% of CDFS (7.3 log kills). In grades III–IV, on the other hand, both pre- and postoperative adjuvant chemotherapy are considered to be effective for metastatic disease as well as for primary tumor; consequently, the log tumor cell kill per course of BCD combination was calculated to be 0.92 by applying the previous log kill potential of HD-MTX, the recovery of tumor cell population during intervals of courses (0.176 logs/week), and the CDFS rate of 84% (7.3 log kills). In addition, since the therapeutic effects of ADR ($\times2$) and CDDP on osteogenic sarcoma appeared to be similar [5, 6], the log tumor cell kill per course of both agents was estimated to be one-half the value of their combination, regardless of their favorable interaction (synergism was suggested by Vogl et al. [7]). The potential of cyclophosphamide (CPM) given for 2 successive days was estimated from the results of grades I–II (CDFS 38%, 2.3 log kills) of Rosen's T-5 protocol [8], by assuming that the therapeutic effect of CPM at a single high dose (40 mg/kg) would be similar to that of 2 successive daily doses (20 mg/kg per day). This is due to its unavoidable microsomal activation in the liver [9], the limitation (10 mg/kg) of metabolic activation in humans [10], as well as the relatively long half-life of the activated CPM in the blood [11].

In terms of the dose and tumor cell kill relationship [12], a single dose of the 2 daily doses in the protocol was estimated to have a one-half log kill potential of the individual regimens; thus, for example, a regimen of an ADR ($\times1$) and CDDP combination was estimated to have a log tumor cell kill per course of 1.25.

Cumulative Maximal Log Tumor Cell Kill and Prognosis

Forty-eight patients with osteogenic sarcoma were analyzed with respect to the cumulative maximal log tumor cell kill during or after treatment with adjuvant chemotherapy. The outcomes of these patients were CDFS for 21 patients, ANED (alive with no evidence of disease) for 6, while 21 died. Nine log tumor cell kills were achieved in only 5 out of 21 CDFS (Table 2). However, almost all the remaining 16 CDFS survived for longer than 5 years, indicating that the numbers of tumor cells deposited in these patients might be less than the individual maximal log tumor cell kills.

Table 2. Cumulative maximal log kill of tumor cells and prognosis

Outcome	Case	Sex	Age (Years)	Survival (Months)	Before the first thoracotomy	After the last thoracotomy
CDFS	J.M.	M	11	34	12.10 (22)[b]	
(21)[a]	H.Y.	M	24	38	9.38 (19)	
	M.U.	F	20	38	9.21 (23)	
	N.M.	M	24	34	9.16 (14)	
	T.T.	M	18	33	9.15 (21)	
	A.K.	M	18	96	8.58 (28)	
	K.M.	M	12	63	6.95 (29)	
	T.K.	M	10	100	6.74 (22)	
	M.M.	F	16	72	6.30 (21)	
	Y.A.	M	13	105	6.24 (29)	
	H.H.	M	20	153	6.10 (14)	
	A.T.	F	18	42	5.24 (13)	
	T.O.	F	15	91	5.24 (15)	
	R.O.	F	17	99	4.86 (22)	
	M.H.	M	13	140	4.16 (18)	
	H.O.	M	8	113	3.94 (13)	
	H.S.	F	12	64	3.72 (30)	
	H.U.	F	14	71	3.12 (14)	
	A.S.	F	12	140	2.93 (16)	
	I.S.	M	9	66	1.91 (5)	
	A.K.	F	49	75	0.37 (5)	
ANED	K.A.	M	13	114	5.40 (11)	5.61 (18)[b]
(6)	M.I.	F	11	164	0.90 (2)	3.66 (15)
	H.S.	M	14	89	5.51 (15)	3.62 (12)
	K.O.	M	13	75	2.85 (11)	2.67 (23)
	H.I.	F	16	97	4.82 (17)	2.43 (13)
	K.I.	F	27	102	3.81 (28)	2.42 (11)
Deceased	M.T.	F	12	7	5.45 (10)	
(21)	K.T.	M	16	28	6.04 (22)	5.02 (7)
	K.K.	F	10	12	1.72 (7)	2.47 (7)
	K.K.	F	11	7	2.29 (4)	
	K.I.	M	19	20	2.55 (7)	2.18 (23)
	M.O.	M	32	11	5.24 (10)	1.78 (4)
	Y.G.	F	14	10	1.44 (5)	1.69 (3)
	C.S.	F	9	26	4.52 (19)	1.56 (2)
	K.K.	M	14	9	2.64 (4)	1.55 (3)
	N.S.	M	14	20	10.82 (20)	1.25 (1)
	S.N.	F	7	41	6.01 (19)	1.25 (1)
	S.K.	M	15	72	7.46 (24)	1.11 (3)
	C.S.	M	11	6	1.04 (2)	
	Y.U.	M	12	11	4.39 (10)	1.00 (2)
	Y.U.	M	12	19	6.97 (11)	0.87 (1)
	M.T.	F	63	6	0.86 (2)	
	Y.M.	M	12	6	4.22 (8)	0.83 (1)
	T.K.	M	12	9	3.67 (9)	0.71 (4)
	M.O.	M	9	10	4.10 (10)	0.45 (2)
	M.F.	F	7	14	3.45 (10)	0.21 (1)
	K.I.	F	14	7	0.12 (2)	

[a] Number of patients, [b] course number at the maximal log kill
CDFS, Continuous disease-free survival; *ANED*, alive with no evidence of disease

Table 3. Course number required to accomplish 9 log tumor cell kills in function of cell kill potentials and course intervals

Log kill/course (L)	Course interval							
	1	2	3	4	5	6	7	8
1.60	7	7	8	10	12	15	21	39
	(7)[a]	(14)	(24)	(40)	(60)	(90)	(147)	(312)
0.90	13	16	23	42	368	?[b]		
	(13)	(32)	(69)	(168)	(1840)	(—)		
0.72	17	24	44	415	?			
	(17)	(48)	(132)	(1660)	(—)			
0.54	25	46	640	?				
	(25)	(92)	(1920)	(—)				

[a] Total weeks, [b] impossible to determine

In the ANEDs and non-surviving cases, the maximal log tumor cell kill after the last thoracotomy was calculated and compared between the 2 groups since it appeared that adjuvant chemotherapy before the first and succeeding thoracotomies had been ineffective for all the macroscopic and microscopic metastases of tumor cells. The results showed that the maximal log tumor cell kill was significantly higher ($P < 0.01$) in the ANEDs (3.40 ± 1.22, mean $\pm$ SD) than in the non-surviving groups either including (1.60 ± 1.36) or excluding (1.50 ± 1.12) five patients who had not undergone thoracotomy (Table 2). However, the reason why the patient with the least tumor cell kill in the ANED group survived while the patient with a higher tumor cell kill in the non-surviving group died is unclear. At present, it seems more likely to assume that the prognosis of patients in these 2 groups was determined by the factor of whether or not the maximal tumor cell kill exceeded the number of tumor cells in the patients.

Course Number Required to Attain 9 Log Cell Kills

In the present analysis, no clear correlation between the cumulative maximal log tumor cell kill and the prognosis of patients could be observed. Other prognostic factors must be considered in evaluating all of the therapeutic effects. However, it appears to be inevitable that similar results would be obtained in the analysis of therapeutic effects on any kind of malignancy since the microscopic deposits of tumor cells are assumed to be distributed from a 10^8-10^0 order. In spite of these considerations, patients should be treated with adjuvant chemotherapy until attaining 9 log tumor cell kills since the number of tumor cells in a patient with a microscopic disease cannot be ascertained. Consequently, it is important to assume that the tumor burden is of a 10^8 order.

The course number required in the function of various cell kill potentials and course intervals were estimated in order to achieve 9 log tumor cell kills (Table

3). The effects of dose modifications are also shown. HD-MTX was estimated to have about 0.90 of the log tumor cell kill per course. When this course was conducted at 3-week intervals, 23 courses (a total of 69 weeks) were needed to achieve 9 log kills. On the other hand, when this course was performed in a weekly schedule, only 13 courses (a total of 13 weeks) sufficed. Moreover, when the HD-MTX regimen was carried out at weekly intervals for 10 courses, the log tumor cell kill remained at 7 logs, resulting in 82% of the CDFS rate (data not shown). A dose reduction by 20% (L = 0.72) or by 40% (L = 0.54) showed a significant influence on the course number required to attain 9 log tumor cell kills. Alternatively, enhancement of log kill potential of a regimen, such as the combination of ADR (×2) and CDDP (L ≃ 1.60), required only a small number of courses to accomplish the same results.

The estimations which have been described are clearly oversimplified because the existence of drug-resistant clones in the tumor cell populations was not taken into account [13]. However, these figures may turn out to be even more probable when 2 or more effective drugs are employed in the adjuvant chemotherapy [14].

References

1. Rosen G, Caparros B, Huvos AG, Kosloff C, Nirenberg A, Cacavio A, Marcove RC, Lane JM, Mehta B, Urban C (1982) Preoperative chemotherapy for osteogenic sarcoma: Selection of postoperative adjuvant chemotherapy based on the response of the primary tumor to preoperative chemotherapy. Cancer 49:1221–1230
2. Skipper H, Schabel FM Jr, Wilcox WS (1964) Experimental evaluation of potential anticancer agents. XIV. Further study of certain basic concepts underlying chemotherapy of leukemia. Cancer Chemother Rep 45:5–28
3. Rosen G (1985) Preoperative (neoadjuvant) chemotherapy for osteogenic sarcoma: A ten-year experience. Orthopedics 8:659–664
4. Frei E, Jaffe N, Gero M, Skipper H, Watts H (1978) Adjuvant chemotherapy of osteogenic sarcoma: Progress and perspectives. J Natl Cancer Inst 60:3–10
5. Cortes EP, Holland JF, Wang JJ, Glidewell O (1975) Adriamycin (NSC-123127) in 87 patients with osteosarcoma. Cancer Chemother Rep 6 (Part 3):305–313
6. Ochs JJ, Freeman AI, Douglass HO Jr, Higby DS, Mindell ER, Sinks LF (1978) Cis-dichlorodiammine-platinum (II) in advanced osteogenic sarcoma. Cancer Treat Rep 62:239–245
7. Vogl S, Ohnuma T, Perloff M, Holland J (1976) Combination chemotherapy with Adriamycin and cis-diamminedichloroplatinum in patients with neoplastic disease. Cancer 38:21–26
8. Rosen G, Marcove RC, Caparros B, Nirenberg A, Kosloff C, Huvos A (1976) Primary osteogenic sarcoma. The rationale for preoperative chemotherapy and delayed surgery. Cancer 43:2163–2177
9. Colvin M, Brundrett RB, Kan MNN, Jardine I, Fenselau C (1976) Alkylating properties of phosphoramide mustard. Cancer Res 36:1121–1126
10. Shimoyama M, Niitani H, Kimura K (1975) Chemotherapeutic effect of cyclophosphamide and its related active compounds. 3. A design of optimal therapeutic schedules of these compounds (in Japanese). Jpn J Cancer Chemother 2:889–901

11. Bagley CM Jr, Bostick FW, DeVita VT Jr (1973) Clinical pharmacology of cyclophosphamide. Cancer Res 33:226–233
12. Frei E III, Freireich EJ (1965) Progress and perspectives in the chemotherapy of acute leukemia. Adv Chemother 2:269–298
13. Goldie JH, Coldman AJ (1979) A mathematic model for relating the drug sensitivity of tumors to their spontaneous mutation rate. Cancer Treat Rep 63:1727–1733
14. Goldie JH, Coldman AJ, Gudauskas GA (1982) Rationale for the use of alternating non-cross-resistant chemotherapy. Cancer Treat Rep 66:439–449

Principles for Designing Scientific Investigations of Orthopedic Malignancies

MASANORI FUKUSHIMA[1]

Introduction

Chemotherapy is presently at an investigational stage, and the findings of ordinary clinical practitioners are an integral part of these investigations. Since tumors of the bone or soft tissue are rare, multi-institutional study is indispensable. One example, chemotherapy of osteosarcoma, is reviewed and principles for conducting a clinical investigation are described.

Chemotherapy of Osteosarcoma

Table 1 summarizes a history of chemotherapy for osteosarcoma during the past decade [1–5]. Most of these studies were directed by medical oncologists. Since osteosarcoma is a systemic disease, as are other malignant tumors, it is impossible to manage this disease without a fundamental understanding of medical oncology. Unfortunately, there are only a small number of medical oncologists in Japan and they are usually affiliated with major cancer centers. Therefore, orthopedists must collaborate with medical oncologists in order to manage patients with this disease as well as to pursue investigations of the disease. It should be emphasized that the T-10 protocol [1] has been repeatedly used by different investigators (Table 1). If each investigator changes the regimen arbitrarily, however, reproducibility of the outcome of T-10 cannot be established, making it difficult to improve the accuracy of treatment. The author believes that Japanese orthopedists can learn a great deal from a precise review of publications. At present, substantial cure rates are achieved in several malignant tumors. This is due to sophisticated treatment programs created mainly by American clinical scientists. Such rapid progress of therapeutics occurred during the past 25 years, and was derived not only from

---

[1] Aichi Cancer Center, Nagoya, 464 Japan

Table 1. Adjuvant chemotherapy for osteosarcoma of the extremity — summary of randomized controlled trials

Report	n	DFS at 2y	Protocol	Eligibility	
		(%)		Age (years)	TNM Stage
1982 Rosen et al. [1]	57	90[a]	T-10	N.S.	I, II
1984 Edmonson et al. [2]	38	52 both	HDMTX	9–62	I, II
1986 Link et al. [3]	36 + 77	66 vs 17	T-10	<30	I, II
1987 Eilber et al. [4]	59	55 vs 20	T-10	4–59	I
1988 Winkler et al. [5]	141	60 ~ 70	T-10	<40	I, II

DFS, Disease free survival; *n*, number of patients registered; *N.S.*, not stated; *TNM*, TNM classification of tumors of bone
[a] Phase II study

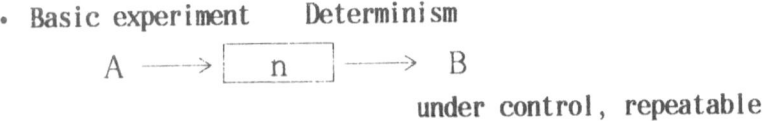

- Basic experiment   Determinism

  A ⟶ [n] ⟶ B

      under control, repeatable

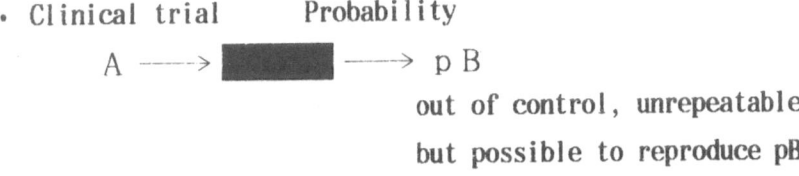

- Clinical trial   Probability

  A ⟶ ▇▇▇▇ ⟶ p B

      out of control, unrepeatable

      but possible to reproduce pB

Fig. 1. Logic in medicine. Reproducibility is ensured by determinism in basic experiments and by probability in clinical trials. *PB*, probability B

development of antitumor agents but also from carefully designed prospective randomized studies.

Logic and Decision-Making in Clinical Science

Science maintains its objectivity by requiring reproducibility. In basic experiments, reproducibility is ensured by determinism. For example, one can obtain output B under controllable conditions consisting of (n) kinds of factors through input A and this procedure is, of course, usually repeatable (Fig. 1). However, in clinical science, the experimental condition "patient" is usually uncontrollable, having innumerable unknown factors — almost a kind of a black box — and one can get output B only as a certain probability. Further complicating matters, the black box changes in the course of time, and even input A sometimes differs among doctors or institutions. Therefore, in clinical investigations, researchers look at the varied gain factor in heterogenous

Table 2. Clinical decision-making

• Scientific	Benefit/risk
• Ethical	Quality of life
• Economical	Cost/benefit

objects through standardized input. Indeed, reported response rates of colon cancer to 5-fluorouracil are distributed from several percent to 80% [6]. As a result, even if one takes a simple response parameter, such as tumor regression, it is quite difficult to establish reproducibility of probability B in clinical science. This is mainly due to a bias of patient selection, different criteria of response determination, and administered dose intensity. This is the reason why we need carefully designed prospective randomized controlled studies. So, for example, when the report of an excellent phase II result appears, such as that by Rosen et al. [1], further trials should be carried out to determine whether or not it is reproducible. In doing so, some investigators repeat phase II with the same protocol and others try using controlled randomized trials. Table 1 shows a typical process of this and how it can usually take a long time. As mentioned above, a patient's condition changes with time and the physician is obliged to do some hard decision-making. The clinical decision-making process consists of scientific, ethical, and economial aspects (Table 2), and the doctor arrives at an optimal decision by weighing these three points in order to maximize the patient's benefit. From this point of view, if the data from the clinical investigation do not provide any objective and quantitative evidence for clinical decision-making, they are of no clinical value.

Design of Clinical Trials

The benefit a patient can receive by the intended therapy is the first and most important question to be addressed. This tells us what are the ultimate goals of the study. Unquestionably, the target is effective therapy, but in some cases we need to compare toxicity, cost, convenience, and quality of life with the results of conventional treatment. Therapeutic efficacy is a relative concept and is judged with reference to some other treatment or to an untreated course of the disease; improvement can be defined in terms of success in reaching the defined goals of the program. Therefore, if a treatment with unknown efficacy is chosen as a control, it is obvious that no conclusion can be drawn from the trial. From an ethical viewpoint, the prospective therapy should be superior than or at least equivalent to the available standard therapy. In terms of interpreting the efficacy, the category of patients who can benefit should be strictly defined. Therapeutic efficacy is generally the center of concern and should ultimately be assessed in terms of overall survival. Since complete regression of the tumor is a prerequisite of survival, tumor shrinkage, disease-free survival, or time to progression are all taken as practical goals. In a study such as that on osteosarcoma, in which the efficacy of adjuvant chemotherapy

Table 3. Reliability of phase II trials

1. Patient eligibility   TNM, PS, Prior therapy.
2. Response criteria
3. Interobserver variability in response assesment
4. Dosage modification and protocol compliance
5. Reporting procedures
6. Sample size

TNM, TNM classification of malignant tumors; *PS*, performance status

is assessed, disease-free survival is a desirable goal because if salvage therapy has only some impact, assessment of overall survival becomes biased. At present, since a multi-institutional study system has not yet been established in Japan, the T-10 protocol should [1] be tried first as a phase II trial [7]. Before pursuing prospective randomized controlled trials to improve therapeutic efficacy, Japanese orthopedists should discipline their practice of treatment based on protocol, i.e., with a view toward prospective trials. During the course of a prospective phase II study, the doctor can experience first-hand the determination of the reliability of clinical trials (Table 3). Study of adjuvant chemotherapy in the orthopedic field requires an extremely high level of standards in clinics, including those not only in surgery but also in patient management after chemotherapy. The study's objective is most important in the phase III trial. If the objective is trivial, the loss is irreparable. A comparative trial should be carefully designed for patient eligibility, number of patients, goals, and study period on the basis of the phase II experience. Particularly, when the treatment program involves surgery, the outcome should be expected to differ according to levels of the surgeons' skills and facilities of the institution. Therefore, before launching a multi-institutional trial, standardization of surgical competence should be attempted through exchanges of information or mutual education [7, 8]. No clinical trial is valid without reproducibility. Therefore, every clinical trial should be written in a comprehensive manner to allow for it to be repeated by others.

Protocol and Quality Control of Clinical Trials

In order to correctly carry out an intended study, protocol must be prepared in advance. A clinical trial without protocol is not an acceptable study. Preparation of protocol is the first step of a clinical trial and only an expert clinician can accomplish it. In repeating a T-10 protocol, a precise agreement on such factors as operative procedure, margin of resection, dose modification, etc. is indispensable for conducting the trial. Currently, informed consent must be obtained from the patient before being entered into a trial. According to the report by Link et al. [3], although 113 out of the 156 registered patients were eligible for the trial, only 36 accepted randomization. However, Link et al. analyzed the results of the remaining 110 patients and found them to agree well with those obtained in the randomized group. Thus, informed consent is not an obstacle to carrying out a randomized clinical trial. Leading international journals require approval of the study by an institutional review board as well as documentation that informed consent has been properly obtained before reviewing the paper.

Quality control is a system to ensure carrying out a trial accurately according to protocol and achieving data collection correctly based on facts. The quality control process is listed below:

1. Qualification of the participants in a clinical trial
   a) Initial screening of institution
   b) Education of the participating investigators
   c) Quality control in diagnosis — central pathological review
2. Data collection and submission at the institutional level
3. Data management at the control office
   a) Formal registration mechanism
   b) Formal second party review
   c) Independent statistical center

Without concern for quality control, no trial can attain any measure of success. The quality control process begins with selection of the institution to be involved. Survival curves for pertinent tumor patients in each institution should be reviewed and differences in patient management should be weighed. Since osteosarcoma is a biologically heterogenous tumor, in order to arrive at the correct diagnosis, a central pathological reviewing system or confirmation of the diagnosis of a specimen by a second pathologist is necessary. Secondly, objectivity in data collection and analysis must be ensured by a formal registration mechanism, an independent statistical center, and by carrying out a second party review for determining whether or not the practice is accurately based on protocol [9, 10]. The clinician can learn about the importance of the above-mentioned points during the actual conducting of a prospective study.

Summary

Responsiveness of tumor of the bone or soft tissue to chemotherapeutic agents is generally low except in childhood Ewing' sarcoma and rhabdomyosarcoma. At present, chemotherapy is considered to be investigational, implying that chemotherapy for patients with such tumors should be administered in a manner conducive for use in prospective studies. The author describes a systematic approach to clinical science and fundamental knowledge for use in a design of clinical trials, protocol, and quality control of scientific investigations which are indispensable for pursuing prospective studies.

In any study, the factors of purpose and rationale can not be over-emphasized. The key to a successful study is to design it to be accurately repeatable by other investigators. Even if the results are negative, it should be of clinical value to the extent that the facts are correctly observed. It has been said that the ideal design is known only at the end of an experiment when more information is available for planning. Accumulating experience in this field allows us to discipline our clinical practice on cancer chemotherapy and to develop effective therapeutics.

Acknowledgments. The author thanks Prof. K. Ono (Osaka University, Osaka, Japan) for his kind support and Ms. Masako Kato for her excellent secretarial assistance.

References

1. Rosen G, Caparros B, Huvos AG, Kosloff C, Nirenberg A, Cavavio A, Marcove R, Lane JM. Mehta B, Urban C (1982) Preoperative chemotherapy for osteogenic sarcoma: Selection of postoperative adjuvant chemotherapy based on the response of the primary tumor to pre-operative chemotherapy. Cancer 49:1221–1230
2. Edmonson JH, Green SJ, Invins JC, Girchrist GS, Creagan ET, Pritchard DJ, Smithson WA, Dahlin DC, Taylor WF (1984) A controlled pilot study of high-dose methotrexate as postsurgical adjuvant treatment for primary osteosarcoma. J Clin Oncol 2:152–156
3. Link MP, Goorin AM, Miser AW, Green A, Pratt CB, Belasco JB, Pritchard J, Malpas JS, Baker AR, Kirkpatrick JA, Ayala AG, Shuster JJ, Abelson HT, Simone JV, Vietti TJ (1986) The effect of adjuvant chemotherapy on relapse-free survival in patients with osteosarcoma of the extremity. New Engl J Med 314:1600–1606
4. Eilber F, Gialiano A, Eckardt J, Patterson K, Moseley S, Goodnight J (1987) Adjuvant chemotherapy for osteosarcoma: A randomized prospective trial. J Clin Oncol 5:21–26
5. Winkler K, Beron G, Delling G, et al. (1988) Neoadjuvant chemotherapy of osteosarcoma: Results of a randomized cooperative trial (COSS-82) with salvage chemotherapy based on histological tumor response. J Clin Oncol 6:329–337
6. Moertel GG, Thyrne GS (1982) Large bowel. In: Holland JF, Frei E III (eds) Cancer medicine, 2nd edn. Lea and Febiger, Philadelphia, pp 1830–1859
7. Yamawaki S, Isu K, Ubayama Y, Takeda N, Yagi T, Usui M, Ishii S (1990) Adjuvant chemotherapy for osteosarcoma (in Japanese). Jpn J Cancer Chemother 17:180–188
8. NIH Consensus Development Conference on Limb-Sparing Treatment of Adult Soft Tissue Sarcoma and Osteosarcoma, U.S. Department of Health and Human Services, 1985
9. Simon R, Wittes RE (1985) Methodologic guidelines for reports of clinical trials. Cancer Treat Rep 69:1–3
10. Zelen M (1983) Guidelines for publishing papers on cancer clinical trials: Responsibilities of editors and authors. J Clin Oncol 1:164–169

Preoperative Chemotherapy for the Treatment of Osteosarcoma

HIDEKI HAMADA,[1] YOSHITAKA SHINTO, TAKAFUMI UEDA,
HIDEKI YOSHIKAWA, ATSUMASA UCHIDA, and KEIRO ONO[2]

Introduction

At present, preoperative chemotherapy preceding limb-salvage surgery, is indispensable therapy for patients with osteosarcoma, in addition to being the most important prognostic factor. The aims of preoperative chemotherapy are (1) to control micrometastasis, (2) to control the primary tumor, and (3) to assess the effectiveness of the drugs used by grading of primary tumor necrosis.

Since 1979, the regimen of chemotherapy (protocol-A) with preoperative intra-arterial Adriamycin (ia-ADR) in fusion for 13 patients with osteosarcoma was administered, but good results could not be obtained. Then, a new regimen (protocol B), designed in 1983, was introduced in 26 patients. In this paper, we describe the results of treatment with either protocol A or protocol B for these 2 groups of patients with osteosarcoma.

Materials and Methods

Patients

Thirty-nine patients with primary high-grade osteosarcoma were treated between 1977 and 1988. The criteria for patients eligible for this study were as follows: (1) under 25 years of age, (2) primary tumor in an extremity, (3) administration of scheduled preoperative and postoperative chemotherapy, (4) radical resection of the primary tumor, (5) no evidence of distant metastasis at the time of the initial treatment, and (6) exclusion of parosteal osteosarcoma, periosteal osteosarcoma, and small cell osteosarcoma (Table 1).

---

[1] Department of Orthopaedic Surgery, Osaka Prefectural Hospital, Sumiyoshi, Osaka, 558 Japan
[2] Department of Orthopaedic Surgery, Osaka University Medical School, Fukushima 1-1-50, Osaka, 553 Japan

Table 1. Evaluable patients with osteosarcoma treated with preoperative chemotherapy

Regimen	Cases (n)	Sex		Age		Location of tumor			Follow-up (months)	
		Male	Female	Range	Median	Femur	Tibia	Humerus	Range	Median
Protocol A	13	10	3	7–17	13	7	6	0	93–132	110
Protocol B	26	16	10	8–24	14	15	9	2	32–88	56
Total	39	26	13	7–24	14	22	15	2	32–132	72

Preoperative Chemotherapy

Protocol A. Ia-ADR infusion (0.8 mg/kg per day) for 3 consecutive days, was administered with an infusion pump, and was repeated 3 weeks later in addition to 2 weekly treatments with high-dose methotrexate with citrovorum factor (HD-MTX-CF). HD-MTX-CF (200 mg/kg) was administered for 6h together with intravenous hydration and alkalization of urine using intravenous sodium bicarbonate. At 3h after administration of HD-MTX, citrovorum factor (CF) was given intravenously at a dose of 15 mg every 6h for a total of up to 20 doses. The level of urine pH of patients was maintained at more than 7.5. Concentration of the methotrexate (MTX) level in the blood was monitored at 6, 12, 24, 48, and 72h after administration of HD-MTX. One week following the HD-MTX-CF infusion, ia-ADR was again administered prior to radical surgery (Fig. 1).

Protocol B. After ia-ADR (1 mg/kg per day) infusion for 2 consecutive days, *cis*-platinum (CDDP) (100 mg/m^2) was administered over 6h on the 3rd day, together with intravenous normal saline hydration and mannitol diuresis. Three weeks later, 2 weekly treatments of HD-MTX-CF (200 mg/kg) were given. Then, a second course of ia-ADR and CDDP was started prior to radical surgery (Fig. 1).

Surgery

Our indications for limb-salvage procedures were (1) the presence of a primary tumor involving the bone of an extremity with the possibility of performing radical resection, (2) that the patients are over the age of 10 years, in whom a length discrepancy of under 5 cm in a lower extremity is expected in the future, and (3) that pulmonary metastasis at the time of tumor diagnosis does not exclude en bloc resection, and provided that the pulmonary lesion is resectable or controllable by chemotherapy.

Out of 39 patients, 9 were treated by amputation, all having received protocol A regimen. All the patients who were given protocol B underwent limb-salvage surgery. Pulmonary metastasis occurred in 17 out of 39 patients, all of whom with one exception, underwent thoracotomies.

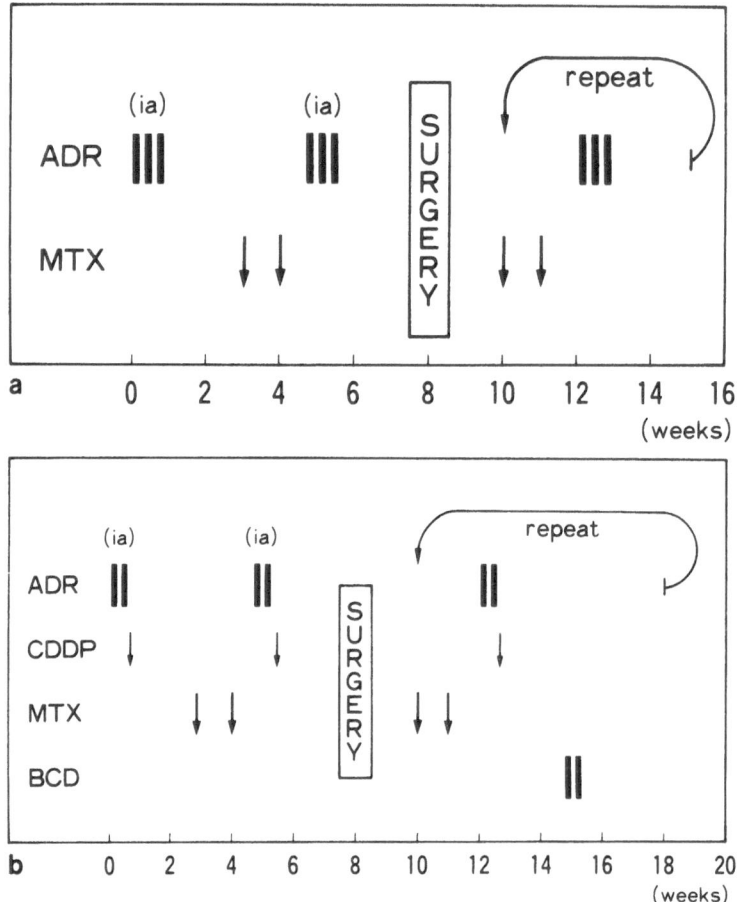

Fig. 1. a Protocol A. Two ia-ADR infusions (0.6–0.8 mg/kg per day) for 3 consecutive days and 2 weekly HD-MTX-CF infusions (100–200 mg/kg) were given prior to radical surgery. Two weeks after radical surgery, the cycle of systemic HD-MTX-CF and ADR was reinstituted and continued for 44 weeks after radical surgery. **b** Protocol B. Ia-ADR infusion (1.0–1.2 mg/kg per day) for 2 consecutive days, CDDP (100–120 mg/m²) on the 3rd day, and 2 weekly HD-MTX-CF (300 mg/kg) were given. Two weeks after radical surgery, the cycle of systemic HD-MTX-CF (300 mg/kg), ADR (0.8 mg/kg per day), CDDP (100 mg/m²), and BCD (bleomycin: 10 mg/m² per day, cyclophosphamide: 600 mg/m² per day, actinomycin D: 0.4 mg/m² per day) was started and continued for 44 weeks. *ia-ADR*, Adriamycin; *HD-MTX-CF*, high-dose methotrexate with citrovorum factor; *CF*, citrovorum factor; *BCD*, bleomycin + cyclophosphamide + actinomycin D; *(ia)*, intra-arterial infusion; *bars* and *arrows*, one drug administration

Table 2. Response of primary tumors to preoperative chemotherapy

Grade	1	2	3	4
		(Poor)		(Good)
Protocol A	4	5	2	2
Protocol B	1	5	17	3
Total	5	10	19	5

Pathological Examination

The percentage of the necrotic area in the resected tumors was evaluated by histological examination of an entire coronal slice. The responses were divided into four grades — grade 1 having a necrotic rate of less than 69%, grade 2 with 70%–89% necrosis, grade 3 with 90%–99% necrosis, and grade 4 with 100% necrosis. Grades 1 and 2 are considered "poor" responses, and grades 3 and 4 "good" responses.

Results

Responses to Preoperative Chemotherapy

Table 2 summarizes the results of histological responses to preoperative chemotherapy. Among 13 patients treated with protocol A, only 4 (30.8%) had good response, whereas the good response rate was 76.9% in the 26 patients treated with protocol B.

Continuously Disease-Free Survival (CDFS)

Out of 13 patients who received protocol A, 2 have remained free of disease for 93 and 110 months. The remaining 11 patients developed pulmonary metastasis. The 5-year CDFS rate of this group was 15.4%. Of the 26 patients treated with protocol B, 20 patients no longer had evidence of disease. The remaining six patients developed pulmonary metastasis. The 5-year CDFS rate of those 26 patients was 76.9% (Table 3).

Out of the 15 patients who had a poor response to preoperative chemotherapy (histological grade 1 or 2) 3 (20%) have been free of disease. Out of the 24 patients who had a good response (histological grade 3 or 4) 19 (79%) remained free of disease (Table 4).

Local Recurrence

Only one patient with osteosarcoma in the proximal humerus treated with protocol B had a local recurrence and simultaneous pulmonary metastasis. The histological grade of this primary tumor to protocol B was grade 2 (necrosis rate; 70%). The local recurrence rate was 2.6% (1/39).

Table 3. Survival rate related to protocols A and B

	Cases	Metastasis		CDF		
		(n)	(months)	n	Months	Rate (%)
Protocol A	13	11	2–28	2	93, 110	15.4
			(median, 14)		(median, 102)	
Protocol B	26	6	7–32	20	32–88	76.9
			(median, 20)		(median, 59)	

CDF, Continuously disease-free

Table 4. Survival rate of good and poor responders

Response	Cases	Metastasis		CDF		
		(n)	(months)	n	Months	Rate (%)
Poor (grade 1 or 2)	15	12	2–30	3	36–65	20.0
			(median, 15)		(median, 51)	
Good (grade 3 or 4)	24	5	7–32	19	32–110	78.9
			(median, 20)		(median, 62)	

CDF, Continuously disease-free

Discussion

In judging the histological effectiveness (good response) of a primary tumor after preoperative chemotherapy with ADR, CDDP, HD-MTX-CF, and bleomycin-cyclophosphamide-actinomycin D (BCD) in malignant bone tumors, it is generally recognized that the tumor necrosis rate is higher than 90%. Good responders clearly showed a better prognosis than poor responders [1, 2], making the response rate of preoperative chemotherapy a good indicator of prognosis [2, 3].

The limb-salvage strategy for the patients who had poor response to pre-operative chemotherapy was first introduced in the Rosen T_{10} protocol, in which alteration of the chemotherapeutic agents for poor responders is made in the postoperative regimen [2]. Although Rosen et al. have reported good results by the T_{10} protocol, no other postoperative strategies with alternative agents for limb-salvage in poor responders have been successful [1, 4, 5]. The difference in the results between the Rosen protocol and those of others seems to result from different histological evaluations in preoperative chemotherapy and from a different chemotherapeutic regimen [6]. There is much debate on postoperative chemotherapeutic strategies for a poor responder. At present, it appears that the best method is that which uses all effective drugs in full doses and in a short period of time, in order to obtain a higher rate of good responders.

There were no significant differences in disease-free survival rates between neoadjuvant chemotherapy (pre-and postoperative chemotherapy) and postoperative chemotherapy alone, although these studies were not randomized [1, 4]. Bacci et al. [1] described that the most prominent advantage for pre-operative chemotherapy was the possibility of controlling the primary tumor in order to enable a safer and easier limb-salvage resection. Since the introduction of preoperative chemotherapy, limb-salvage surgery has become more common [7]. At present, more than 70% of these patients undergo limb-saving procedures.

There are several problems in limb-salvage surgery, the most significant of which is local recurrence. Because local recurrence is related to the size of the surgical margins and to the response rate of the tumor to the chemotherapy [8], wider surgical margins for tumor resection in patients with poor responses to preoperative chemotherapy are needed. On the other hand, Picci et al. [9] reported that viable cells were found with a higher frequency in the region of soft tissue invaded by tumor cells than that in bone involvement. This may mean that the tumor cells in satellite regions are more drug-resistant. In order to achieve a safer and easier limb-salvage procedure, we must concentrate our studies on accurate preoperative detection of satellite regions of the tumor.

Despite the findings that the prognosis of patients with osteosarcoma has greatly improved since the introduction of protocol B, the patients who developed pulmonary metastasis are not cured even by thoracotomy and/or salvage chemotherapy. In addition, the number of patients who developed extra-pulmonary multiple metastases have increased after introduction of intensive chemotherapy. For those cases, there is an urgent need for the development of an effective second line chemotherapeutic regimen.

References

1. Bacci G, Picci P, Ruggieri P, Mercuri M, Avella M, Capanna R, Brach Del Prever A, Mancini A, Gherlinzoni F, Padovani G, Leonessa C, Biagini R, Ferraro A, Ferruzzi A, Cazzola A, Manfrini M, Campanacci M (1990) Primary chemotherapy and delayed surgery (neoadjuvant chemotherapy) for osteosarcoma of the extremities. Cancer 65:2539–2553
2. Rosen G, Caparros B, Huvos AG, Kosloff C, Nirenberg A, Cacavio A, Marcove RC, Lane JM, Mehta B, Urban C (1982) Preoperative chemotherapy for osteogenic sarcoma: Selection of postoperative adjuvant chemotherapy based on the response of the primary tumor to preoperative chemotherapy. Cancer 49:1221–1230
3. Goldie JH, Coldman AJ (1979) A mathematic model for relating the drug sensitivity of tumors to their spontaneous mutation rate. Cancer Treat Rep 63:1727–1733
4. Winker K, Beron G, Delling G, Heise U, Kabisch H, Purfurst C, Berger J, Jurgens H, Gerin V, Graf N, Russe W, Gruemayer ER, Ertelt W, Kotz R, Preusser P, Prindull G, Brandeis W, Landbeck G (1988) Neoadjuvant chomotherapy of osteosarcoma: Results of randomized co-operative trial (COSS-82) with salvage chemotherapy based on histological tumor response. J Clin Oncol 6:329–337
5. Provisor A, Nachman J, Krailo M, Ettinger L, Hammond D (1987) Treatment of non-metastatic osteogenic sarcoma (os) of the exremities with pre- and postoperative chemotherapy. Proc Am Soc Clin Oncol 6:217

6. Rosen G (1988) The current management of malignant bone tumours: Where do we go from here? Med J Aust 148:373–377

7. Eilber FR, Mirra JJ, Grant TT, Weisenburger T, Morton DL (1980) Is amputation necessary for sarcoma?: A seven-year experience with limb salvage. Ann Surg 192:431–438

8. Rosen G (1986) Neoadjuvant chemotherapy for osteogenic sarcoma: A model for the treatment of other highly malignant neoplasms. Recent Results Cancer Res 103:148–157

9. Picci P, Bacci G, Campanacci M, Gasparini M, Pilotti S, Cerasoli S, Bertoni F, Guerra A, Capanna R, Albisinni U, Galletti S, Gherlinzoni F, Calderoni P, Sudanese A, Baldini N, Bernini M, Jaffe N (1985) Histologic evaluation of necrosis in osteosarcoma induced by chemotherapy. Cancer 56:1515–1521

Intra-Arterial Cisplatin Chemotherapy for Osteogenic Sarcoma

SOO-YONG LEE, CHIN YOUB CHUNG, GOO HYUN BAEK, and
HONG SIK BYUN[1]

Introduction

The classical method for treating osteogenic sarcoma had been amputation followed by chemotherapy for about 1 year. Recently, preoperative chemotherapy has been tried in many cancer centers [1–3], with the resultant benefits of controlling micrometastasis, permitting the analysis of the response of the tumor to chemotherapy, and providing a better chance to save the endangered limb by reducing and consolidating the tumor volume [4]. Intra-arterial preoperative chemotherapy has been shown to control local lesions very effectively [3].

Ochs et al. tried *cis*-platinum (CDDP) for advanced cases of osteogenic sarcoma [5], and Jaffe et al. tried it intra-arterially for osteogenic sarcoma and malignant fibrous histiocytoma [6], both groups reporting relatively good response.

Stine et al. administered preoperative chemotherapy with systemic adriamycin and intra-arterial CDDP for osteogenic sarcoma, and their regimen showed good responses [3].

We describe the use and results of systemic adriamycin and intra-arterial CDDP as a preoperative chemotherapeutic modality. This therapy could allow the patient and clinician the choice of limb salvage or amputation while avoiding any delay in initiating systemic therapy.

Materials and Methods

Patient Selection

From June, 1987 to December, 1989, 17 patients who were diagnosed as having osteogenic sarcoma of the extremities, and who had not received any chemo-

---
[1] Department of Orthopedic Surgery, Korea Cancer Center Hospital, 215–4, Gongneung-Dong, Rowon-Ku, Seoul 139-240, Korea

therapy or undergone surgery other than open biopsy, were selected after confirmation of the absence of metastasis with simple radiography, bone scan, and computed tomography of the chest and sites of lesion. Additionally, normal renal function, determined by urinalysis consisting of urinary cell count, blood urea nitrogen (BUN), creatinine, and creatinine clearance, along with normal liver function tested by serum protein, albumin, bilirubin, glutamate oxalate transferase (SGOT), and glutamic pyruvate transferase (SGPT), were prerequisites for entering this protocol.

Treatment Protocol

Once the diagnostic evaluations were confirmed, patients received more than 2,000 ml prehydration with electrolyte solution for at least 12 h before intra-arterial CDDP chemotherapy. Sedation was done with $10 \, mg/m^2$ intravenous diazepam injection 30 min before arteriography. With percutaneous insertion of the catheter into the contralateral (in the case of lower extremity) or right (in the case of upper extremity) femoral artery, CDDP was infused for 2 h at a dosage of $100 \, mg/m^2$ in 300 ml 3% saline solution with 3,000 units heparin. The catheter tip was located just proximal to the feeding vessels, confirmed by initial arteriography.

Intravenous adriamycin was given after completing CDDP infusion at a dosage of $60 \, mg/m^2$.

Intravenous hydration during and after CDDP infusion was achieved with more than 3,500 ml electrolyte solution. For diuresis, 100 ml 20% mannitol was infused 20 min before CDDP infusion, and 10 mg furosemide was infused simultaneously. With an indwelling Foley catheter, the urine output was monitored closely, and if there were less than 60 ml/h of urine output we used 40 mg furosemide intravenously.

Nausea and vomiting were controlled by intravenous injection of 20 ml metaclopramide before the 30 min CDDP infusion and then at 1, 3, and 5 h after starting CDDP infusion. Twenty minutes before CDDP infusion, 20 mg dexamethasone was infused. Ten milligrams diazepam was given for sedation for severe nausea or vomiting when necessary.

Preoperatively, for prepuberty patients (under 14 years for males, under 12 years for females), we tried 7 cycles of intra-arterial CDDP biweekly, 6 cycles of intravenous adriamycin and cyclophosphamide every 3rd week, 5 cycles of intra-arterial CDDP every 3rd week, 2 cycles of intra-arterial CDDP every 3rd month, and then intra-arterial CDDP every 6 months until near puberty. For those patients who were near or post-puberty, 7 cycles of intra-arterial CDDP biweekly combined with intravenous adriamycin every 4th week was tried preoperatively.

Toxicity was closely monitored after intra-arterial chemotherapy. Before starting each intra-arterial chemotherapy, we checked renal function with measurements of blood urea nitrogen, creatinine, creatinine clearance, myelo-suppression with whole blood cell counts with differential counts. Liver function was determined by SGOT, SGPT, and bilirubin.

Table 1. Chemotherapy schedule

1. Preoperative
a) Near or postpubertal
IA Cisplatin q̄ 2 weeks ×7
IV Adriamycin q̄ 4 weeks ×4
b) Prepubertal
IA Cisplatin q̄ 2 weeks ×7
→ IV Adriamycin and cytoxan q̄ 3 weeks ×6
→ IA Cisplatin q̄ 3 weeks ×5
→ IA Cisplatin q̄ 3 months ×2
→ IA Cisplatin q̄ 6 months until puberty
2. Postoperative: Bleomycin, cyclophosphamide and actinomycin-D for 2 days q̄ 3 weeks ×5

IA, Intra-arterial, IV, intravenous
Dosage: Cisplatin $100\,mg/M^2$, adriamycin $60\,mg/M^2$ in 2 days, bleomycin $15\,mg/M^2$, cyclophosphamide $800\,mg/M^2$, actinomycin-D $0.5\,mg/M^2$

Response to treatment was determined by (1) changes in clinical symptoms during chemotherapy such as subsidence of pain and/or reduction of the circumference of the tumor site, (2) preoperative radiological findings compared with serial angiograms in relation to the tumor vessels or tumor staining, and (3) postoperative pathological findings in relation to tumor necrosis.

Postoperative chemotherapy included 5 cycles of bleomycin ($15\,mg/m^2$), cyclophosphamide ($800\,mg/m^2$), and actinomycin-D ($0.5\,mg/m^2$) every 3rd week, irrespective of response rate.

The overall chemotherapy schedule is shown in Table 1.

Results

Patients' Characteristics

The characteristics of the patients are illustrated in Table 2. The mean age of the 11 males and 6 females was 16.2 years (range: 9–26). The most common site of the lesion was the distal femur (7 cases), followed by the proximal tibia (4 cases), proximal humerus (3 cases), proximal femur (2 cases), and proximal fibula (1 case).

According to Enneking's classification of musculoskeletal neoplasm [7], 2 cases were IIA and 15 were IIB. Twelve out of 17 patients underwent limb salvage and the remainder had amputation or disarticulation. A limb salvage technique was chosen when the tumor was confined under the periosteum. Amputation or disarticulation was performed when the tumor invaded over the periosteum. The average duration from the onset of symptoms to diagnosis was 3.1 months (range: 1–13 months).

Radiological Response

All 17 cases showed a good radiological response which was confirmed by using serial angiograms. This was defined by complete disappearance of the tumor

Table 2. Characteristics of the patients

Case	Sex/age (years)	Location of tumor	Stage	Number of IA courses	Rate of necrosis	Type of surgery	Duration between symptoms and diagnosis (months)	Site of metastasis	Duration between diagnosis and metastasis (months)	Duration of follow-up (months)	Current status
1	M/17	Proximal tibia	IIA	7	95%	Amputation	2			36	CDF
2	F/14	Distal femur	IIB	7	100%	Arthrodesis	13	Lung	19	21	Deceased
3	F/14	Proximal humerus	IIB	7	95%	Arthroplasty	2			20	CDF
4	M/20	Proximal tibia	IIB	7	100%	Arthroplasty	2	Bone	5	10	Deceased
5	F/20	Proximal fibula	IIA	7	95%	Arthroplasty	3			34	CDF
6	M/15	Distal femur	IIB	7	100%	Amputation	2			15	CDF
7	M/14	Proximal tibia	IIB	7	100%	Amputation	1			17	CDF
8	M/14	Proximal humerus	IIB	7	100%	Arthroplasty	2	Bone	13	19	AWD
9	M/15	Distal femur	IIB	7	100%	Arthroplasty	1	Bone	14	17	AWD
10	F/ 9	Proximal tibia	IIB	7	100%	Amputation	1	Lung, bone	8	17	Deceased
11	M/18	Distal femur	IIB	7	100%	Arthroplasty	1	Lung, bone	11	22	AWD
12	M/16	Distal femur	IIB	7	50%	Arthroplasty	1	Lung	7	12	AWD
13	M/26	Proximal humerus	IIB	7	50%	Arthroplasty	12			30	CDF
14	M/17	Proximal femur	IIB	7	50%	Arthroplasty	3			28	CDF
15	M/13	Proximal femur	IIA	13	50%	Disarticulation	4	Lung	16	19	Deceased
16	F/16	Distal femur	IIB	7	100%	Arthroplasty	2	Lung	14	15	Deceased
17	F/18	Distal femur	IIB	7	100%	Arthroplasty	1	Lung	18	28	Deceased

IA, Intra-arterial; *CDF*, continuously disease-free; *AWD*, alive with disease

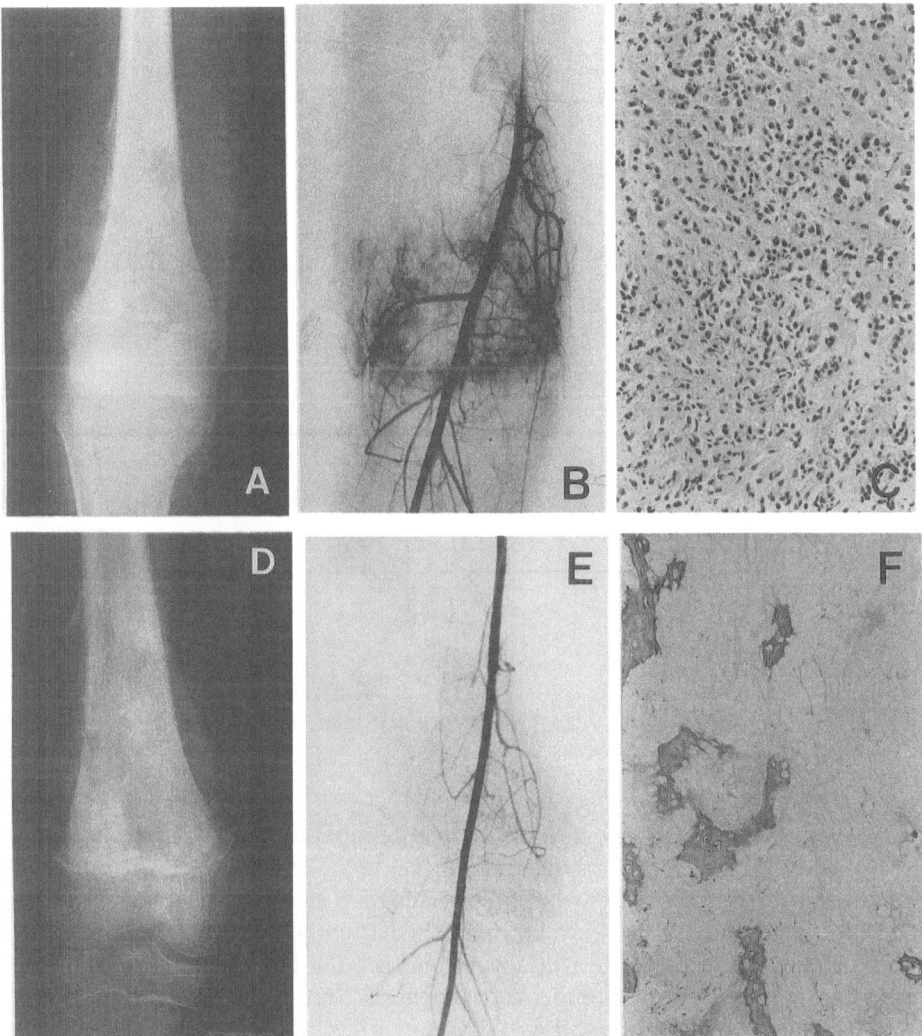

Fig. 1. Initial findings of tumor. **A** The border of the tumor mass is indistinct on simple X-ray. **B** Tumor vessels and stainings are noted in the angiogram. **C** Pathological findings show typical malignant osteoid formation (H and E, ×56). **D–F** Findings after intra-arterial chemotherapy. The border of the tumor mass is distinctly calcified, especially along the medial side (**D**). Marked loss of tumor vessels and stainings are seen (**E**). Resected specimen after chemotherapy showed complete necrosis with no viable tumor cells (**F**). H and E, ×56

vessels and staining which was usually seen at the time of the 4th or 5th session of intra-arterial CDDP chemotherapy (Fig. 1). Simple X-ray showed marginal sclerosis of the tumor and calcification of the tumor itself. Additionally these cases showed a good clinical response based upon symptoms and signs, such as reduction of pain and circumference of the tumor region.

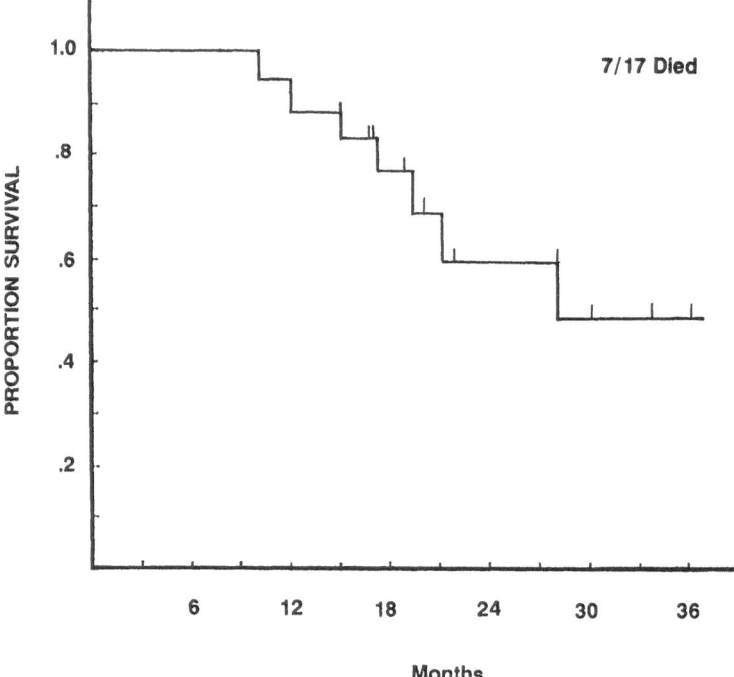

Fig. 2. The estimated 3-year survival rate by Kaplan-Meier method was 46.9% in all 17 patients

In cases of long-term chemotherapy for prepubertal subjects (cases 10 and 15), there was also a good initial radiological and clinical response, but there was regrowth of the tumor during maintenance therapy with intra-arterial CDDP. Therefore we performed a disarticulation of the hip after the 13th cycle of intra-arterial CDDP infusions in case 15, but this patient died of pulmonary metastasis 19 months from diagnosis. In case 10, early amputation was inevitable because of the regrowth after 7 cycles of intra-arterial CDDP infusions.

Pathological Response

In our series, 10 out of 17 patients showed no viable tumor cells (58.8%), and 3 cases showed tumor necrosis of more than 95% of the lesion. According to the grading system of Huvos et al. [8], this result means that 76.5% of the cases showed complete response to this intra-arterial chemotherapy (Fig. 1). There was one each of the chondroblastic and fibroblastic type, but these cases responded with less than 50% of tumor necrosis.

Survival

The duration of follow-up was from 10 months to 36 months (average: 21.2 months). Ten patients (58.8%) survived and 7 (41.2%) expired. Among the ten living patients, 7 (41.2%) remain continuously disease-free, and three (17.6%) are surviving with metastasis. The estimated Kaplan-Meier's [9] 3-year survival rate was 46.9% (Fig. 2).

Metastasis

Ten out of 17 patients showed metastasis (58.8%). The average duration from diagnosis to metastasis was 12.5 months (range: 5–19 months). Three cases showed metastasis within 1 year after diagnosis. Of the five patients who survived more than 2 years, only one showed metastasis. There were 5 cases of bone metastasis (50% of metastasis) of which 3 showed only bone metastasis without any evidence of lung or other visceral metastasis.

Local Recurrence

There was one case of local recurrence (case 12). This patient was treated with radiotherapy, but pulmonary metastasis appeared during this time and death occurred 5 months later.

Complications and Toxicity

No difficulty was met in the placement of the intra-arterial catheters.

Nausea and vomiting persisted for 2 or 3 days after injection of CDDP, and were more severe when combined with adriamycin.

One case showed local soft tissue reactions, such as erythema, swelling, pain, and tenderness to heat sensation, from intra-arterial chemotherapy, but these disappeared within 1 week with conservative treatment. However, local induration remained in the area that had been tender.

There was no significant hematologic change in response to CDDP, except for mild anemia, but one patient showed alteration of renal function evidenced by oliguria and increased BUN and creatinine after the 3rd cycle of intra-arterial CDDP. This patient recovered after 2 weeks of conservative measures. CNS symptoms due to hypomagnesia or hypocalcemia were experienced by four patients. These reactions were controllable by oral magnesium and sedation in mild cases or intravenous injection of magnesium, calcium, and sedation when the symptoms were severe.

Neutropenia, thrombocytopenia, and anemia, all of which were reversible within 2 weeks, resulted from the administration of adriamycin.

Operation-related complications were found in 2 cases (cases 5 and 8). These were superficial wound infections which were controlled with dressing and systemic antibiotics given for about 4 weeks.

Miscellaneous

Bone resection or amputation was done at least 7 cm above or below the hot uptake lesion as measured with a bone scan. To assure accuracy of measurement, we applied an indicator for measurement of the length of the hot lesion on the bone scan.

Case 2, a 14-year-old female, underwent arthrodesis with intramedullary nailing and bone cement for spacer.

Kotz's modular tumor prosthesis was used for all arthroplasty cases of the lower extremities.

For shoulder arthroplasty in an upper humerus lesion, one patient (case 8) received a custom-made ceramic prosthesis, and two patients (cases 3 and 13) received autoclaved bone grafts combined with Neer's shoulder prosthesis.

Discussion

Several groups have reported their results on intra-arterial chemotherapy using *cis*-platinum (CDDP) for osteogenic sarcoma [6, 10–14]. Because this approach permits higher cytotoxic concentrations to be directed to the target lesion [3], it was claimed that this type of therapy is very effective in controlling local lesions, making limb salvage easier without jeopardizing the patient's chances of recovery.

Previously, only less than 20% of the patients of the amputated group had survived more than 5 years when there was no chemotherapy [15–19]. This shows that there can be micrometastasis even when there is no evidence of metastasis from routine X-rays, bone scan, or other laboratory results.

Patients with metastasis at diagnosis make the success of chemotherapy more difficult to achieve than those without metastasis. Even if there is no metastasis, if the tumor extends outwards into the extracompartment from the original site, the expectation of effective response to chemotherapy and limb salvage is more limited because of the large volume of tumor to be controlled.

These facts convinced us to use preoperative chemotherapy for earlier control of systemic and local lesions. Furthermore, it was thought that the resultant quality of life of patients undergoing limb-salvage surgery was better than that of those undergoing amputation. There were also several reports of there being a higher local level in the tumor tissue of the chemotherapeutic agent when it was used intra-arterially [3, 6]. The response rate with intravenous CDDP alone was approximately 30% [5, 20–22], but when it was used in the intra-arterial route [11], especially when combined with adriamycin [10], the effect was enhanced even in the presence of metastasis.

In our patients, CDDP was administered by percutaneous femoral catheterization with a dose of $100\,mg/m^2$ per course at the site proximal to the feeding vessel of the tumor. A CDDP-associated complication in 1 case was found to be oliguria with increased BUN and creatinine. This was controlled with conservative treatment.

Nausea and vomiting were minimal with CDDP alone, but there were 4 cases of CNS signs due to hypomagnesia and hypocalcemia, which were controllable by oral or intravenous magnesium and calcium administration with sedation.

Adriamycin was delivered for 2 days (with a total of $60\,mg/m^2$) every 4 weeks after intra-arterial CDDP infusion for each course.

Preoperatively, 4 courses of adriamycin were administrated for adolescents and adults. The adriamycin-associated toxicities were neutropenia and thrombocytopenia.

Radiologically, we could see calcification and consolidation of the tumor mass throughout the course of therapy, which were confirmed during surgery. When compared at the time of preparation of pathological examination, the margin of the tumor was bony-hard and the dissection was somewhat easier than that of a specimen retrieved by amputation without any preoperative chemotherapy.

In cases of regrowth during chemotherapy, pathologic examination showed viable tumor cells at the periphery of the original tumor mass.

Chondroblastic or fibroblastic osteosarcoma showed less tumor vascularity and staining as seen from the first angiogram, and the pathological response was not as good (only 50% of tumor necrosis in cases 13 and 14). However, the prognosis looked better than that for classical osteosarcoma. From these findings, we suggest that tumor characteristics and responses to each treatment protocol would be different according to the type of osteosarcoma. Our group of patients appears to be too small to draw any conclusions, but a study including more cases of chondroblastic of fibroblastic variants of osteosarcoma which can be compared with classical osteosarcoma under the same protocol could provide more conclusive information.

The typical site of metastasis in osteosarcoma before the introduction of successful chemotherapy had been the lung. Presently, extrapulmonary metastasis to bone, brain, heart, and other atypical sites [23–26] are common with adjuvant chemotherapy. In our series, 5 out of 10 patients with metastasis showed bone metastasis, and 3 of them had only bone metastasis without lung involvement.

Considering that the majority of patients (15/17) were classified as having IIB lesions, the survival rate was similar to that of UCLA. In that study, the estimated Kaplan-Meier's 2-year survival rate was 65%, and the 5-year survival rate was 36% in the IIB osteosarcoma category [27].

Although our cases were few in number and the follow-up period was rather short, we suggest that intra-arterial CDDP chemotherapy may be one of the more effective methods of treating osteosarcoma, especially in view of radiological and pathological responses.

Summary

Since adriamycin and *cis*-platinum (CDDP) are two very effective chemotherapeutic agents for treating osteogenic sarcoma, we tried using intra-arterial CDDP to control local lesions, and intravenous adriamycin to control systemic lesions preoperatively.

From June, 1987 to December, 1989, we gave this preoperative chemotherapy to 17 cases. The average follow-up period was 21.2 months (range: 10–36.months). Long-term chemotherapy was used in two prepubertal cases to minimize postoperative limb length discrepancy. Among the 17 cases, 2 were designated as being IIA and 15 as IIB according to Enneking's classification of musculoskeletal neoplasm. The types of operation were limb salvage in 12 cases and amputation in 5 cases.

Radiologically, the response of this preoperative chemotherapy were good in all the cases. Pathologically, 76.5% showed tumor necrosis of more than 95%.

The estimated 3-year survival rate by the Kaplan-Meier method was 46.9% in all 17 patients. There was one local recurrence after the limb-salvage operation. Distant metastases developed in 58.8%. The average duration from diagnosis to metastasis was 12.5 months (range: 5–19 months). Fifty percent of the metastasis involved bone.

Regrowth occurred during the maintenance period in prepubertal children who underwent long-term chemotherapy.

Acknowledgments. Our appreciation is extended to Dr. Jang for his review of pathological specimens, Ms. Bechtel for her excellent assistance with the manuscript, and Ms. Kim for her clerical assistance.

References

1. Eilber F, Grant T, Morton D (1978) Adjuvant therapy for osteosarcoma: Preoperative and postoperative treatment. Cancer Treat Rep 62:213–216
2. Rosen G, Caparros B, Huvos A, Kosloff C, Nirrenberg A, Cacavio A, Marcove R, Lane J, Metha B, Urban C (1982) Preoperative chemotherapy for osteogenic sarcoma. (Selection of postoperative adjuvant chemotherapy based on the response of the primary tumor to preoperative chemotherapy). Cancer 49:1221–1230
3. Stine KC, Hockenberry MJ, Harrelson I, Miner D, Falletta JM (1989) Systemic doxorubicin and intraarterial cisplatin preoperative chemotherapy plus postoperative adjuvant chemotherapy in patients with osteosarcoma. Cancer 63:848–853
4. Simon MA, Aschliman M, Thomas N, Mankin HJ (1986) Limb salvage treatment versus amputation for osteosarcoma of the distal end of the femur. J Bone and Joint Surg [Am] 68:1331–1337
5. Ochs J, Freeman A, Douglass HJ, Hingby D, Mindell E, Sinks L (1978) Cis-diamminedichloroplatinum (II) in advanced osteogenic sarcoma. Cancer Treat Rep 62:239–245
6. Jaffe N, Knapp J, Chuang V, Wallace C, Ayala A, Murray J, Cangir A, Wang A, Benzamin R (1983) Osteosarcoma: Intraarterial treatment of the primary tumor with cis-Diamminedichloroplatinum II (CDP): Angiographic, pathologic and pharmacologic studies. Cancer 51:402–407
7. Enneking WF (1986) A system of staging musculoskeletal neoplasms. Clin Orthop 204:9–24
8. Huvos AG, Rosen G, Marcove CR (1977) Primary osteogenic sarcoma: Pathologic aspects in 20 patients after treatment with chemotherapy, en bloc resection, and prosthetic bone replacement. Arch Pathol Lab Med 101(1):14–18
9. Kaplan EL, Meier R (1958) Nonparametric estimation from incomplete observation. J Am Stat Assoc 53:457–481

10. Benjamin R, Chawla S, Carrasco C (1988) Arterial infusion in the treatment of osteosarcoma. In: Ryan J, Baker L (eds) recent concepts in sarcoma treatment. Kluwer, Dordrecht, pp 269–274

11. Jaffe N (1989) Chemotherapy for malignant bone tumors. Orthop Clin North America 20(3):487–503

12. Jaffe N, Prudich J, Knapp J, Wang Y, Bowman R, Cangir A, Ayala A, Chuang V, Wallace S (1983) Treatment of primary osteosarcoma with intraarterial and intravenous high dose methotrexate. J Clin Oncol 1(7):428–431

13. Jaffe N, Raymond A, Ayala A, Carrasco C, Wallace S, Robertson R, Griffiths M, Wang Y (1989) Effect of cumulative courses of intraarterial cis-Diamminedichloroplatinum-II on the primary tumor in pediatric osteosarcoma. Cancer 63:63–67

14. Jaffe N, Spears R, Eftekhari F, Robertson R, Cangir A, Takaue Y, Carrasco C (1987) Pathologic fracture in osteosarcoma: Impact of chemotherapy on primary tumor and survival. Cancer 59:27–35

15. Carter SK (1980) The dilemma of adjuvant chemotherapy for osteogenic sarcoma. Cancer Clin Trials 3:29–36

16. Dahlin DC, Coventry MB (1967) Osteosarcoma: A study of 600 cases. J Bone Joint Surg [Am] 49:101–110

17. Friedman MA, Carter SX (1972) The therapy of osteogenic sarcoma: Current status and thoughts for the future. J surg Oncol 4(5):482–510

18. Taylor WF, Ivins JC, Dahlin DC, Edmonson JH, Pritchard DJ (1978) Trends and variability in survival from osteosarcoma. Mayo Clin Proc 53:695–700

19. Weiner M, Harris M, Lewis M, Jones R, Sherry H, Feurer E, Johnson T, Lahman E (1986) Neoadjuvant high dose methotrexate, cisplatin, and doxorubicin for the management of patients with nonmetastatic osteosarcoma. Cancer Treat Rep 70:1431–1432

20. Baum E, Greenberg L, Gaynon P (1978) Use of cisplatinumdiammine dichloride (CPDD) in osteogenic sarcoma (OS) in children (abstract C-315). Proc AACR-ASCO 19:335

21. Nitschke R, Starling KA, Vats T, Bryan H (1978) Cis-Diamminedichloroplatinum (NSC-119875) in childhood malignancies: A southwest oncology group study. Med Pediatr Oncol 4:127–132

22. Pratt C, Hayes F, Green A (1979) Phase II pharmacokinetic study of cis-platinum diamminedichloride (CPDD) in children with solid tumors. Proc AACR-ASCO 20:361

23. Baram TZ, van Tassel P, Jaffe NA (1988) Brain metastasis in osteosarcoma: Incidence, clinical and neurological findings and management options. J Neuro-oncol 6:47–52

24. Giuliano A, Feig S, Eilber F (1984) Changing metastatic patterns of osteosarcoma. Cancer 54:2160–2164

25. McCarten KM, Jaffe N, Kirkpatrick JA (1980) The changing radiographic appearance of osteogenic sarcoma. Ann Radiol 23:203–208

26. Takaue Y, Slopis JM, Anzai T, Robertson R, Jaffe N (1985) Successful treatment of pulmonary and abdominal metastatic osteosarcoma. Med Pediatr Oncol 13:126–128

27. Eckardt II, Eilber FR, Dorey FI, Mirra IM (1987) The UCLA experience in the management of stage IIB osteosarcoma: 1972–1983. In: Enneking WF (ed) Limb salvage in musculoskeletal oncology. Churchill Livingstone, New York, pp 314–326

Clinical Study of Recombinant Human Granulocyte Colony-Stimulating Factor in Patients Undergoing Intensive Chemotherapy for Malignant Bone and Soft Tissue Tumors

Yoshitaka Shinto, Atsumasa Uchida, Ikuo Kudawara, and Keiro Ono[1]

Introduction

In intensive chemotherapy for patients with malignant bone and soft tissue tumors, bone marrow toxicity is one of the most hazardous side effects. Recently recombinant forms of four human hematopoietic colony-stimulating factors have been purified [1–3], and their potential clinical application seem to be very promising for prevention of bone marrow suppression by chemotherapy. Reports on the effect of recombinant human granulocyte colony-stimulating factor (rhG-CSF) on granulocytopenia induced by chemotherapy in patients with solid tumor have been published [4–9], but these studies are still in the experimental stage. In this paper, we evaluated the efficacy and feasibility of the use of rhG-CSF for rescue of chemotherapy in malignant bone and soft tissue tumors.

Materials and Methods

Recombinant Human G-CSF

The rhG-CSF used (KRN8601, Kirin:Amgen), consisting of 174 amino acid residues and in the nonglycosylated form with a moleuclar weight of 18,800, was kindly provided by Kirin and Sankyo Company (Tokyo, Japan) [4]. It was purified from E. coli and its specific activity is 1.0×10^8 units/mg of protein. There is no detectable endotoxin content.

Patients

From 1989–1991, 50 patients with malignant bone and soft tissue tumors were enrolled in this study. The patients' age ranged from 6 to 71 years (average,

[1] Department of Orthopaedic Surgery, Osaka University Medical School, Fukushima-ku, Osaka, 553 Japan

47.5 years), and 23 were male and 27 were female. The eligibility criteria were histologically- or cytologically-proven malignant bone and soft tissue tumors. Other criteria included a normal peripheral blood count before chemotherapy (white blood cells $> 4 \times 10^3$, hemoglobin $> 10\,g/dl$, platelets $> 10^5$), adequate renal functions, and normal hepatic functions. Patients were excluded if they had the following: evidence of repeated infection, hypersensitivity to E. coli-derived preparations, chronic lung disease with resting hypercapnia, disabling congesitive cardiac failure, or a history of unstable angina. Informed consent was obtained from all participating patients.

Chemotherapy

All patients underwent the following chemotherapy regimen: Adriamycin $(30\,mg/m^2)$ on days 1 and 2, and *cis*-platinum $(80\,mg/m^2)$ on day 3. This regimen, being used routinely in our Department in patients with malignant bone and soft tissue tumors, caused severe granulocytopenia (less than $1000/mm^3$) in 60% of the patients but significantly improved the survival rate. Chemotherapy was repeated every 4 weeks up to a total of 6 cycles.

Study Design

Patients were divided three groups. The historical control group consisted of 20 patients who underwent 58 courses of chemotherapy; 9 were males and 11 were females and ages ranged from 8–65 years. The partial rhG-CSF administration group (P group) consisted of 18 patients who received injections of rhG-CSF only from the 4th–6th cycles of chemotherapy. Nine of these patients underwent 22 courses of chemotherapy that comprised intravenous injection (iv) of rhG-CSF in 100 ml of 5% glucose solution 24–48 h after intensive chemotherapy for 14 consecutive days. The remaining 9 patients underwent 18 courses of chemotherapy and were injected subcutaneously (sc) for the same period. The initial starting dose in this study was $50\,\mu g/m^2$, and after evaluating the toxicity and change of neutrophil counts, the doses of G-CSF were escalated to $75\,\mu g/m^2$ and $100\,\mu g/m^2$. The third group were administered rhG-CSF at every cycle of chemotherapy (C group). This group consisted of 32 patients; 16 patients underwent 62 courses of chemotherapy and received rhG-CSF 24–48 h after intensive chemotherapy, and the remaining 16 patients underwent 78 courses of chemotherapy after occurrence of granulocytopenia (less than $1500/mm^3$). In both subgroups of 16 patients, each 8 patients had iv administration and 8 patients sc administration. The concurrent use of steroids or other immunomodulating drugs which might influence the production of leukocytes in bone marrow was prohibited. There were no significant differences in patients' data in these three groups.

Statistics

The two-sample *t*-test was used to compare chemotherapy-induced granulocytopenia with or without rhG-CSF, the method and timing of rhG-CSF ad-

Y. Shinto et al.

Table 1. Patient characteristics

Sex	
Male	23 (cases)
Female	27
Age	6–71 years (average: 47.5)
Bone tumor	
Osteosarcoma	14 (cases)
Ewing's sarcoma	5
Chondrosarcoma	4
MFH	2
Soft tissue tumor	
Liposarcoma	5
Synovial sarcoma	5
MFH	3
Fibrosarcoma	2
Chordoma	2
Malignant schwannoma	1
Rhabdomyosarcoma	1
Hemangiopericytoma	1
Clear cell sarcoma	1
Metastatic bone tumor	
Nasopharyngeal carcinoma	1
Mammary carcinoma	1
Lung cancer	2

MFH (malignant fibrous histiocytoma)

Table 2. Response of granulocyte to rhG-CSF

rhG-CSF ($\mu g/m^2$)	Numbers of cases	Granulocyte nadir counts (/mm^3)	Duration of granulocytopenia (day)		Duration of febrile period (day)	
			1,000>	2,000>	37C°<	38C°<
0	58	345 ± 436	3.2 ± 2.5	5.7 ± 7.2	4.6 ± 5.3	2.6 ± 3.4
50	59	1264 ± 846*	1.1 ± 0.8*	4.1 ± 3.6	3.9 ± 2.9	1.0 ± 0.8*
75	59	1586 ± 1463*	0.4 ± 0.4**	1.8 ± 1.5**	1.4 ± 1.2**	0.5 ± 0.4**
100	60	2200 ± 1643*	0.04 ± 0.5**	0.5 ± 0.6**	0.5 ± 0.4**	0.01 ± 0.02**

* $P < 0.05$; ** $P < 0.01$
Values are mean ± SD

Table 3. Comparison of rhG-CSF effect between subcutaneous and intravenous administration

rhG-CSF route	Number of cases	Duration of granulocytopenia (day)		Duration of febrile period (day)	
		1,000>	2,000>	37C°<	38C°<
Subcutaneous administration	88	0.3 ± 0.7**	1.7 ± 2.2*	1.4 ± 2.0**	0.3 ± 0.8**
Intravenous administration	92	2.1 ± 1.9	4.7 ± 2.7	4.2 ± 2.2	1.2 ± 1.7

* $P < 0.05$; ** $P < 0.01$
Values are mean ± SD

Table 4. Comparison of the timing of rhG-CSF administration. In early group, rhG-CSF was injected within 48 hours after chemotherapy and in late group, the administration of rhG-CSF started at the time below 1500/mm³ granulocyte counts

Timing of rhG-CSF administration	Number of cases	Duration of granulocytopenia (day)		Duration of febrile period (day)	
		1,000>	2,000>	37C°<	38C°<
Early	62	0.1 ± 0.4**	0.9 ± 1.4**	0.6 ± 1.0**	0.1 ± 0.4**
Late	78	1.0 ± 1.6	5.1 ± 2.4	4.2 ± 2.2	1.2 ± 1.7

* $P < 0.05$; ** $P < 0.01$
Values are mean ± SD

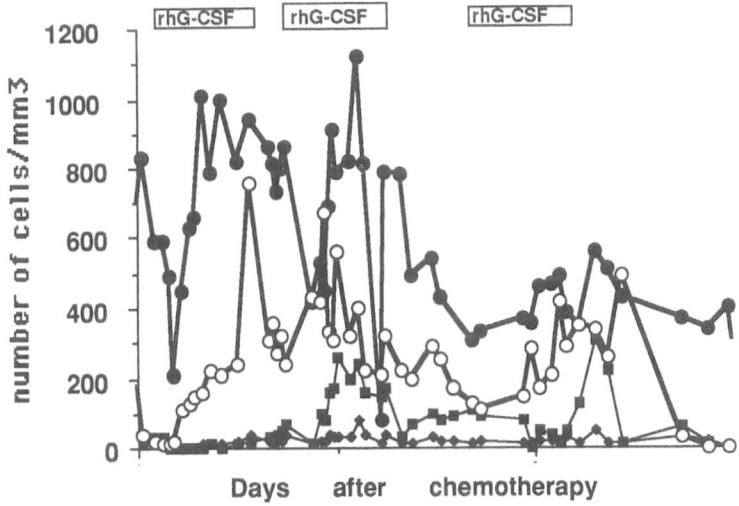

Fig. 1. Cell counts before and after administration of rhG-CSF. *Solid square*, eosinophil; *solid diamond*, basophil; *solid circle*, lymphocyte; *open circle*, monocyte

ministration, and the effect of rhG-CSF on neutrophil activity. The Wilcoxon test was used for comparison of the escalated dose effects of rhG-CSF.

Results

The characteristics of the patients enrolled in this study are shown in Table 1.

As shown in Table 2, administration of rhG-CSF showed a significant improvement ($P < 0.05$) in the nadir count of granulocytes, the duration of granulocytopenia, and the febrile period, as compared to the control group

In the P and C groups, the duration of granulocytopenia and the febrile period were studied in relation to three different doses of rhG-CSF (50, 75, 100 μg/m²). The rhG-CSF doses of 75 μg/m² and 100 μg/m² significantly shortened the duration of granulocytopenia and the febrile period compared to the dose of $50\,\mu g/m^2$ ($P < 0.05$). When the duration of granulocytopenia and the febrile period were studied in relation to iv and sc administration of rhG-CSF, the subcutaneous route showed stronger effects than the intravenous one (Table 3). When the duration of granulocytopenia and the febrile period were studied in relation to early and late administration of rhG-CSF, early administration of rhG-CSF following chemotherapy produced significantly better results than late administration (Table 4).

There were no significant changes in lymphocyte, monocyte, basophil, and eosinophil levels before and after administration of rhG-CSF (Fig. 1). In addition, rhG-CSF increased the migratory potential of neutrophil, but did not change the phagocytotic potential.

Discussion

Dose intensity of chemotherapeutic regimens is important in achieving their full potential. In order to preserve a high dose intensity, it is necessary to develop new methods for preventing the side effects of chemotherapy.

There seem to be three major advantages in the use of rhG-CSF: (1) increased absolute nadir count of granulocytes after chemotherapy, (2) shortened duration of granulocytopenia and the febrile periods and (3) increased activity of neutrophils.

Some studies have already shown that the neutrophil count increased in a dose-dependent manner and the duration of neutropenia by chemotherapy significantly shortened with rhG-CSF [4–6]. In our study, rhG-CSF also increased the absolute nadir count of granulocytes, and shortened the duration of granulocytopenia and the febrile period. The most effective dose was $100\,\mu g/m^2$.

In the patients who had undergone repeated chemoradiotherapy treatment before the administration of rhG-CSF, there was some tendency toward a prolonged duration of granulocytopenia, as compared to those who did not undergo previous chemotherapy. It may be necessary to escalate the dose level of rhG-CSF in patients with previous repeated chemotherapy.

Ohsaki et al. has reported that rhG-CSF enhanced the proliferation of human nonhematopoietic tumor cell lines in a study using the double-layer clonogenic assay [10]. In our previous study [11], rhG-CSF increased the growth of an osteosarcoma cell line and synovial sarcoma. Therefore, we should examine the sensitivity of rhG-CSF to the tumor cells in tumor-bearing patients.

We conclude that the most appropriate method for administration of rhG-CSF in patients undergoing intensive chemotherapy for malignant bone and soft tissue tumor is $75–100\,\mu g/m^2$ by sc injection within 48 h of chemotherapy for 14 consecutive days. In patients who have undergone previous repeated chemotherapy, the recommended dose of rhG-CSF is $100\,\mu g/m^2$ because of the possibility of a lower bone marrow response.

References

1. Souza LM, Boone TC, Gabrilove J, Lai PH, Zsebo KM, Murdock DC, Chazin VR, Bruszewski J, Lu H, Chen K, Barendt J, Platzer E, Moore MAS, Mertelsmann R, Welte K (1986) Recombinant human granulocyte colony-stimulating factor: Effects on normal and leukemic myeloid cells. Science 232:61–65

2. Kawasaki ES, Ladner MB, Wang AM, Arsdell JV, Warren MK, Coyne MY, Schweickart VL, Lee MT, Wilson KJ, Boosman A, Stanley ER, Ralph P, Mark DF (1985) Molecular cloning of the complementary DNA encoding human macrophage colony-stimulating factor (CSF-1). Science 230:291–296

3. Nagata S, Tsuchiya M, Asano S, Kaziro Y, Yamazaki T, Yamamoto O, Hirata Y, Kubota N, Oheda M, Nomura H, Ono M (1986) Molecular cloning and expression of cDNA for human granulocyte colony-stimulating factor. Nature 319:415–418

4. Morstyn G, Campbell L, Souza LM, Alton NK, Keeth J, Green M, Sheridan W, Metcalf D (1988) Effect of granulocyte colony-stimulating factor on neutropenia induced by cytotoxic chemotherapy. Lancet 2:667–671

5. Bronchud MH, Scafle JH, Thatcher N, Crowther D, Souza LM, Alton NK, Testa NG, Dexter TM (1987) Phase I/II study of recombinant human granulocyte colony-stimulating factor in patients receiving intensive chemotherapy for small cell lung cancer. Br J Cancer 56:809–813

6. Gabrilove JL, Jakubowski A, Scher H, Sternberg C, Wong G, Grous J, Yagota A, Fain K, Moore MAS, Clarkson B, Oettgen H, Alton K, Welte K, Souza LM (1988) Effect of granulocyte colony-stimulating factor on neutropenia and associated morbidity due to chemotherapy for transitional-cell carcinoma of the urothelium. N Engl J Med 318:1414–1422

7. Brandt SJ, Peters WP, Atwater SK, Kurtberg J, Borowitz MJ, Jones RB, Shapall EJ, Bast RG, Gilbert CJ, Oette DH (1988) Effect of recombinant human granulocyte-macrophage colony-stimulating factors on hematopoietic reconstitution after high-dose chemotherapy and autologous bone marrow transplantation. N Engl J Med 318:869–876

8. Vadhan-Raj S, Buescher S, LeMaistre A, Keating M, Walters R, Ventura C, Hittelman W, Broxmeyer HE, Gutterman JU (1988) Stimulation of hematopoiesis in patients with bone marrow failure and in patients with malignancy by recombinant human granulocyte-macrophage colony-stimulating factors. Blood 72:134–141

9. Antman KS, Griffin JD, Elias A, Socinski MA, Ryan L, Cannistra SA, Oette D, Whitley M, Frei E III, Schnipper LE (1988) Effect of recombinant human granulocyte-macrophage colony-stimulating factors on chemotherapy-included myelosuppression. N Engl J Med 319:593–598

10. Ohsaki Y, Bungo M, Horichi N, Fujiwara Y, Minato K, Niimi S, Nakagawa K, Ohe Y, Sasaki S, Eguchi K, Sasaki Y, Saijo N (1989) Effects of recombinant human colony-stimulating factors on colony formation of lung cancer cell lines. Jpn J Cancer Chemother 16:431–433

11. Shinto Y, Uchida A, Araki N, Ono K (1991) Enhancement of cell activity in malignant bone and soft tissue tumors by granulocyte colony stimulating factor. J Jpn Orthop Assoc 65:S1259

Future Directions in the Management of Malignant Bone Tumors

Robert L. Souhami[1]

Introduction

In spite of the considerable improvements produced by combination chemo-therapy, there remain many problems still to be tackled in order to enhance the survival rate of patients with primary malignant bone tumors. There is some evidence that current chemotherapy programs have reached a plateau in their effect on survival, and that further improvements are going to be difficult both to obtain and to detect. This chapter describes some of the remaining problems and discusses some possibilities for advancement. The increasing specialization of the treatment of primary malignant bone tumors has had the advantage that, in many countries, the expertise has been concentrated in a few major centers. This means that national and international collaboration in clinical trials should become easier if agreement can be reached on the nature of the questions to be posed.

Osteosarcoma

It is now apparent that adjuvant chemotherapy prolongs disease-free intervals in operable osteosarcoma. Two studies [1, 2] have shown that the disease-free interval in patients treated immediately with chemotherapy is considerably greater than those in whom chemotherapy is given only if and when metastases occur. Although, in the study of Link et al., there was no difference in overall survival in the two arms at the time of the report, it seems likely that such a difference will occur if follow-up is prolonged. One problem with this study was that the number of randomized patients (36) was so small that even large differences in survival were more likely to have been missed than detected. Both these studies have illustrated the need for adjuvant chemotherapy and also the weakness of small-scale studies in answering questions of survival.

[1] Department of Oncology, University College and Middlesex School of Medicine, London, W1P 8BT, UK

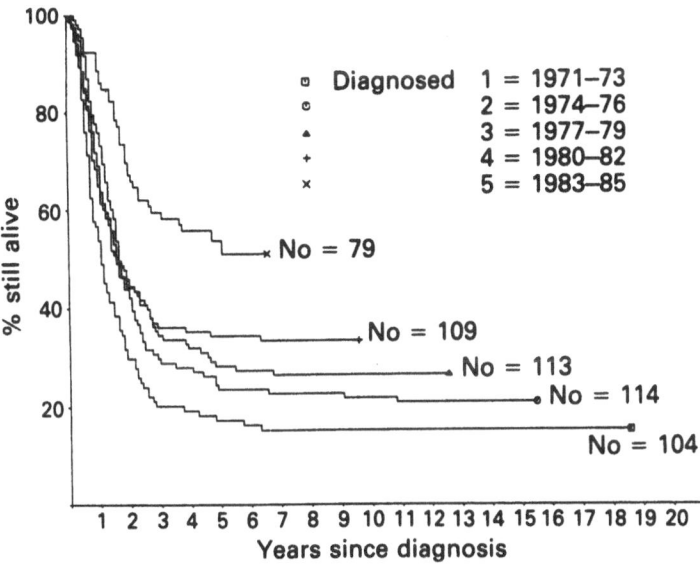

Fig. 1. Survival of pediatric osteosarcoma in the United Kingdom between 1972 and 1985 (From [3] with permission)

Recent data from the United Kingdom [3] have shown that, in the 3-year cohorts from 1972 through 1985, national survival in the pediatric age range has steadily improved. The largest gain is shown in the data from the early 1980s when intensive combination chemotherapy was widely introduced as part of national programs in the treatment of osteosarcoma (Fig. 1). Similar data are available from the COSS studies [4, 5]. In COSS-80, the disease-free survival at 3 years was approximately 60%. Longer term follow-up of these patients suggested that only a few patients are relapsing after this time. This study consisted largely of pediatric cases and may not be truly representative of all osteosarcoma in pediatric, adolescent, and early adult life. Survival data from the Southwestern Oncology Group (SWOG) indicated that relapse occurs beyond 5 years and the survival curves do not become stable until 10 years or more [6]. The problem of late recurrence has become more apparent in recent years and it is clear that, for some patients, chemotherapy is delaying metastasis but not preventing it.

At the same time, the toxicity of chemotherapy is increasingly being recognized. Cisplatin causes high-tone hearing loss, renal impairment which may be long lasting, and peripheral neuropathy [7]. Doxorubicin is associated with cardiomyopathy in a dose-dependent manner although the schedule of administration of doxorubicin may also be important in its cardiac effects. It is increasingly apparent that ifosfamide causes renal tubular damage which, like that of cisplatin, may be long lasting. These effects, occurring in children and young adults, are serious problems for the future. They argue for dose reduction where possible.

Could we, then, identify those patients who are at low risk of metastasis and who may be cured by short and intensive, less toxic, chemotherapeutic programs, and those patients who have a poor prognosis wherein the likelihood of death is so high that the toxicity of treatment is of secondary importance? This is possible to some extent. It is clear that the prognosis of patients who already have metastatic disease at presentation is poor [8]. Similarly, patients with large inflammatory tumors and a very high level of alkaline phosphatase are also at high risk of metastasis and early death [8, 9]. Between these extremes there are many patients who cannot be clearly identified as falling into one prognostic category or another. Although the histological appearances of telangiectatic osteosarcoma were thought to be a poor prognostic feature, there is increasing evidence that these tumors, like others, are responsive to chemotherapy and do not necessarily have a worse outcome [10]. The small cell variant of osteosarcoma is rare [11] and appears to be a highly malignant variety. However, for the majority of patients, a clear statement of prognosis cannot be made on the basis of histological subtype. For the time being, therefore, our major efforts must be directed towards trying to improve chemotherapy.

The most active drugs used in the treatment of osteosarcoma are cisplatin, doxorubicin, high-dose methotrexate (HDMTX), and ifosfamide. Of these, ifosfamide is the newest agent and its activity in osteosarcoma is rather less well documented than those of the other drugs. There has been widespread use of the program introduced by Rosen et al. [12], known as the T10 protocol. This is heavily reliant on intensive pre-operative treatment with HDMTX, but there is increasing evidence to suggest that it is not a good policy to omit cisplatin and doxorubicin from the early treatment of patients [5]. Currently, the European Osteosarcoma Intergroup (EOI) has achieved results comparable with multicenter use of the T10 program using doxorubicin and cisplatin alone. The EOI is now conducting a randomized trial of this two-drug intensive regimen against the T10 programme. It seems probable that optimum results will be achieved by the intensive use of most of the active agents over a relatively short period of time. Such an approach would lend itself to attempts to increase dosage by the use of agents, such as colony stimulating factors to spare bone marrow suppression.

The intra-arterial (IA) route has been widely used in the treatment of osteosarcoma [13–15]. While high responses are observed to IA cisplatin and although this may be useful for increasing the success of limb-preservation surgery, the main problem in osteosarcoma is survival and, for this, systemic chemotherapy is essential. Randomized comparisons of intra-arterial and intravenous chemotherapy have seldom been undertaken, and the value of the IA route has not been convincingly demonstrated.

The management of pulmonary metastasis presents particular problems in osteosarcoma. Unlike most cancers, it is undoubtedly true that some patients with pulmonary metastases may be cured by metastasectomy. Several studies have shown that if the thorax can be made disease-free by surgery, there is an approximately 30% chance of long-term survival [16]. The choice of patients

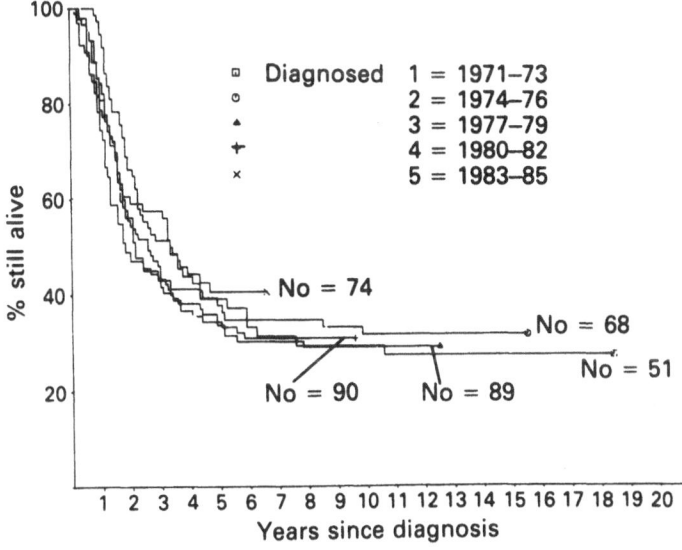

Fig. 2. Survival of Ewing's sarcoma in the United Kingdom between 1972 and 1985 (From [3] with permission)

who are suitable for thoracotomy has been examined in several retrospective studies. It seems that the prognosis is related to the disease-free interval [17, 18], the number of pulmonary metastases [19], and whether the metastases are unilateral or bilateral [19]. It is, of course, common sense to assume that patients who suffer a relapse after a long period free of disease with few metastases are more likely to be cured than those who have a relapse with multiple bilateral recurrences shortly after chemotherapy has been finished. Nevertheless, between these extremes there are very difficult clinical choices to make. The value of pre-thoracotomy chemotherapy is inadequately studied. It will depend on the treatment-free interval and on the amount of previous chemotherapy as well as the drugs which have previously been employed. Radiological responses to second-line chemotherapy in osteosarcoma are infrequent and usually short-lived. Similarly, the value of post-thoracotomy chemotherapy and radiation are poorly substantiated. These questions remain important areas for further study in the disease.

Ewing's Sarcoma

Because of its rarity, it has always been difficult to amass enough cases to carry out randomized comparisons of treatment in Ewing's sarcoma. For this reason, knowledge for determining the best form of treatment has proceeded rather slowly. In recent years, the prognostic factors predictive of outcome have become clearer. It has been recognized that small round cell tumors arising in bone may not be a homogeneous group, and the importance of intensive combination chemotherapy has been widely understood. In the United Kingdom there has been little advance in the prognosis of Ewing's sarcoma in children under the age of 16 in the years 1972 to 1985 [3] (Fig. 2). More recent studies in the UK have indicated that, as with other childhood cancers, the prognosis of Ewing's sarcoma is improving as a result of a national effort in clinical trials of intensive treatment.

Chemotherapy

Alkylating agents were shown to be effective in Ewing's sarcoma almost 30 years ago [20]. Shortly afterwards, vincristine was shown to produce responses [21]. Actinomycin D and doxorubicin were later shown to be effective [22–24]. More recently, ifosfamide has been shown to be an extremely effective agent [25], and VP16 has also been demonstrated to have activity [26].

Numerous studies have been carried out with multidrug regimens. The Intergroup Ewing's Sarcoma Study (IESS) showed, in a randomized study, that doxorubicin significantly added to the antitumor effect of vincristine, actinomycin, and cyclophosphamide used in combination [27]. A longer term follow-up has substantiated this conclusion [28].

The most recent studies have used various combinations of doxorubicin, actinomycin, cyclophosphamide, and vincristine, and have reported disease-free survival rates of approximately 40%–50% at 3 years. Typical of these studies are those by Hayes et al. [29] and Jürgens et al. [30], reporting on the Cooperative Ewing's Study (CESS) in pediatric cases. In Italy, Bacci et al. [31] used chemotherapy for 2 years (vincristine, doxorubicin, and cyclophosphamide) with comparable results. Rosen et al. [32] has reported on patients treated with a variety of multidrug regimens incorporating vincristine, doxorubicin, actinomycin, and cyclophosphamide in the early studies, and then bleomycin, BCNU, and/or methotrexate were added in the later studies. A later report [33] indicated a disease-free survival of 65% for axial skeletal lesions and 76% and 90% for proximal and distal long bone lesions, respectively. Longer-term follow-up figures have not been supplied.

Prognostic Factors in Ewing's Sarcoma

It has long been apparent that pelvic tumors have a worse prognosis than those in the long bones. However, much of this prognostic information lies in the volume of the tumor rather than in the site. Several studies have shown that the larger the tumor size the shorter the disease-free interval and overall survival [29, 30]. Indeed, when tumor size is taken into account, the site of the tumor has much less prognostic importance. The tumor volume predicts not only the occurrence of pulmonary metastasis but also local recurrence after radiation treatment.

It has also become clear that some patients presenting with a round cell tumor in bone do not have the typical histopathological features of Ewing's sarcoma. Kissane et al. [34] reported that, in the IESS studies, a filigree appearance was associated with a worse prognosis than that of typical Ewing's sarcoma. More recently, several reports of round cell tumors of bone with neuroectodermal features have appeared [35, 36]. These neuroectodermal features include expression of neuron-specific enolase, chromogranin, and dense core granules seen on electron microscopy. In a recent report, Hartman et al. [37] have presented data to show that the expression of neuroectodermal characteristics is associated with a worse prognosis in round cell tumors in bone. These authors also described an appearance which they called "atypical Ewing's sarcoma" characterized histologically by a lobular and alveolar pattern. These tumors tended to show a high mitotic rate and cellular pleomorphism (including nuclear pleomorphism). These "atypical" Ewing's tumors were also associated with a worse prognosis, although they did not express typical neuroendocrine markers. It remains to be seen, in larger prospective studies, whether there is prognostic information in these pathological appearances over and above that obtained from clinical manifestations such as tumor size.

Local Recurrence in Ewing's Sarcoma

Radiation has been the established treatment for the local control of Ewing's sarcoma for many years [38]. Typically, in a limb, a radiation dose of 44 Gy is given in daily fractions of 200 cGy. The majority of the bone is treated to this dose and the fields are then shrunk to allow an additional boost of 10–20 Gy to the main tumor. It does not appear that increasing the dose over 55 Gy is beneficial. There are considerable uncertainties about the fractionation schedule to be employed, and there has been recent interest in hyperfractionated and accelerated radiation.

The local recurrence rate after radiation varies from 10%–30%, depending on the site, and distant metastasis is more common in those patients in whom local recurrence occurs. With the advent of more powerful systemic chemotherapy, solitary local recurrence is not common and local recurrence is increasingly a feature of a failure of systemic as well as local tumor control.

Nevertheless, local recurrence remains a problem in Ewing's sarcoma and is much more frequent in large tumors [29, 30]. For this reason, there is considerable interest in conservative surgery as an adjunct to radiotherapy. The problem here is that the most difficult tumors, and those most likely to recur locally, are bulky lesions located particularly in the axial skeleton. It is precisely in these sites that surgical approaches remain most difficult.

It may be possible to further reduce local recurrence rates by the combination of fractionated radiation and concurrent chemotherapy. However, many of the chemotherapeutic agents which are most effective in this disease are also radiation sensitizing. The long-term sequelae of radiation include failure of linear bone growth, muscular atrophy, fibrosis and edema distally in the limb, and radiation sarcoma. The latter complication is increasingly reported but it is difficult to estimate the risk precisely. Ewing's sarcoma was the primary site in several of the 91 cases of bone sarcoma recently reported as second malignant neoplasms following treatment of cancer in childhood [39]. These complications are reasons for considering the additional role of surgery. However, endoprostheses do not always give a perfect functional result and they may not be stable or reliable over a lifetime of use. We need much more information and longer follow-up before we can decide on firm recommendations for the local treatment of Ewing's sarcoma.

Other Future Directions

The prognosis of the Ewing's sarcoma which is metastatic at diagnosis remains poor [40]. Although some patients (approximately 25%) may be long-term survivors when they present with pulmonary metastases at diagnosis, the majority of patients die quickly. Approximately 30% of patients present in this way and new chemotherapeutic strategies need to be considered for this group. Such strategies will probably include intensification of chemotherapy using hemopoietic growth factors, the addition of drugs (such as etoposide) to standard chemotherapy regimens, and the use of high-dose chemotherapy with autologous bone marrow transplantation following induction of complete remission. At the moment, there is only anecdotal evidence to support each of these approaches in the treatment of the disease. Because of the rarity of Ewing's sarcoma, collaborative groups will be necessary to make progress quickly in these categories of patients.

Malignant Fibrous Histiocytoma and Other High-Grade Spindle Cell Sarcomas

Malignant fibrous histiocytoma of bone (MFHB) accounts for approximately 5% of all primary malignant bone tumors. The traditional treatment has been surgical excision of the tumor, usually by amputation. Several reports have indicated that the survival of this approach to treatment is approximately 30% at 5 years [41]. These poor figures have led several groups to use adjuvant chemotherapy in addition to surgical resection. Several of these studies have indicated that when chemotherapy has been given pre-operatively, histopathological responses in the form of tumor necrosis have been frequently observed [42, 43]. These reports indicate chemosensitivity of MFHB. In our own institution, we have treated 15 such patients with pre-operative chemotherapy, including ifosfamide, doxorubicin, and high-dose methotrexate, and have seen histopathological responses of 90% or more in 13 patients. It is difficult to know if pre-operative and post-operative chemotherapy will add to survival rates in MFHB and other spindle cell sarcomas. The rarity of these tumors makes collaboration in studies essential if reliable data are to be obtained not only on MFHB but on other high-grade spindle cell sarcomas. Such studies have been started by the European Osteosarcoma Intergroup.

References

1. Link MP, Goorin AM, Miser AW (1986) The effect of adjuvant chemotherapy on relapse-free survival in patients with osteosarcoma of the extremity. N Engl J Med 134:1600–1606

2. Eiber F, Giuliano A, Eckardt J, et al. (1987) Adjuvant chemotherapy for osteo-sarcoma: A randomized prospective trial. J Clin Oncol 5:21–26
3. Stiller CA, Bunch KJ (1990) Trends in survival for childhood cancer in Britain diagnosed 1971–85. Br J Cancer 62:806–815
4. Winkler K, Beron G, Kotz R (1984) Neoadjuvant chemotherapy for osteogenic sarcoma: Results of a cooperative German/Austrian study. J Clin Oncol 2:617–624
5. Winkler K, Beron G, Delling G (1988) Neoadjuvant chemotherapy of osteo-sarcoma: Results of a randomized cooperative trial (Coss-82) with salvage chemo-therapy based on histological tumor response. J Clin Oncol 6:329–337
6. Ryan J, Baker L, Benjamin R (1990) Long-term follow-up in the cure of osteogenic sarcoma. Chir Organi Mov 75 (Supp 1):48
7. Ochs JJ, Freeman AI, Douglass HO (1978) Cis-dichlordiammineplatinum (II) in advanced osteogenic sarcoma. Cancer Treat Rep 62:239–245
8. Taylor WF, Ivins JC, Unni K (1989) Prognostic variables in osteosarcoma: A multi institutional study. J Natl Cancer Inst 81:21–30
9. Bacci G, Picci P, Orlando M, et al. (1987) Prognostic value of serum alkaline phosphatase in osteosaracoma. Tumori 73:331–336
10. Rosen G, Huvos AG, Marcove R, Nirenberg A (1986) Telangiectatic osteogenic sarcoma. Clin Orthop 207:164–173
11. Sim FH, Unni KK, Beabout JW, Dahlin DC (1979) Osteosarcoma with small cells simulating Ewing's tumor. J Bone Joint Surg [AM] 61A:207–215.
12. Rosen G, Caparros B, Huvos AG (1982) Preoperative chemotherapy for osteogenic sarcoma: Selection of postoperative adjuvant chemotherapy based on the response of the primary tumor to preoperative chemotherapy. Cancer 49:1221–1230
13. Eckardt JJ, Eiber FR, Grant TT, et al. (1985) Management of stage IIB osteogenic sarcoma: Experience at the Unviersity of California, Los Angeles Cancer Treat-ment Symposia 3:117–130
14. Jaffe N, Robertson R, Ayala A (1985) Comparison of intra-arterial cis-diammine-dichloroplatinum II with high dose methotrexate and citrovorum factor rescue in the treatment of primary osteosarcoma. J Clin Oncol 3:1101–1110
15. Benjamin RS (1989) Regional chemotherapy for osteosarcoma. Semin Oncol 16:323–327
16. Goorin AM, Delorey MJ, Lack EE, et al. (1984) Prognostic significance of com-plete surgical resection of pulmonary metastases in patients with osteogenic sarcoma: Analysis of 32 patients. J Clin Oncol 2:425–431
17. Burgers JHV, Brair K, van Dobbenburgh AO, et al. (1980) Role of metastatectomy without chemotherapy in the management of osteosarcoma in children. Cancer 45:1664–1668
18. Han M-T, Telander RL, Pairolero PC, et al. (1981) Aggressive thoracotomy for pulmonary metastatic osteogenic sarcoma in children and young adolescents. J Ped Surg 16:928–933
19. Meyer WH, Schell MJ, Kumar APM (1987) Thoracotomy for pulmonary meta-static osteosarcoma. An analysis of prognostic indicators of survival. Cancer 59:374–379
20. Sutow WW, Sullivan MP (1962) Cyclophosphamide therapy in children with Ewing's sarcoma. Cancer Chemother Rep 23:55–60
21. Selawry OS, Holland JF, Wolman IJ (1968) Effect of vincristine on malignant solid tumors in children. Cancer Chemother Rep 53:497–500
22. Wang JJ, Cortes E, Sinks L, Holland JF (1971) Therapeutic effect and toxicity of adriamycin in patients with neoplastic disease. Cancer 28:837–843

23. Senyszyn JJ, Johnson RE, Curran RE (1970) Treatment of metastatic Ewing's sarcoma with Actinomycin D (NSC-3053). Cancer Chemother Rep 54:103–107

24. Oldham RK, Pomeroy TC (1972) Treatment of Ewing's sarcoma with adriamycin (NSC-123127). Cancer Chemother Rep 56:635–639

25. Magrath I, Sandlund J, Raynor A (1986) A phase II study of ifosfamide in the treatment of recurrent sarcomas in young people. Cancer Chemother Pharmacol 18 (Suppl 2):S25–S28

26. Hayes FA, Green A, Thompson E (1983) Phase II trial of VP 16-213 in pediatric solid tumors (Abstract No C-256). Proc Am Soc Clin Oncol

27. Nesbit ME, Perez CA, Tefft M (1981) Multimodal therapy for the management of primary non metastatic Ewing's sarcoma of bone: An Intergroup Study. Nat Cancer Inst Monogr 56:255–262

28. Nesbit ME, Gehan EA, Burgert EO (1990) Multimodal therapy for the management of primary, non-metastatic Ewing's sarcoma of bone: A long-term follow-up of the first Intergroup study. J Clin Oncol 8:1664–1674

29. Hayes FA, Thompson E, Meyer W, et al. (1989) Therapy for localized Ewing's sarcoma of bone. J Clin Oncol 7:208–213

30. Jürgens H, Exner U, Gadner H (1988) Multidisciplinary treatment of primary Ewing's sarcoma of bone. A 6-year experience of a European cooperative trial. Cancer 61:23–32

31. Bacci G, Picci P, Gherlinzoni F, et al. (1985) Localized Ewing's sarcoma of bone: Ten years' experience at the Instituto Orthopedico Rizzoli in 124 cases treated with multimodal therapy. Eur J Cancer Clin Oncol 21:163–173

32. Rosen G, Caparros B, Nirenberg A (1981) Ewing's sarcoma: Ten-year experience with adjuvant chemotherapy. Cancer 47:2204–2213

33. Rosen G (1982) Current management of Ewing's sarcoma. Progr Clin Cancer 8:267–282

34. Kissane JM, Askin FB, Foulkes M, Strattan LB, Shirley SF (1983) Ewing's sarcoma of bone: Clinico-pathological aspects of 303 cases from the Intergroup Ewing's Sarcoma Study. Hum Path 14:773–779

35. Jaffe R, Santamaria M, Unis EJ (1984) The neuroectodermal tumor of bone. Am J Surg Pathol 8:885–898

36. Daugaard S, Kamby C, Sunde LM, et al. (1989) Ewing's sarcoma: A retrospective study of histological and immunohistochemical factors and their relation to prognosis. Virchows Arch [A] 414:243–251

37. Hartman KR, Triche TJ, Kinsella TJ, Miser JS (1991) Prognostic value of histopathology in Ewing's sarcoma. Long-term follow-up of distal extremity tumors. Cancer 67:163–171

38. Suit HD (1975) Role of therapeutic radiology in cancer of bone. Cancer 35:930–935

39. Newton WA, Meadows AT, Shimada H (1991) Bone sarcomas as second malignant neoplasms following childhood cancer. Cancer 67:193–201

40. Cangir A, Vietti TJ, Gehan EA, et al. (1990) Ewing's sarcoma metastatic at diagnosis. Results and comparisons of two Intergroup Ewing's sarcoma studies. Cancer 66:887–893

41. Earl HM (1987) Chemotherapy of rare malignant bone tumours. In: Souhami RL (ed) Bone Tumours. Ballières Clinical Oncology, vol 1. Ballières Tindall, London, pp 223–241

42. den Heeten GJ, Schraffordt-Koops H, Kamps WA, et al. (1985) Treatment of malignant fibrous histiocytoma of bone. A plea for primary chemotherapy. Cancer 56:37–40
43. Urban C, Rose C, Huvos AG (1983) Chemotherapy of malignant fibrous histiocytoma of bone. A report of five cases. Cancer 51:795–802

Part 3

Radiotherapy

Fast Neutron Radiotherapy for Sarcomas of the Bone and Soft Tissue

HIROSHI TSUNEMOTO, SHINROKU MORITA, TAKASHI NAKANO, and
SHINICHIRO SATOH[1]

Introduction

It has been generally accepted that sarcomas of the bone and soft tissue are radioresistant compared with other tumors, such as squamous cell carcinoma and adenocarcinoma. Therefore, patients with sarcoma of the bone and soft tissue have been usually referred to radiation therapy after removal of the tumor in order to manage residual tumor cells. On the other hand, there is support for the role of preoperative irradiation for those sarcomas in order to preserve function of the involved extremities.

Radiation therapy has made marked progress since the introduction of megavoltage machines, while efforts have been made to improve the effects of radiation and to sensitize hypoxic tumor cells. Fast neutrons, which are characterized by a low oxygen enhancement ratio as well as by a low repair capability of the irradiated cells, have been introduced in the treatment of radioresistant and locally advanced cancers. Clinical trials with fast neutrons was introduced in 1968 at the Hammersmith Hospital in London. In Japan, the trials were initiated at the National Institute of Radiological Sciences (NIRS) on November, 1975.

In this study, results of treatment with fast neutrons performed at the NIRS were evaluated for sarcomas of the bone and soft tissue.

Materials and Methods

Materials

Between November, 1975 and December, 1989, 78 patients who had osteosarcoma of the extremities and 105 patients who had soft tissue sarcoma were treated with fast neutrons at the NIRS. The results of the treatment were

---

[1] Hospital Division, National Institute of Radiological Sciences, Chiba, 260 Japan

Table 1. Histologic characteristics of patients with soft tissue sarcoma receiving fast neutron therapy

Histology	Patients (n)
Liposarcoma	30
Leiomyosarcoma	11
Rhabdomyosarcoma	10
Synovial sarcoma	10
Fibrosarcoma	9
Malignant fibrous histiocytoma	9
Malignant schwannoma	8
Angiosarcoma	5
Neurogenic sarcoma	3
Others	10
Total	105

evaluated for the patients who were followed more than 6 months after receiving radical irradiation. Histological classification of the soft tissue sarcoma in the patients who participated in the clinical trials is shown in Table 1.

Methods

The fast neutrons used in this clinical trials were obtained by bombarding a thick Beryllium target with 30 MeV deuterons accelerated by a medical cyclotron installed at the NIRS.

The maximum build-up of the beam was seen at 6 mm below the surface and the depth-dose curves obtained at a source-to-surface distance (SSD) of 175 cm were almost the same as those for Tele-cobalt gamma rays measured at SSD 75 cm.

Fast neutron therapy was performed by applying a vertical beam obtained by a bending deuteron beam through a magnet. The dose rate in a tissue-equivalent phantom was 42 rad (n, γ)/min per 30 μA for 11.4 × 11.4 cm field at a source-to-tumor distance (STD) of 200 cm. Gamma ray contamination was estimated to be less than 4% in the beam. Treatment was performed by using regimens for which fast neutrons alone, a mixture, and fast neutrons with a boost were provided. For therapy of fast neutrons alone, a total dose of 16.2 Gy was delivered with 18 fractions throughout 6 weeks, which was equivalent to a time dose and fractionation factor (TDF) of 100. When the mixed schedule was used, fast neutrons were irradiated on Tuesdays and Fridays and for the other 3 days, Monday, Wednesday, and Thursday, photon beam irradiation was provided. Boost irradiation with fast neutrons was usually followed by a shrinking field technique after 40 Gy of photons. For the patients suffering from osteosarcoma, treatment was provided by using fast neutron irradiation combined with chemotherapy, in which drugs were prescribed by either intravenous injection or infusion through a regional artery. Infusion of the drugs was usually scheduled prior to irradiation. Some of the patients

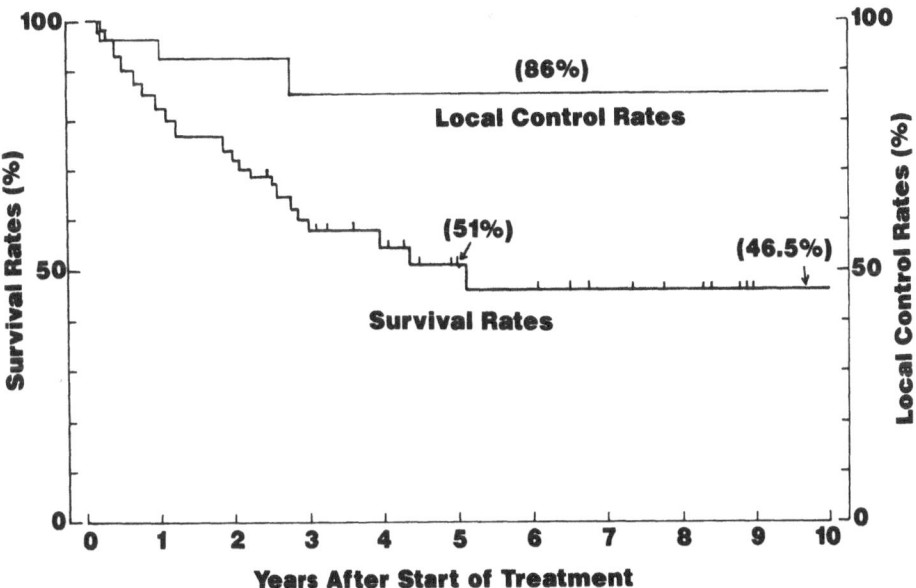

Fig. 1. Survival rates and local control rates of patients with osteosarcoma receiving fast neutron therapy; (*NIRS*; National Institute of Radiological Sciences, Chiba, Japan)

receiving combined therapy were referred for acquisition of a prosthesis in order to replace the bone affected by an artificial one. Evaluation was made for the patients receiving irradiation where doses at the lowest were equivalent to TDF 80 for fast neutrons alone, TDF 70 for postoperative irradiation, and TDF 60 for preoperative irradiation.

Results

Osteosarcoma

Of the 78 patients with osteosarcoma who received fast neutron therapy, 39 were evaluated in this study. Out of these 39 patients, 35 achieved local control, the durations of which were 6–123 months. Survival rates of the patients evaluated by the Kaplan-Meier method showed that the 5-year survival rate was 51% and 46.5% at 10 years (Fig. 1).

Soft Tissue Sarcoma

Fast neutron therapy was provided for 105 patients suffering from soft tissue sarcoma. Out of the 72 who were evaluated, 48 had previously untreated sarcomas, and the remaining 24 had recurrent sarcomas.

Local control rates. Out of 48 patients who had previously untreated sarcoma, 34 (70.8%) achieved local control. A regimen of fast neutrons alone was

Table 2. Results of fast neutron therapy for patients suffering from previously untreated soft tissue sarcoma

	Patients evaluated (n)	Local control	Complications	Deceased	Follow-up (months)	Doses (TDF)
Radiation alone	7	2 (28.5%)	0	5	12–240	>80
Preoperative radiation therapy	11	9 (81.8%)	0	3	13–168	>60
Postoperative radiation therapy	30	23 (76.6%)	1	7	10–144	>70
	48	34 (70.8%)	1	15		

(National Institute of Radiological Sciences, Chiba, Japan, July 1990)
TDF, Time dose and fractionation factor

Table 3. Results of fast neutron therapy for patients suffering from recurrent disease of soft tissue sarcoma

	Patients evaluated (n)	Local control	Complications	Deceased	Follow-up (months)	Doses (TDF)
Radiation alone	8	2 (25%)	1	5	7–126	>80
Preoperative radiation therapy	3	3	0	—	60–106	>60
Postoperative radiation therapy	13	9 (69.2%)	0	5	15–113	>70
	24	14 (58.3%)	1	10		

(National Institute of Radiological Sciences, Chiba, Japan, July 1990)
TDF, Time dose and fractionate factor

prescribed for seven patients suffering from locally advanced soft tissue sarcoma, of whom two achieved local control. Local control rates of the patients receiving either preoperative irradiation or postoperative irradiation were 81.8% (9/11) and 76.6% (23/30), respectively (Table 2). Complications were seen in 1 out of 48 patients.

Twenty-four patients who had postoperative recurrence of soft tissue sarcoma received fast neutron irradiation, of whom 14 (58.3%) achieved local control. Postoperative irradiation was provided for 13 patients who had recurrent sarcoma, of whom 9 (69.2%) achieved local control. Local control rate of the patients receiving fast neutrons alone was 25% (2/8). Complications were observed in 1 out of the 24 patients who participated in the study (Table 3).

Survival rates. Five-year survival rates of the patients who had previously untreated sarcoma and received fast neutron therapy were found to be 90% for those who had received preoperative irradiation, 76% for postoperative irradiation, and 17% for fast neutrons alone (Fig. 2).

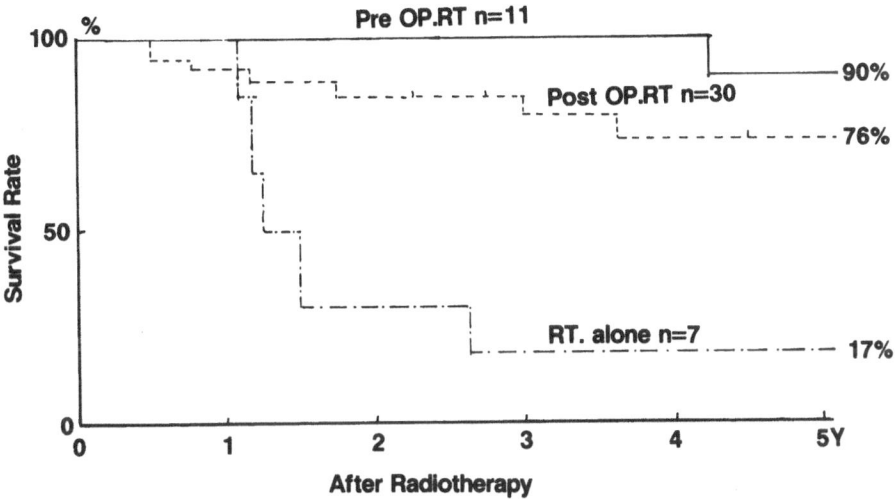

Fig. 2. Survival rates of patients with soft tissue sarcoma treated with fast neutrons-previously untreated disease. *RT*, Radiotherapy, *Pre OP.*, preoperative; *Post OP.*, postoperative

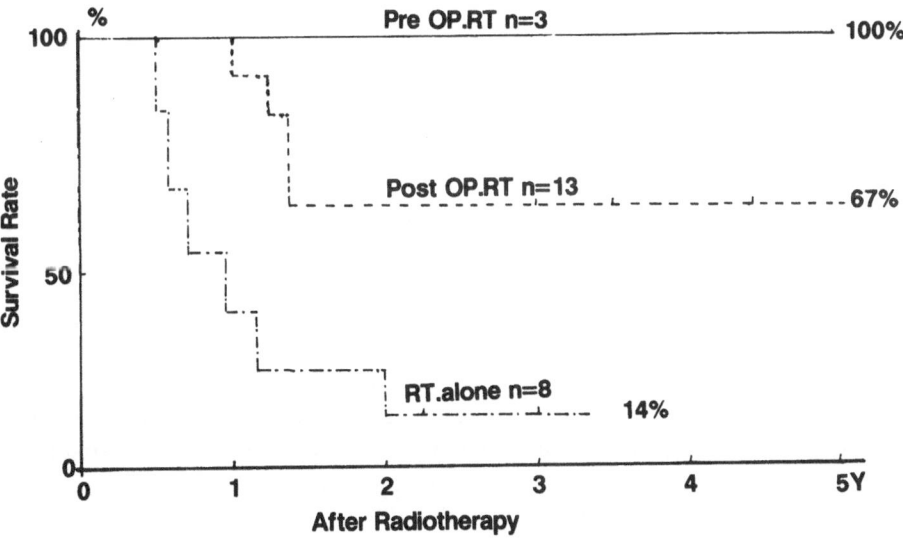

Fig. 3. Survival rates of patients with soft tissue sarcoma treated with fast neutrons-recurrent disease. *RT*, Radiotherapy; *Pre OP.*, preoperative; *Post OP.*, postoperative

For the patients who had recurrent soft tissue sarcoma following surgery, fast neutron therapy was also provided. Five-year survival rates were found to be 100% for the patients receiving preoperative irradiation, 67% for postoperative irradiation, and 14% for fast neutrons alone (Fig. 3).

It was emphasized that preoperative irradiation with fast neutrons was of great value in the treatment of soft tissue sarcoma in order to improve local control, while maintaining function of the involved limbs without complications from radiation, even in patients with recurrence of sarcomas after surgery.

Discussion

Clinical trials with fast neutrons are being performed in 17 institutions world-wide as of 1990. There were 15,000 patients who were treated with fast neutrons since 1968. Results of the trials have shown that carcinoma of the salivary gland, carcinoma of the prostate, osteosarcoma, and soft tissue sarcoma are indications for fast neutron therapy. Recently, the effects of fast neutrons have been confirmed in the treatment of Pancoast's tumor. However, the merits of fast neutrons have not been confirmed in the treatment of tumors such as carcinoma of the uterine cervix, esophagus, and lung.

The Role of Fast Neutron Therapy in the Treatment of Osteosarcoma

At the beginning of the studies, response of osteosarcoma to fast neutrons was investigated by using the specimens obtained from open biopsy performed after irradiation or amputation. Results of the histopathological studies showed that viable tumor cells were scarcely found in the specimens obtained from 15 out of 17 patients who had osteosarcoma, while degenerated tumor cells were seen in one out of the two patients who had chondrosarcoma [1]. Results of biological studies have shown that relative biological effectiveness (RBE) of fast neutrons relative to photons was found to be five for human osteosarcoma subcutaneously inoculated into the hind leg of nude mice [2]. Results of worldwide clinical trials showed that in the treatment of osteosarcoma, the local control rate of the patients receiving fast neutron therapy was 54% (52/97), while the rate was 21% (15/73) for those receiving photon beams [3].

On the other hand, it was emphasized that in the treatment of osteosarcoma, doses delivered to the target volume have to be prescribed in consideration of permitting the future use of a prosthesis after irradiation of fast neutrons. Finally, the doses to be irradiated have been reduced from equivalent of TDF 100 to TDF 80. It was also recommended that when the patients suffering from osteosarcoma are referred for radiation therapy, the type of treatment, such as combined chemotherapy, must be considered in light of recent developments in chemotherapy for osteosarcoma.

The Role of Fast Neutron Therapy in the Treatment of Soft Tissue Sarcoma

Results of worldwide clinical trials with fast neutrons showed that of 297 patients suffering from soft tissue sarcoma, 157 (53%) achieved local control, while the local control rate for those receiving photon beam irradiation was found to be 38% (49/128) [3].

The results were also evaluated according to the status of the patients referred for fast neutron therapy. It was reported that when the tumors were completely excised, the local control rates, confirmed after treatment with fast neutrons (mean energy: 7.5 MeV or 5.8 MeV), were found to be 94% or 75%, respectively. The rates were 52% for gross tumors and 75% for palpable tumors. The rates of complications were 40.9% (7.5 MeV) and 28.6% (5.8 MeV) for fast neutrons. Another clinical trial performed with fast neutrons (mean energy: 21 MeV) showed that the local control rate for unresectable sarcoma was 32%, and that the rate of complications was 13%, which are lower scores than the rates observed when low-energy fast neutrons were used [4−6].

It is recommended that an optimal schedule of fast neutron therapy should be explored for the treatment of soft tissue sarcoma, in light of the evidence showing that biological effects of irradiation are enhanced as the energy of fast neutrons decreases.

Conclusions

The role of fast neutrons in the treatment of sarcomas of the bone and soft tissue was investigated. It was confirmed that osteosarcoma is an indication for fast neutron therapy. Merits of fast neutron therapy were evaluated in the treatment of osteosarcoma in which the local failure rate was improved.

In order to improve local control and to preserve limb function, preoperative irradiation with fast neutrons must be introduced in the treatment of patients suffering from soft tissue sarcoma.

It was concluded that the role of high linear energy transfer (LET) radiations will be more precisely confirmed in the treatment of cancer and sarcoma by using charged particles, characterized by the Bragg peak as well as by high LET.

References

1. Tsunemoto H, Morita S, Arai T, Kutsutani Y, Kurisu A, Umegaki Y (1979) Results of clinical trials with 30 MeV d-Be neutrons at NIRS. In: Abe M (eds) Treatment of radio-resistant cancers. Elsevier, North Holland, pp 115−126
2. Tatezaki S (1979) Systemic multi-modal treatment of osteosarcoma, with special reference to the role of fast neutron radiotherapy, J Jpn Orthop Assoc 53:831−846
3. Wambersie A (1989) The future of high LET radiation in cancer therapy. Justification of the heavy-ion therapy program. In: Chaubel P (ed) Proceedings of the EULIMA Workshop on the Potential Value of Light Ion Beam Therapy (CAL edn). Commission of the European Communities, Brussels, Publn. No. EUR 12165 EN, pp XIX−LIII
4. Pickering DG, Stewart JS, Rampling R, Errington RA, Stamp G, Chia Y (1987) Fast neutron therapy for soft tissue sarcoma. Int J Radiat Oncol Biol Phys 13: 1489−1495

5. Schmitt G, Sassow JS, Schnabel, K, Bormann R, Bamberg M (1984) Radiotherapy of soft tissue sarcoma with neutrons or a neutron boost. Br J Radiol 57:247–250
6. Slater JD, Marsha D, Peters LT (1986) Radiation therapy for unresectable soft tissue sarcomas. Int J Radiat Oncol Biol Phys 12:1729–1734

Future Directions of Proton Beam Radiotherapy for Bone and Soft Tissue Tumors

HIROHIKO TSUJII and HIROSHI TSUJI[1]

Introduction

Bone and soft tissue tumors frequently recur locally when treated with surgery alone. Therefore, in an effort to improve treatment outcome, combined surgery and radiotherapy has been advocated as an effective modality. However, with conventional radiation, these tumors can usually be given only a moderate dose of radiation with the result that most recur locally. In this regard, proton beam radiotherapy offers potential advantages with respect to dose distribution characterized by Bragg-peak formation, which allows precise delivery of high radiation doses to a tumor while avoiding irradiation to adjacent normal tissues [1, 2].

We discuss the rationale for the use of proton beam radiotherapy in bone and soft tissue tumors as well as the clinical experience at University of Tsukuba (Tsukuba, Japan).

The Role of Radiotherapy in Bone and Soft Tissue Tumors

Rationale for using radiotherapy. It is a widely accepted concept that the first choice of treatment for bone and soft tissue tumors is surgery. However, over the years there has been a major change in the management strategy from reliance on surgery alone to that of combined modality treatment [3–5]. The rationale behind this is to reduce the extent of surgery in order to improve the functional and cosmetic results at a comparable or higher local control rate. It has been reported that the local recurrence rate after simple excision is greater than 80% and about 30% after radical excision, but conservative excision followed by postoperative radiotherapy gave a local recurrence of about 25% with a more functional anatomy than after radical excision [6].

A number of investigators have indicated a benefit in high-dose radiotherapy for bone and soft tissue tumors. Some patients with a very radiosensitive tumor

---

[1] Proton Medical Research Center, University of Tsukuba, Tsukuba, Ibaragi, Japan

could be effectively treated with only radiotherapy. However, treatment with radiotherapy alone is usually reserved mainly for patients with recurrent or inoperable tumors. This is because bone and soft tissue tumors usually require high doses of radiation which may induce such unavoidable sequelae as subcutaneous fibrosis or delayed wound healing.

Tepper and Suit [5] reported the results of treatment with radiotherapy alone for 51 patients with soft tissue sarcoma. The overall 5-year survival and local control rates were 25.1% and 33%, respectively, and for patients treated to a dose of 6400 cGy or greater they were 28.4% and 43.5%, respectively. Slater et al. [6] reported on 72 patients with unresectable soft tissue sarcomas treated with photons alone or combined photons and neutrons. The 5-year tumor control rate was 29% and the malignancy grade was the only factor which significantly affected tumor control. No apparent improvement in tumor control was observed in patients receiving fast neutron therapy or combined modality treatment with chemotherapy. Greiner et al. [7] reported on 21 patients with unresectable retroperitoneal soft tissue sarcoma where the actuarial 5-year local tumor control rate was 60%, and the actuarial 5-year survival rate was 33%.

Timing of radiotherapy. Regarding the timing of radiotherapy relative to surgical excision, radiation can be given pre-, post- or intra-operatively. Suit et al. [3, 4] indicated that the major advantage of preoperative radiation was that the target area irradiated preoperatively could be made smaller than that irradiated postoperatively, resulting in higher radiation tolerance with a lower incidence of later sequelae. Although preoperative radiation reduces tumor volume before surgery and thus facilitates conservative excision, the disadvantage is that some patients will have delayed wound healing and a few will require skin grafting.

The advantage to surgery being carried out first is that an entire specimen can be made available to the pathologist for histopathological study. Therefore, for a small tumor clinically equivocal as being benign or malignant, it is advisable to begin by making a local excision.

Suit et al. [3] reported the results of 220 patients with M_0 soft tissue sarcoma of the extremities, torso, and head and neck region managed by radiation and resectional surgery. The local control rates were 85% for 131 patients treated with postoperative radiation and 90% for 89 patients treated with preoperative radiation (Table 1). Treatment by preoperative radiation appeared to have a major advantage for patients with a very large sarcoma, i.e., >15 cm in maximum dimension.

There has been an increased interest in the use of intraoperative radiation, but its potential applicability has not yet been well understood because only limited experience has been accumulated for this modality.

Proton Beam Radiotherapy

Characteristics of proton beams. The physical characteristics of proton beams which make them attractive in radiation therapy are finite ranges in tissue and

Table 1. Five-year results by treatment methods in soft tissue sarcoma (Massachusetts General Hospital) [3]

AJC Stage	Post-operative (n)	LC (%)	Pre-operative (n)	LC (%)
I				
A	12	100	3	100
B	17	100	8	70
II				
A	25	83	7	100
B	25	72	28	100
III				
A	25	95	6	83
B	26	68	35	83
IV				
A	1	100	2	100
Total	131	85%	89	90%

AJC, American Joint Committee; *LC*, local control

Table 2. Results of treatment with charged-particle radiotherapy for chordoma and chondrosarcoma at the base of the skull or cervical spine [2, 12]

Institution	Particle (RBE)	GyE Total	GyE Fraction size	Category	Patient No.	Five-year results Local control	Survival
Massachusetts General Hospital	Proton (1.1)	57–74	1.8–2.0 (5 × /W)	All	136	73%	88%
				Skull base	110	74%	
				Spine	26	61%	
Lawrence Berkeley Laboratory	He ion (1.2)	59–80	2.0–2.5 (4 × /W)	All	45	59%	62%
				<20 cc	26	80%	
				20–35 cc	6	33%	
				>35 cc	13	33%	

RBE, Relative biological effectiveness; *GyE*, cobalt Gy equivalent

sharply defined lateral beam edges. These features provide the basis for the proton dose distributions that are superior to those obtainable with photons in terms of tumor to normal tissue relationships. The relative biological effectiveness (RBE) of protons is similar to or about 10% higher than ^{60}Co. This feature makes them easy for clinical use because almost the entire accumulated radiobiological data for conventional irradiation can be used in proton radiotherapy.

Clinical indications for proton beam radiotherapy. Chordoma and chondrosarcoma are uncommon, locally aggressive tumors which have a similar biological behavior when occurring at the base of the skull. With conventional radiation techniques, the local recurrence rate is 64%, and the local control rate at 5 years is 35% [8–10]. Surgery is often incomplete because of the close proximity of the tumor to critical structures. It was felt, therefore, that the superior dose-localizing properties of protons or helium ions would be advantageous in treating these lesions. They are effectively treated with protons at the Massachusetts General Hospital-Harvard Cyclotron Laboratory and with helium ions at the Lawrence Berkeley Laboratory (Table 2).

According to Austin-Seymour et al. [2], surgical resection combined with high-dose proton radiation therapy represented the current best management for chordoma or low-grade chondrosarcoma at the base of the skull. Proton beams were used to treat 88 patients with these tumors, with the median tumor dose of 69 CGE (cobalt Gy equivalent). Protons allowed the delivery of high doses of radiation to the residual tumors following initial surgical removal, resulting in a 5-year actuarial control rate of 82% and a disease-free survival rate of 76%. These figures are significantly superior to the 5-year local control rate of less than 35% by conventional irradiation [8].

Similar results were also obtained with helium ion beam [12]. Definitive helium therapy following subtotal resection of chordoma and chondrosarcoma led to very favorable results with acceptable complications. The actuarial survival and local control rates at 5 years were 62% and 53%, respectively. Heavier ions, however, did not provide favorable results. It was initially felt that potential biological advantages of neon ions (similar to that of neutrons) would be useful in the treatment of these slow-growing tumors, but due to the high RBE for central nervous system damage, use of this ion was discontinued [13].

Results from the Massachussetts General Hospital of treatment with proton beam radiotherapy for 66 patients with soft tissue sarcoma have been reported [11]. The overall control rate was 85.7% (54/63), and the best result was observed in paraspinal tumors: the local control rate was 93.3% (14/15). The patients were irradiated with a mean proton dose of 66 Gy, and no radiation myelopathy had been observed after the treatment.

From the data available in the literature, it appears that the most important factor in obtaining long-term local control for retroperitoneal soft tissue sarcoma is the ability to perform a complete surgical resection. However, most retroperitoneal tumors are located adjacent to critical organs, hence a complete resection is often difficult and high-dose radiation with conventional irradiation can be performed only in a minority of patients. In light of such difficulties, favorable dose distribution with charged particles should yield good results in this type of tumor [7].

Proton beam radiotherapy at our institution. The clinical study of cancer treatment using 500 MeV proton beams produced by the booster synchrotron of the National Laboratory for High Energy Physics was initiated in 1983 at Tsukuba University [14]. The primary energy for use in cancer treatment is degraded to 250 MeV by passing the beams through a graphite absorber. The maximum range of protons thus obtained is 36.7 cm in water. For generating a spread-out Bragg peak (SOBP), an aluminum ridge filter or range-modulator made of an acryl plate 5 mm in thickness is used. The oil-bath degrader is also used for modulating the depth of beam penetration.

Thus far, 147 patients received partial or full treatment with definitive proton therapy; 92 patients (63%) were treated with proton beams alone, and 55 patients (37%) with combined proton and photon beams. Satisfactory results have been achieved in tumors of the lung, esophagus, liver, uterine cervix, bladder, prostate, as well as in the skin and head and neck areas. These accomplishments have stimulated us to design a dedicated proton therapy facility.

We have only limited experience for the treatment of muskculo-skeletal diseases. This includes treatment of one patient with chordoma at the clivus and one patient with giant cell tumor of the tibia, both with satisfactory results. We suggest that proton therapy should be considered as a valuable method when used alone or combined with conservative resection.

Conclusions

Proton beams possess a physical characteristic allowing the delivery of high doses of radiation to deep-seated lesions while giving lesser doses to the surrounding healthy tissues. In the conservative therapy of bone and soft tissue tumors, this favorable feature of proton beams should be useful in reducing the extent of surgery in order to improve the functional and cosmetic results at comparable or higher local control rates. Among various type of tumors, chordoma and chondrosarcoma at the base of the skull or cervical spine have been treated most effectively with proton beams. Other types of muskulo-skeletal tumors, however, have been rarely treated with protons, but accumulated data strongly indicate that a conservative surgical resection combined with high-dose proton radiation therapy may represent the best management currently available for these tumors. Further clinical study to confirm this is warranted.

References

1. Munzenrider JE (1987) Clinical results of proton beam radiotherapy in Boston. In: Proc of 8th ICRR (vol 2). Taylor and Francis, New York, pp 916–922
2. Austin-Seymour M, Munzenrider JE, Goitein M (1989) Fractionated proton radiation therapy of chordoma and low-grade chondrosarcoma of the base of the skull. J Neurosurg 70:13–17
3. Suit HD, Mankin HJ, Wood WC (1988) Treatment of the patient with Stage M0 soft tissue sarcoma. J Clin Oncol 6:854–862
4. Suit HD (1982) Soft tissue sarcomas: The role of radiation therapy. Hospital Practice, July, pp 114–120
5. Tepper JE, Suit HD (1985) Radiation therapy alone for sarcoma of soft tissue. Cancer 56:457–479
6. Slater JD, McNeese MD, Peters LJ (1986) Radiation therapy for unresectable soft tissue sarcoma. Int J Radiat Oncol Biol Phys 12:1729–1734
7. Greiner RH, Blattmann H, Thum P (1989) Dynamic pion irradiation of unresectable soft tissue sarcoma. Int J Radiat Oncol Biol Phys 17:1077–1083

8. Cummings BJ, Hodson DI, Bush RS (1983) Chordoma: The results of megavoltage radiation therapy. Int Radiat Oncol Biol Phys 9:633–642

9. Heffelfinger MJ, Dahlin DC, MacCarty CS, Beabout JW (1973) Chordomas and cartilaginous tumors at the skull base. Cancer 32:410–420

10. Higinbotham NL, Phillips RF, Farr HW, Hustu HO (1967) Chordoma. Cancer 20:1841–1850

11. Austin-Seymour M, Urie M, Munzenrider JE, Willett C (1989) Consideration in fractionated proton radiation therapy: Clinical potential and results. Radiother Oncol 70:13–17

12. Berson AM, Castro JR, Petti P (1988) Charged particle irradiation of chordoma and chondrosarcoma of the base of skull and cervical spine: Lawrence Berkeley Laboratory Experience. Int J Radiat Oncol Biol Phys 15:559–565

13. Linstadt D, Castro JR, Phillips TL (to be published) Neon ion radiotherapy: Results of the phase I–II clinical trials. Int J Radiat Oncol Biol Phys

14. Tsujii H (1989) Clinical results of high energy proton radiotherapy at Tsukuba. In: Proc of Int Heavy Particle Therapy Workshop, pp 90–94

3.3

Treatment of Malignant Bone Tumors Using Radioisotopes

Rikushi Morita[1]

Introduction

Metastatic spread to the bone occurs in a variety of tumors. Basically, any malignant tumor may metastasize to bone and the lesions may cause osteolytic or osteoblastic destruction.

In most patients, bone metastases cause such intense pain that the ultimate use of morphine and its derivatives can not be avoided. At this stage, chemotherapy and hormonal management are usually not effective, and the use of external radiation is limited in number and sites of treatments.

Although the radionuclide is the last possible treatment mode for bone metastasis, the presently existing treatments only have a limiting palliative effect on bone pain without effecting any prolongation of survival.

Therapeutic Use of Radioisotopes

The effect of therapeutic radiation on a malignant lesion depends on two factors: (1) the radiation dose to which the tumor is exposed and (2) the radiation sensitivity of the tumor. Therefore, the techniques for delivering adequate amounts of radioisotopes specifically to the tumor and avoiding normal tissue are the most important objectives in radioisotope treatment.

^{131}I treatment for thyroid carcinoma and ^{131}I-MIBG (Metaiodobenzyl-guanidine) for malignant pheochromocytoma and neuroblastoma are the specific treatments aiming at tumor regression of the particular tumor, whereas other treatments using several bone-seeking agents, such as ^{32}P, ^{89}Sr, ^{186}Re, ^{153}Sm, and ^{90}Y, are being used as palliative measures for bone pain relief.

^{131}I Treatment for Bone Metastasis from Thyroid Carcinoma

Well differentiated thyroid carcinomas most commonly metastasize to the lung and bone, and ^{131}I has been used for the treatment of these distant matastasis

[1] Department of Radiology, Shiga University of Medical Science, Otsu, Japan

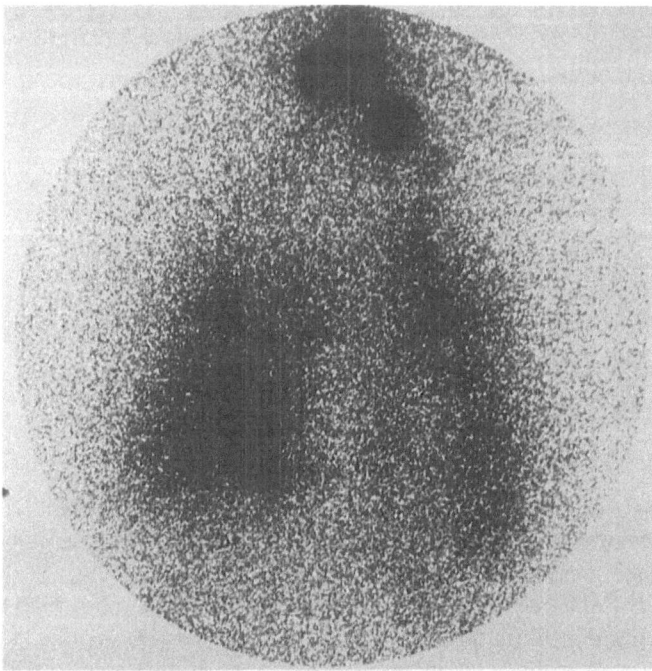

Fig. 1. Scintigram of the lung fields at 7 days after administration of 1.8 GBq of ^{131}I in a patient with lung metastasis (25% reduction)

for more than 30 years. Increased survival and decreased tumor recurrence are now well known to occur in patients who have received ^{131}I treatment after total thyroidectomy [1].

The efficacy of ^{131}I-therapy is directly related to success in increasing the uptake of ^{131}I by the metastatic lesions and prolonging its retention in the tumors. Although the uptake of ^{131}I by the thyroid carcinoma was originally poor compared to normal thyroid tissue, ^{131}I uptake is enhanced in 50%–80% of adenocarcinoma of the thyroid under appropriate procedures. [131]I therapy will deliver a tumor dose of about 5 times the absorbed dose that can be achieved by external radiation.

Benua et al. [2] reported significant remission in 16 cases and temporary remission in 11 cases of 48 ^{131}I-treated patients with metastases to lungs and bones. Varma et al. [3] reported a significant increase in survival in patients older than 40 years after ^{131}I treatment. Brown et al. [4] stated that 54% of patients with lung metastases were alive and free of disease for 10 years after ^{131}I treatment, whereas no patient with bone matastasis was alive at 10 years after the treatment.

Figure 1 shows a scintigram obtained at 7 days after the administration of 1.8 GBq of ^{131}I to a 35 year-old female with lung metastasis from thyroid carcinoma whose chest X-ray film showed dense snowflake-like metastasis over

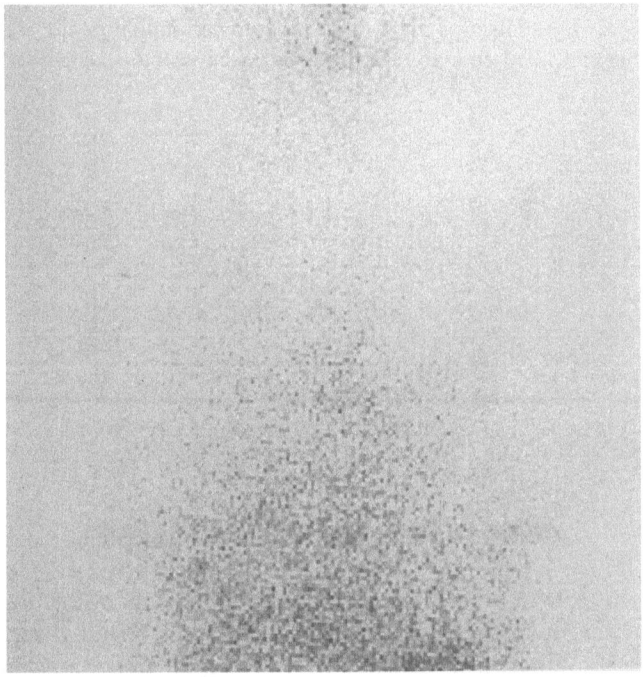

Fig. 2. Scintigram of the lung fields in the same patient as Fig. 1, after the 3rd ^{131}I therapy (25% reduction)

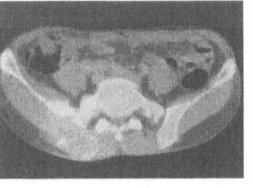 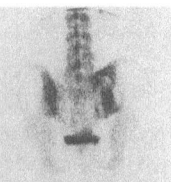

Fig. 3. CT scan and scintigram in a patient with a pulsative mass in the right buttock (50% reduction)

both lung fields. Remarkable amounts of ^{131}I are distributed over both the lungs and thyroid bed after total thyroidectomy. After the 3rd ^{131}I therapy, lung metastases were seen to completely disapper on both the ^{131}I scintigram (Fig. 2) and chest X-ray film.

Figure 3 shows the CT scan and scintigram of the pelvis of a 45-year-old male who noted a pulsative mass in the right buttock. Destruction of the right ilium and sacrum is evident on CT and an irregular uptake of ^{99m}Tc-MDP by that area is on evident the bone scintigram. Since the biopsy revealed differentiated carcinoma, a dose of 3.7 GBq of ^{131}I was given after total thyroidectomy. On the whole body scintigram (Fig. 4), a markedly increased accumulation of ^{131}I was observed in the areas of the thyroid bed and the metastatic lesion in the pelvis. Two additional ^{131}I treatments were performed on this patient during the following 2 years and his condition is now being monitored.

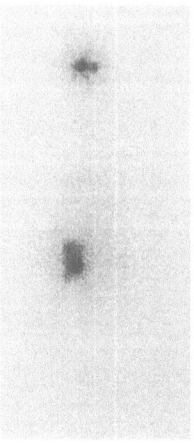

Fig. 4. Whole body scintigram of the same patient as in Fig. 3, showing a markedly increased accumulation of ^{131}I in the thyroid bed area and a metastatic lesion in the pelvis (50% reduction)

Control of Pain from Bone Metastasis

Control of pain from bone metastasis and maintenance of a functional status is an important task in the management of patients with terminal carcinoma. At these stages, chemotherapy is usually ineffective even after the primary lesions are controlled, external radiation is limited to focal areas, and dose is limited as well.

Several kinds of radioisotopes, especially bone-seeking radiopharmaceuticals, such as ^{32}P, ^{89}Sr, ^{186}Re, ^{153}Sm, and ^{90}Y, have been used for pain relief from extensive bone metastasis.

Radioactive Phosphorus (^{32}P)

The use of ^{32}P for pain relief from bone metastasis dates back to the early 1950s [5, 6]. ^{32}P emits a moderatly penetrating β particle (1.79 MeV), with no associated γ emission and has a half-life of 14.3 days. Since ^{32}P-diphosphonate (EHDP) and ^{32}P-polymetaphosphate are physiologically and avidly concentrated into the site of new bone formation, any metastasis that evokes an osteoblastic response, as indicated by bone scan, would be suitable for the treatment.

Generally, 2 mCi (74 MBq) of ^{32}P is administered intravenously every 4 days for a total of 12 mCi (888 MBq) or until hemopoietic depression emerges. Pain relief is effective in about 50% of the patients. The relief usually begins after several doses and persists for several months to a year. Survival, however, is not prolonged, probably due to the other visceral metastases which are not affected by this therapy.

As for the side effects, myelosuppression is inevitable and thrombocytopenia is a real risk factor.

Strontium 89 ^{89}Sr

Strontium 89 is a pure β emitter (1.46 MeV) and has a half-life of 50.4 days. ^{89}Sr is incorporated into the hydroxyapatite of the newly formed bone by a mechanism similar to that of calcium. For pain relief, ^{89}Sr has proved to be as effective as ^{32}P with less consequent marrow suppression than ^{32}P because of its longer half-life and decreased dose rate requirements.

Generally, 2.0 MBq/kg of ^{89}Sr is administered intravenously and treatment is repeated with an interval of 3–4 months if necessary. ^{89}Sr has definite objective effects on bone metastasis. Pain relief is effective in 50%–90% of the patients and the relief persists for weeks to months [7].

Bone scinitigraphy shows progressive decrease in ^{99m}Tc-MDP uptake by the metastatic lesions, and X-ray film of these sites shows resolution of the lytic defect and abundant sclerosis [8]. The treatment is not effective for any osteolytic lesion which is not accompanied by reactive new bone formation nor in prevention of developement of new metastasis where ^{89}Sr uptake is absent at the time of the therapy. As for side effects, myelosuppression is limited to a transient fall of platelet counts unaccompanied by hemorrhagic complications.

Conclusions

Treatment with ^{131}I for thyroid carcinoma is specifically aimed at tumor regression. For palliation of severe bone pain, ^{89}Sr is effective in more than 50% of the patients, with the effect persisting for weeks to months from a single intravenous dose. Side effects are minimum and transient, and the treatment can be performed on an outpatient basis, because ^{89}Sr is a pure β emitter and the total body retention exceeds 80% of the dose. Palliation treatment by radioisotope is effective, easily performed, and reasonably safe. With the availability of newer radioisotopes, radioisotope treatment is expected to open new horizons for treatment of bone metastasis.

References

1. Beierwaltes, WH (1987) Radioiodine therapy of thyroid diseases. Nucl Med Biol 14:177–181
2. Bennua RS, Cicale NR, Sonenberg M (1962) The relation of radioiodine dosimetry to result and complications in the treatment of metastatic thyroid cancer. Am J Roentogenol 87:171–182
3. Varma VM, Beierwaltes WH, Nofal MM (1970) Treatment of thyoid cancer: Death rates after surgery and after surgery followed by sodium iodides I-131. JAMA 214:1437–1442
4. Brown AP, Greening WP, McCready VR (1984) Radioiodine treatment of metastatic thyroid carcinoma: The Royal Marsden Hospital experience. Br J Radiol 57:323–327
5. Storaasli JP, Krieger H (1961) Palliations of osseous metastases from breast carcinoma with radioactive phosphorus alone and in combination with adrenalectomy. Radiology 76:422–429

6. Maxfield JR, Maxfield JG, Maxfield WS (1958) Use of radioactive phosphorus and testosterone in metastatic bone lesions from breast and prostate. South Med J 51:320–328
7. Silberstein EB, Williams C (1985) Strontium-89 therapy for the pain of osseous metastases. J Nucl Med 26:345–348
8. Kloiber R, Molnar CP, Barnes M (1987) Sr-89 therapy for metastatic bone disease: Scintigraphic and radiographic follow up. Radiology 163:719–723

Part 4

Surgical Treatment

<u>**4.1**</u>

Optimal Design in Tumor Prostheses: Application of Extracortical Bone Bridging and Ingrowth Fixation Principle

EDMUND Y.S. CHAO[1]

Introduction

The utilization of custom-designed segmental bone and joint replacement prostheses in tumor surgery has been a viable option for quite some time [1–4]. However, the clinical results and prosthetic device performance still require improvements, especially in active patients with greater functional demands. The associated poor clinical results were mainly due to implant failure through fracture, loosening, dislocation, and infection. For conditions of massive bone defect, relatively smooth and straight cortex, and large bending torsional loads, traditional methods of implant fixation face a grim outlook in this class of bone and joint replacement. The lack of normal soft tissue coverage and constraint make the joint less stable, which contributes to poor functional results and increases the propensity of stem loosening. Other problems associated with custom prosthetic replacement include the lack of interchangeability, limited availability of the implant components at the time of surgery, improper size and dimension, length of time required for implant fabrication, and high cost.

Some of these problems can be managed by using a modular system for both hip and knee reconstruction with interchangeable prosthetic components together with cement fixation [5]. However, a new "*composite*" fixation principle employing initial cement fixation of intramedullary stems and extracortical bone bridging and ingrowth over the porous prosthetic segment may provide substantial improvements on both short- and long-term implant fixation to bone [6, 7]. This biological "*composite*" fixation concept is defined as "*extracortical bone bridging and ingrowth*" (EBBI) fixation (Fig. 1). The bone formation over the prosthesis is to be accomplished by applying autogenous iliac grafts. The hypothetical advantages of composite fixation are: (1) cement

[1] Biomechanics Laboratory/Department of Orthopedics, Mayo Clinic/Mayo Foundation, Rochester, MN 55905, USA

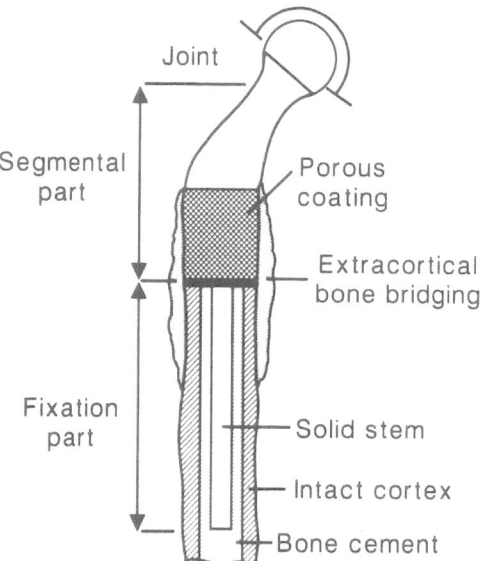

Joint

Segmental
part

Porous
coating

Extracortical
bone bridging

Fixation
part

Solid stem

Intact cortex

Bone cement

Fig. 1. The schematic diagram of a proximal femur segmental bone and hip joint replacement prosthesis utilizing the new composite fixation concept through extracortical bone bridging and ingrowth

provides secure initial fixation for enhancing bone graft incorporation, (2) a solid stem without a porous coating increases its fatigue strength, (3) extracortical bone bridging can provide more effective load transfer from the implant to the remaining bone cortex without relying solely on intramedullary fixation, (4) fewer stem sizes are required to facilitate the design of a modular system, and (5) it allows easier revision when component removal or replacement is deemed necessary. In many revision cases involving the hip and knee in association with a segmental bone defect, this type of implant system and its fixation concept can be readily applied with surprisingly good results.

Different experimental and animal studies were conducted to validate and improve the modular prosthesis system and its composite fixation concept through the process of EBBI. Furthermore, a well-controlled and carefully followed clinical series utilizing such an implant design and fixation principle has been established over the past 14 years not only in order to document successful results, but also to identify potential problems and technical difficulties. This paper will attempt to summarize the fundamental background knowledge related to the composite fixation concept and the associated implant design principles. Finally, both the clinical and basic science factors related to the EBBI principles will be outlined to aid future implant design improvements and clinical applications.

Design of the Prosthesis

Two porous-coated segmental bone/joint replacement prosthetic systems are being developed utilizing the present composite implant fixation concept. One system is based upon a Co-Cr-Mo cast material with a beaded porous sur-

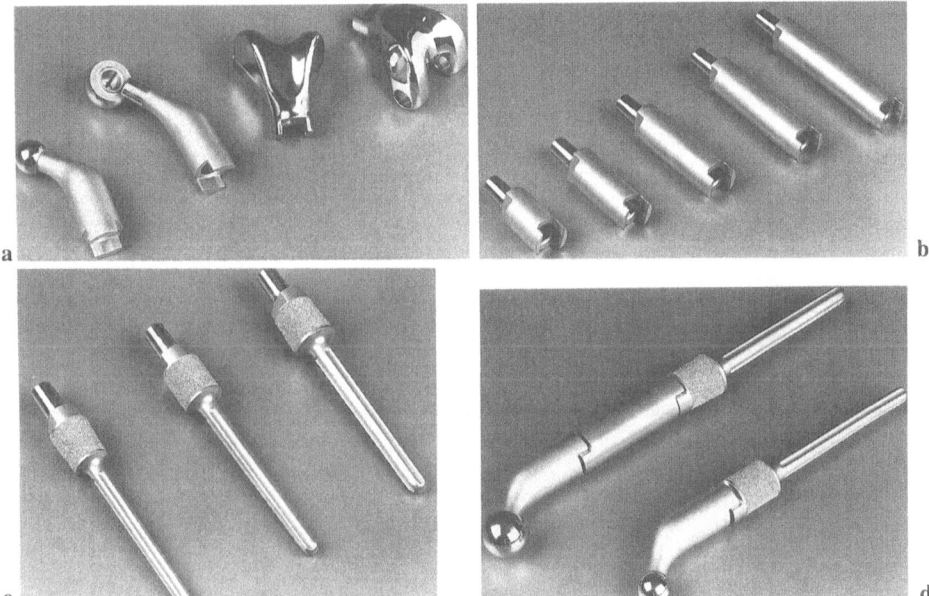

Fig. 2a–d. The Co-Cr-Mo modular segmental bone/joint replacement prosthesis system currently marketed by Howmedica (Rutherford, N.J.). **a** The modular joint components for proximal and distal femur. **b** The stem component with different diameters and lengths. **c** The modular segmental components with the square interference wedge to prevent component rotation. **d** The assembled implant for proximal femur replacement. Note that the porous coating is applied only on the stem component at the shoulder region

face, currently manufactured and marketed by Howmedica Inc. (Rutherford, N.J., USA) (Fig. 2). The other system employs Ti-6Al-4V alloy with pure Ti fibermetal porous coating, manufactured by Zimmer (Warsaw, Ind., USA) (Fig. 3). The general configurations of these systems are similar, but each has specific design features to accommodate the implant material used. The basic prosthetic structure consists of the joint component, the stem component, and segmental components interconnected by conical coupling joints (Morse taper). Both systems contain porous coating at the effective region (prosthetic shoulder of the segmental portion of the prosthesis) to enhance extracortical bone bridging and ingrowth, while the intramedullary stems are solid either for press-fit or for cement fixation. The Ti system relies on offset locking screws and interlocking keyways to prevent possible rotation and distraction of the conical coupling joint. The Co-Cr-Mo system has a wedge-shaped interference coupling outside of the Morse taper to resist component relative rotation. The basic dimensions and incremental lengths of these implant systems were based on the existing anatomical, clinical, and pathological data [8].

The strength of the conical coupling was examined both statically and under cyclic load using experimental models. Compressive, torsional, and four-point

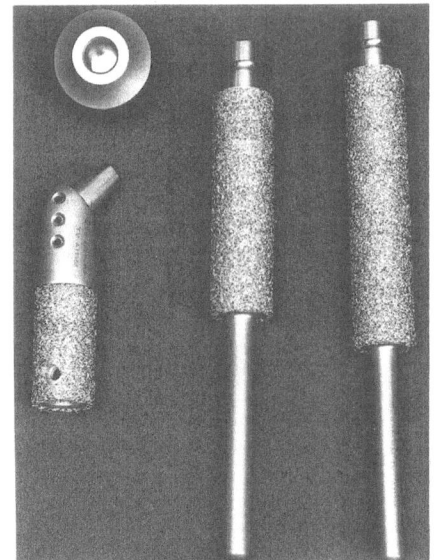

a

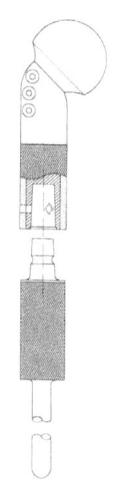

b

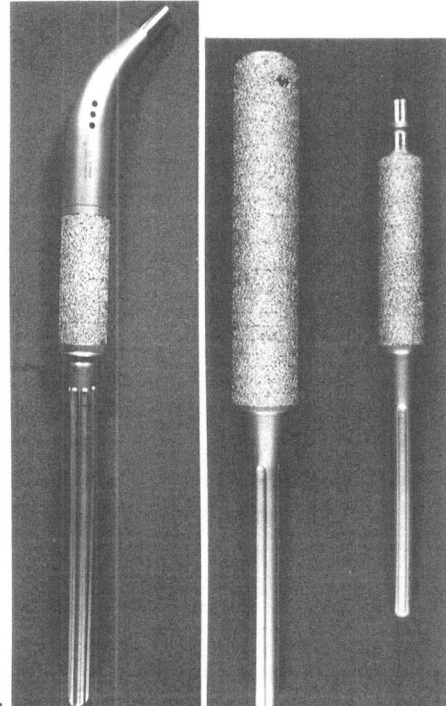

c   d

Fig. 3a–d. The Ti-6Al-4V modular segmental bone/joint replacement prosthetic system for proximal femur and segmental bone replacement (including knee fusion), a product of Zimmer (Warsaw, Ind.). **a** Modular system for proximal humerus replacement with soft tissue attachment holes. **b** Schematic diagram of the proximal humerus prosthesis. **c** Proximal femur replacement prosthesis with modular head and neck composition. **d** Stem components with option for diaphyseal bone segment replacement or joint arthrodesis. Note that the fibermetal coating covers both the prosthetic shoulder section and the conical coupling (Morse taper) section

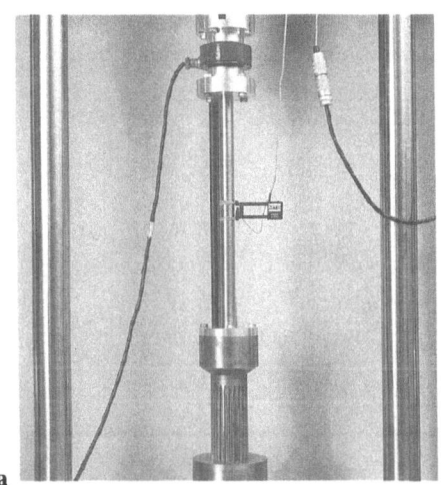
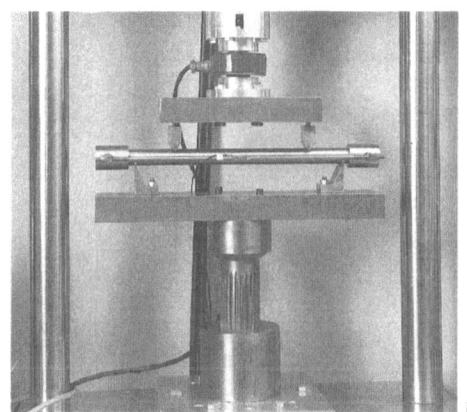

Fig. 4a–b. Experimental models used to test the effect of cone angle, implant material and loading type on conical coupling joint strength. **a** Axial compression and torsion. **b** 4-point bending

bending loads were applied under a known axial preload (Fig. 4). In the static compression and torsion test, decreasing the cone angle increased fixation strength, and titanium provided stronger fixation than that of stainless steel. The joint distraction increased under repetitive compressive loading. Under a cyclic bending load in one direction, the joint initially decreased its distraction force, but as the number of cycles increased, the locking strength of the conical coupling joint recovered. These results suggest that the conical coupling joint alone may not be sufficient to prevent joint rotation, especially when the implant is subjected to distraction and bending in reversed directions. Hence, additional features to resist distraction and rotation were adopted in the present modular implant system design.

Finite element analysis was used to study the high stress distribution in the conical coupling joint. Under axial compression and bending, peak stresses were found at the tip and base of the cone, and around the rim and the base corner of the conical sleeve. These stresses increased exponentially with reduction of the cone angle. Higher stresses occurred under bending. Significant reduction of prosthetic stress was found when tissue bridging across the conical coupling joint occurred (Table 1). The amount of stress reduction was dependent upon the type of bridging tissue. Therefore, when porous coating is available around the conical coupling joint, and bone bridging and ingrowth across the joint becomes complete, distraction or rotation of the coupling joint can be effectively prevented and high implant stress can also be reduced to avoid long-term abrasive wear and fatigue failure.

An additional axisymmetric finite element model was developed to study stress distribution in the implant/cement/bone composite system adjacent to

Table 1. Effect of tissue bridging on conical coupling joint equivalent stress distribution at the critical zones. (Note the location of the critical stress zones defined in the *right diagram*)

Loading mode	Critical zone	Equivalent stress (N/cm²)		
		No tissue bridging	Fibrous bridging	Bony bridging
Axial compression	1	1.05	0.11	0.07
(1 Newton)	2	5.77	1.29	0.18
	3	5.84	1.33	0.30
	4	4.92	1.14	0.33
	5	2.82	0.95	0.31
Bending moment	1	2.18	1.96	1.11
(1 Newton/cm)	2	0.42	0.39	0.26
	3	1.24	1.08	0.55
	4	0.44	0.43	0.36
	5	0.70	0.65	0.40

the prosthetic shoulder region. Extracortical tissue formation was also included in the model with different mechanical properties to simulate either fibrous tissue or bone. It was found that under axial compression, extracortical bone bridging and ingrowth provided significant reduction of stem and cement stress when compared to a no-tissue-bridging condition. If the bridging tissues were fibrous, the stress reduction became less effective. Under bending or torsional load, the reduction of stem and cement stresses became even more significant for both osseous and fibrous tissue bridging (Fig. 5). Although the stresses in the original bone cortex remained unchanged, the newly formed extracortical bone picked up substantial stress which reflected the stress-sharing role of the extracortical bone formation over the prosthetic shoulder region. The current model assumes rigid bonding between bone and cement. When micromovement occurred at such an interface, load transfer from the implant to the bone cortex bypassing the stem and cement was found to be even more effective. This phenomenon represents the fundamental advantage of extracortical bone bridging and ingrowth fixation of the modular porous-coated revision prostheses for the hip and knee.

Biologic Process of Extracortical Formation

A time-sequenced study was designed to elucidate the basic biological processes involved in extracortical bone formation [9]. A 60-mm segment of the femoral diaphysis was resected and replaced by a Ti porous-coated prosthesis in 32 adult mixed-breed dogs. The resected diaphysis and iliac grafts were morselized, mixed with autogenous marrow, and applied around the prosthesis and the opposing cortex. Serial fluorochrome labeling was used to identify newly formed bone. Eight dogs each were euthanized at 2, 4, 8, and 12 weeks. Tissue samples from the extracortical bone were analyzed by light microscopy and transmission electron microscopy (TEM).

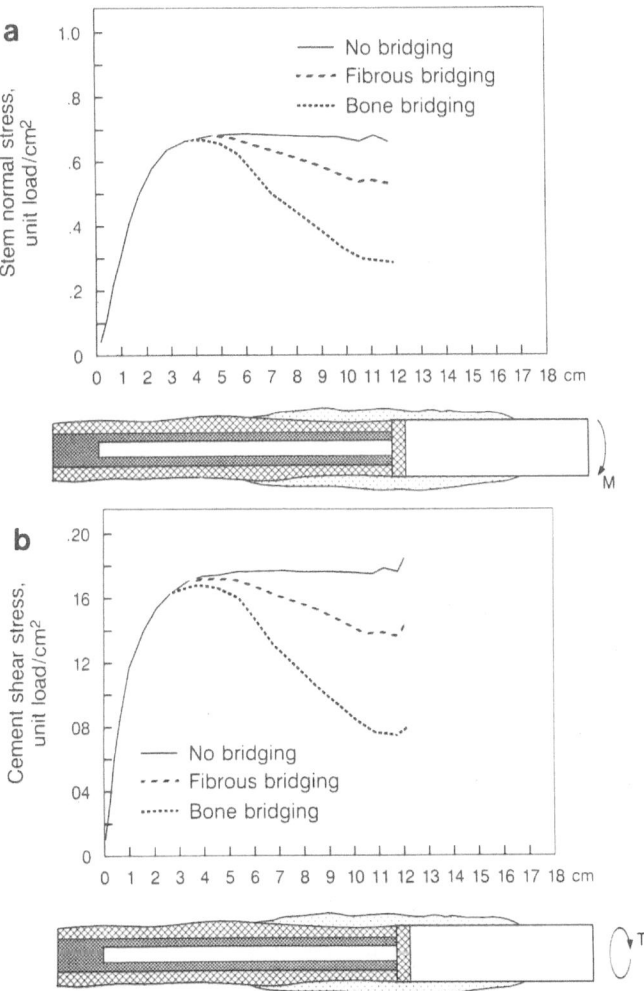

Fig. 5a–b. Effect of tissue bridging extracortically on **a** stem normal stress under unit bending moment, M, **b** cement shear stress under unit torsion, T

At 2 weeks after surgery, cortical and cancellous bone grafts were scattered within a fibrous tissue bed. At this time, there was active bone turnover and new bone formation in and around the graft. Foci of hyaline cartilage were concurrently formed within the fibrous tissue matrix (Fig. 6). Hypertrophic chondrocytes and mineralization of the intercellular matrices were also noted. At 4 weeks, all grafted spongiosa were replaced by newly formed bone through the intramembranous ossification process (Fig. 7). At 8 weeks, hypertrophied and degenerated chondrocytes as well as matrix mineralization were seen between cartilage and bone. At 8 and 12 weeks, new compact bone was gradually established in the outer area of the callus.

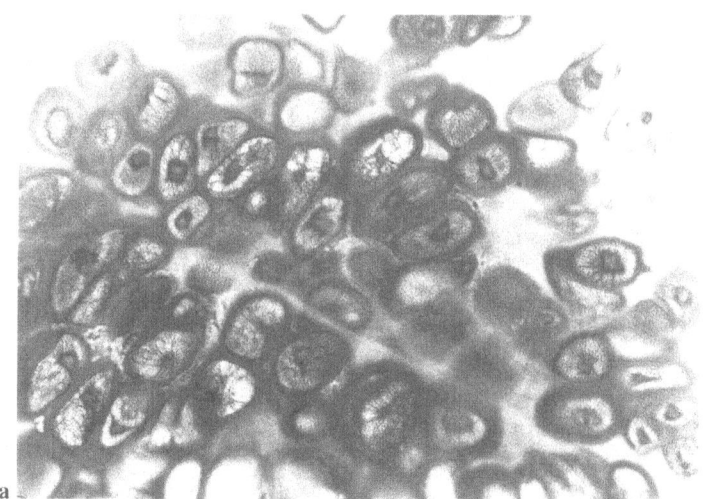

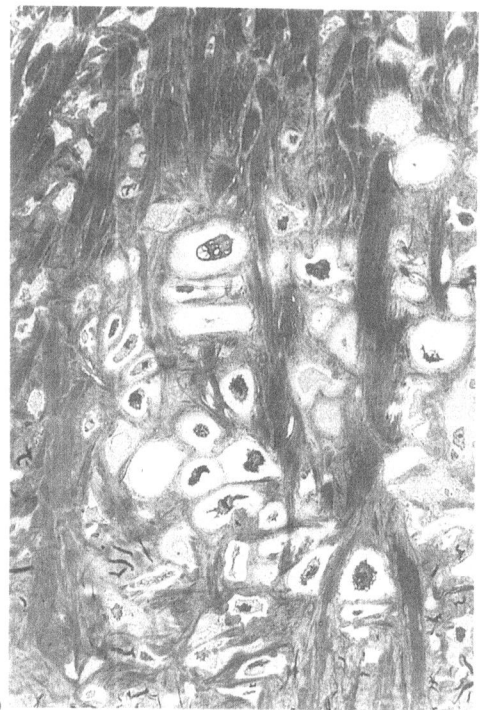

Fig. 6a–b. Foci of hyaline cartilage with hypertrophic and atrophic chondrocytes reflecting the early stage of the endochondral ossification process. **a** Hypertrophic chondrocytes. **b** Atrophic chondrocytes with interlaced fibrous tissue and mineralized tissue

Active appositional bone formation occurred early after graft application and continued through the 12-week period. Parts of the cortical and cancellous grafts were resorbed while forming exuberant callus surrounding the implant shoulder region. The remaining graft survived, but was remodeled in such a

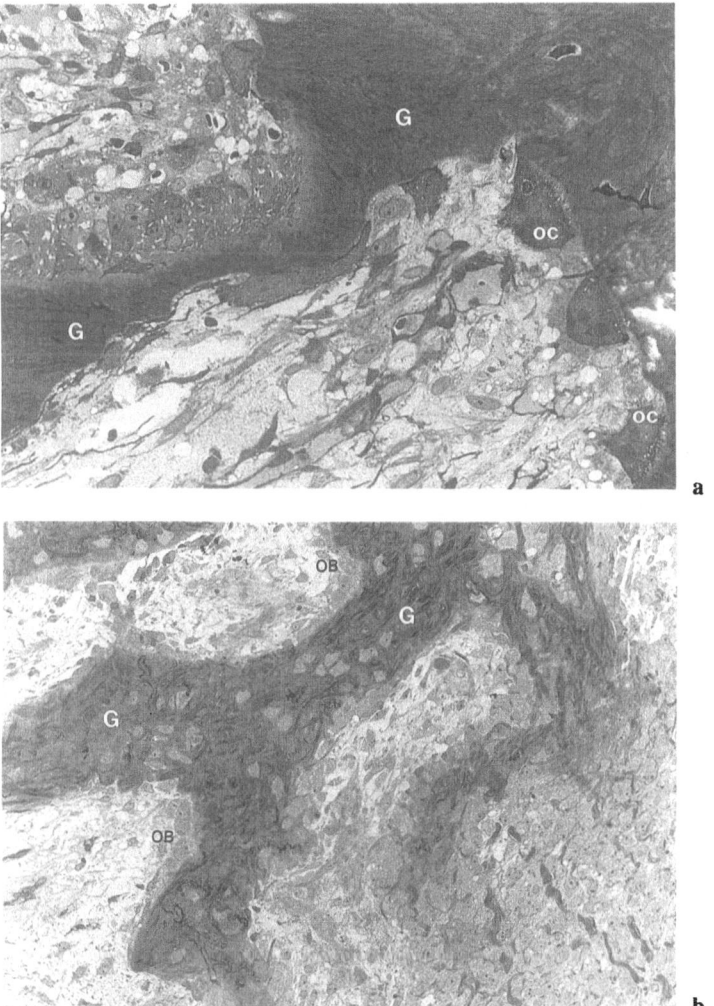

Fig. 7a–b. Bone resorption and new bone formation adjacent to surviving autogenous bone graft through an intramembranous ossification process. **a** Bone resorptive surface on surviving graft (*G*) with active osteoclasts (*OC*). **b** New bone formation adjacent to surviving graft (*G*) laced with osteoblasts (*OB*)

way that the grafts could no longer be identified in the newly formed bone. At 4 weeks, woven bone formation occurred within the matured callus through endochondral ossification. As the callus became reduced in size, woven bone began to fuse with remodeled bone grafts. A cortical shell formed in the outer area of the callus to complete the extracortical bone bridging and ingrowth process. The overall biological mechanisms involved in this biological reaction can be summarized in a simplified flow diagram (Fig. 8).

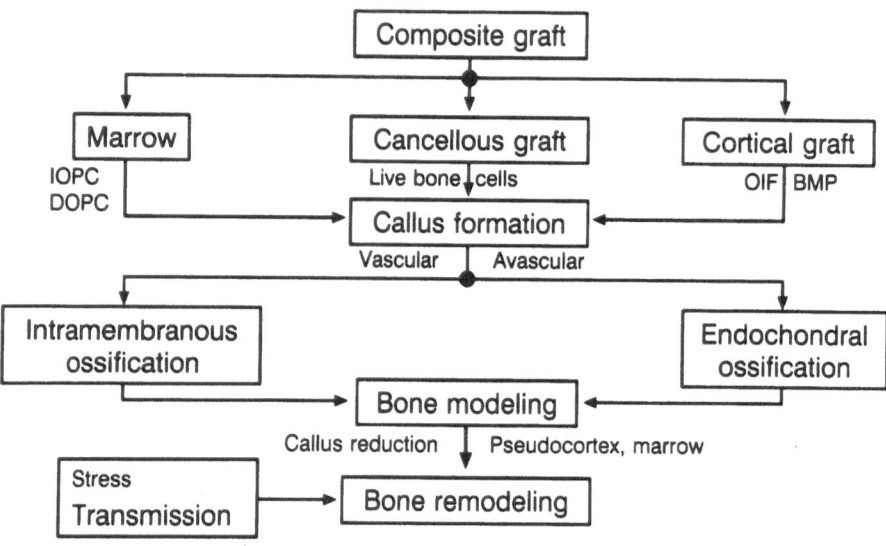

Fig. 8. Flow diagram illustrating the biologic mechanism involved in the *"extracortical bone bridging and ingrowth"* (EBBI) fixation process. *OIF*, Osteoinductive factors; *BMP*, bone morphogenic protein; *IOPC*, inducible osteogenic precursor cells; *DOPC*, determined osteogenic precursor cells

Other Factors Affecting Bone Formation

The effects of immobilization and animal age on bone bridging and ingrowth over the segmental bone replacement prosthesis were investigated using a similar animal model [10, 11]. Initial immobilization was found to have a significant effect on organized fibrous tissue and bone ingrowth in the porous layer. Such tissues appeared to provide strong support against interface shear load. Therefore, in the early stages of prosthetic incorporation, immobilization of the affected limb and implant enhance bone and organized fibrous tissue ingrowth. The quality of implant stability appears to be more important than age in enhancing bony incorporation of the prosthesis. The conical coupling joint provided adequate fixation strength which was further reinforced by biological tissue bridging the joint line. The quality of extracortical bone bridging was found to be independent of the type of porous coating [12]. Radiographically, maximum extracortical bone formation occurred 2–4 weeks after grafting in the canine model and gradually decreasing thereafter, but with an increase in callus density, reflecting an active remodeling process.

The efficacy of demineralized allogenic bone matrix (DABM) in achieving extracortical bone bridging and ingrowth was investigated in 12 adult mongrel dogs using the same porous canine segmental bone replacement prosthesis [13]. Autogenous cortical grafts alone, without marrow, were also studied in the same model. There was slightly more bone formation on the cortical graft side, but both groups had significantly less bone formation compared to that achieved previously with autogenous corticocancellous graft and marrow. The cortical graft was resorbed with little or no new bone formation. However, both sides had a higher prosthetic failure torque at the bone/implant junction than that produced in the control specimens ($P < 0.05$). This was mainly due to the ingrowth of well-organized fibrous tissue.

The effects of therapeutic radiation on the incorporation of autogenous bone grafts over the porous segment of the prosthesis in order to achieve extra-cortical bone bridging and ingrowth was investigated [14]. Parallel opposed beams were used to compensate the effects of backscatter due to the presence of the metallic implant. The results showed that bone adjacent to the prosthesis involved necrotic changes due to the simulated therapeutic radiation. Extra-cortical bone formation and ingrowth was significantly inhibited by radiation.

Discussion

As in routine joint replacement, implant fixation will dictate the long-term success of segmental bone/joint replacement prosthesis in cases where massive bone defect is involved. However, such application faces three additional challenges. First, the implants are longer and larger, tending to increase the load transmitted to the bone. Second, the intramedullary stems are situated in the straight diaphyseal portion of the long bone, making cement fixation less desirable. Finally, extensive resection of soft tissue or the presence of scar tissue from multiple operative procedures can affect the stability and functional control of the joint. These potential problems are responsible for poor functional results and implant longevity after revision surgery.

It is generally accepted that cement fixation of prosthetic components can achieve long-term success if cement interdigitation with cancellous bone can be achieved. Unfortunately, the diaphyseal segment of the femur, humerus, and tibia contains a relatively straight and smooth intramedullary canal, which cannot provide the optimal interface condition for secured cement fixation. Therefore, the current concept of composite biological fixation appears to be ideal, since bone cement is expected to achieve only the initial phase of implant stability until extracortical bone bridging and ingrowth is successfully accomplished. Such a fixation method and implant design is expected to change the outlook of major revision surgery. The surprisingly good clinical and functional results achieved in the limb-salvage operation involving musculoskeletal neoplasm using this type of prosthesis further supports this new fixation principle [15, 16].

The lack of soft tissue constraint and direct attachment to the segmental implant are the main drawbacks in this type of reconstruction. However, the same principles can be utilized to obtain soft tissue incorporation directly to the prosthesis. This biological "composite" implant fixation concept, when fully established, may well be the ideal solution for limb-salvage procedures after musculoskeletal tumor resection, or in revision surgery after failed joint replacement prosthesis with major bone defect (Fig. 9). The biological process

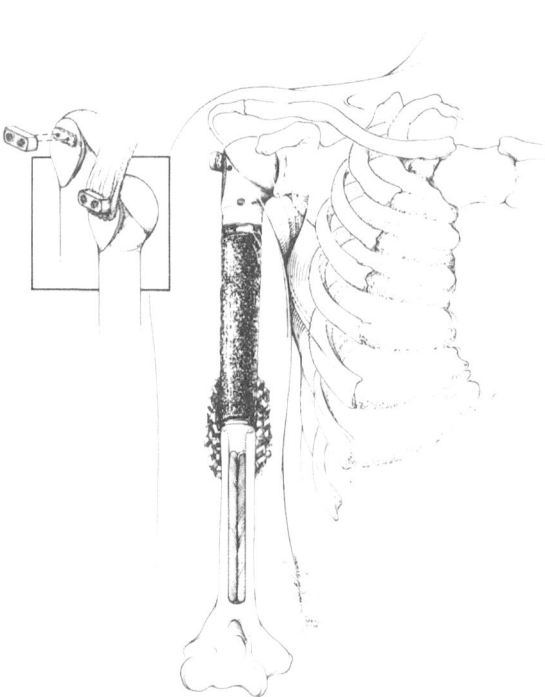

Fig. 9. Artist's rendition of the proximal humerus segmental bone and shoulder joint replacement prosthesis using the composite fixation concept. A proposed soft-tissue attachment technique to the prosthesis is also illustrated

involved in the present method of reconstruction is similar to that which occurs after massive allograft transplantation adjacent to a host segmental defect. The advantage of using a metallic implant is its ability to provide immediate mobility, which is important in patients with tumors who are subject to neoadjuvant therapy and unknown long-term prognosis.

The implants and the composite fixation concept described herein have had successful clinical trials in the reconstruction of large bony defects resulting from tumor resection, metabolic bone disease, and trauma with severe bone loss. Extracortical fixation was achieved in all cases where sufficient bone grafting was used. The clinical results obtained in revision cases are comparable to other methods of reconstruction when large bony defect is involved. The implant-related failures, except for those due to infection, can be minimized through implant modification and improved surgical techniques. Hence, the long-term outlook for such an implant design concept and fixation method seems very promising.

There are several potential improvements which need to be explored before such a composite implant fixation concept can be relied upon as the design of choice for segmental bone and joint defect replacement prostheses. First, the bone grafts tend to migrate away from the critical zone where bone bridging and ingrowth are required, and certain methods of preventing such problems would be desirable. Second, sufficient autogenous corticocancellous grafts are not always available in large quantity. Other bone graft substitutes must be developed to ensure the extracortical bone bridging process. Third, different forms of physical, chemical, or cellular stimulation may be required to accelerate bone formation over the porous-coated segmental bone/joint replacement implants. Finally, attachment of soft tissue directly to the implant is desirable in improving joint functional results and implant stability. This last improvement will help to further increase the acceptability of using prosthetic devices as opposed to the use of massive allograft in limb-salvage surgery involving tumor resection or failed joint replacement arthroplasty with massive bone loss.

Conclusions

A composite fixation method for a porous-coated modular segmental bone/joint prosthetic system was developed to reconstruct segmental bone and joint defects after tumor resection. The porous coating is limited only to the segmental shoulder region of the prosthesis, while bone cement is used to provide initial implant stability. Autogenous bone grafts are applied over the porous-coated region to achieve extracortical bone bridging and ingrowth for long-term biological fixation. Bench tests, theoretical analysis, and animal experiments were performed to validate this fixation concept. Clinical, radiographic, and functional results of patients using these prostheses are very encouraging. A number of limiting factors were identified and further improvements are being investigated to foster this concept as a viable alternative in limb-salvage surgery in patients with resectable musculoskeletal tumor.

Acknowledgments. This developmental work was supported by PHS grant number CA 23751, awarded by the National Cancer Institute. The research results reported in this paper are the work of many research fellows in our laboratory whose contributions to this effort were truly immense and are gratefully acknowledged.

References

1. Campanna R, Van Horn JR, Biagini R, Ruggieri R, Bettelli G, Sola G, Campanacci M (1986) A humeral modular prosthesis for bone tumor surgery. A study of 56 cases. Int Orthop 10(4):231–239
2. Chao EYS, Ivins JC (1983) Tumor prostheses for bone and joint reconstruction. Thieme-Stratton, New York
3. Sim FH, Chao EYS (1981) Hip salvage for proximal femoral replacement. J Bone Joint Surg [Am] 63:1228–1239
4. Sim FH, Chao EYS (1979) Prosthetic replacement of the knee and a large segment of the femur or tibia. J Bone Joint Surg [Am] 61:887–892
5. Kotz R, Ritschl P, Trachtenbrodt J (1986) A modular and tibia reconstruction system. Orthopedics 9(12):1639–1652

6. Chao EYS (1989) A composite fixation principle for modular segmental defect replacement (SDR) prostheses. Bone tumors: Evaluation and treatment. Orthop Clin North Am 20(3):439–453

7. Chao EYS, Sim FH (1985) Modular prosthetic system for segmental bone and joint replacement after tumor resection. Orthopedics 8:641–651

8. Dai KR, An KN, Hein T, Nakajima I, Chao EYS (1985) Geometric and biomechanical analysis of the human femur. Transactions of 31st Annual Meeting of the Orthopedic Research Society, p 99

9. Nakao Y, Dueland RT, Turner RT, Chao EYS (1990) An ultrastructural study of the biologic mechanism of extracortical bone bridging over porous-coated segmental bone prosthesis. Transactions of 36th Annual Meeting of the Orthopedic Research Society, p 482

10. Heck DA, Nakajima I, Chao EYS, Kelly PJ (1986) The effect of immobilization on biologic ingrowth into porous titanium fibermetal prostheses. J Bone Joint Surg [Am] 68:118–126

11. Nakajima I, Dai KR, Kelly PJ, Chao EYS (1985) The effect of age on tissue incorporation into Ti fibermetal segmental bone prostheses — an experimental study in canine models. Transactions of 31st Annual Meeting of the Orthopedic Research Society, p 193

12. Okada Y, Suka T, Sim FH, Gorski JP, Chao EYS (1988) Comparison of bone segmental prostheses with different porous coatings for extracortical fixation. J Bone Joint Surg [Am] 70(2):160–172

13. Wippermann BW, Hsu RWW, Wilkins RM, Chao EYS (1989) Autogenous cortical graft versus demineralized bone matrix in achieving extracortical bone bridging fixation of segmental prostheses. Proceedings of the 5th International Symposium on Limb Salvage, September 6–9, Saint-Malo, France

14. Chin HC, Frassica FJ, Markel MD, Frassica DA, Schray MF, Sim FH, Chao EYS (1989) The effect of therapeutic irradiation on bone ingrowth and extracortical bone formation in porous-coated prosthetic components. Transactions of 35th Annual Meeting of the Orthopedic Research Society, p 555

15. Heck DA, Chao EYS, Sim FH, Pritchard DJ, Shives TC (1986) Titanium fibermetal segmental replacement prostheses. Clin Orthop 204:266–285

16. Sim FH, Beauchamp CP, Chao EYS (1987) Reconstruction of musculoskeletal defects about the knee for tumor. Clin Orthop 221:188–201

4.2

A Limb-Saving Operation for Cases with Malignant Pelvic Bone Tumors

Atsumasa Uchida, Yoshitaka Shinto, Ikuo Kudawara,
Hideki Yoshikawa, Keiro Ono,[1] Takafumi Ueda,[2] and
Hideki Hamada[3]

Introduction

At present, primary malignant tumors involving the pelvic bone are treated with hemipelvectomy. However, a limb-saving operation should theoretically obtain the same surgical margin in tumor resection as that of a hemipelvectomy (Fig. 1). Based on this functional consideration, limb-saving operations have been performed on selected patients. In this paper, we describe the methods of resection and reconstruction, and the functional results in limb-saving operations of primary malignant pelvic tumors.

Materials and Methods

Preoperative studies, such as CT and MRI, indicated that 23 patients were suitable candidates for the limb-saving procedure, which could be expected to result in tumor removal with an adequate margin and without injury to the external iliac artery or sciatic nerve. The group was comprised of 15 males and 8 females whose average age was 32 years (range: 12–73 years). The follow-up period was between 6–78 months (average: 38 months). Eleven cases were followed for over 2 years.

In terms of the 3 divisions of the pelvic bone — the periacetabular bone, the iliac bone away from the acetabulum, and the ischiopubic bone [1] — there were 16 periacetabular tumors, 5 iliac tumors away from the acetabulum, and 2 pubic tumors. Histological diagnosis showed 8 chondrosarcomas, 6 osteosarcomas, 5 Ewing's sarcomas, and various others (Table 1). All but two

[1] Department of Orthopaedic Surgery, Osaka University Medical School, Fukushima 1-1-50, Osaka, 553 Japan
[2] Osaka Prefectural Adult Disease Center, Nakamichi 1-3-3, Higashinari, Osaka, 537 Japan
[3] Osaka Prefectural Hospital, Mandaihigashi 3-1-56, Sumiyoshi, Osaka, 558 Japan

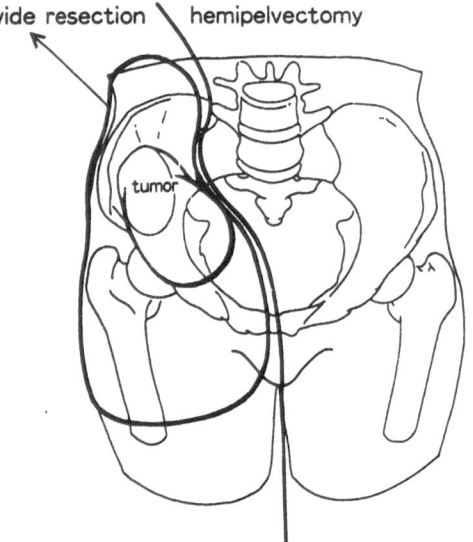

wide resection   hemipelvectomy

tumor

Fig. 1. Illustration of the surgical margin in a wide resection and hemipelvectomy for malignant pelvic tumors. The radical nature of tumor resection is the same for these 2 procedures

Table 1. Histological diagnosis in primary malignant pelvic tumors

Tumor type	Number
Periacetabular	
Osteosarcoma	6
Chondrosarcoma	5
Ewing's sarcoma	2
MFH	2
Parosteal osteosarcoma	1
Iliac (away from the acetabulum)	
Ewing's sarcoma	2
Chondrosarcoma	2
Lymphoma	1
Ishiopubic	
Chondrosarcoma	1
Ewing's sarcoma	1

MFH, Malignant fibrous histiocytoma

patients, one with a periosteal osteosarcoma and one with a grade I chondrosarcoma, received pre- and postoperative chemotherapy with Adriamycin, *cis*-platinum and high-dose methotrexate. Radiotherapy was used postoperatively in only 2 cases with intralesional margin of the tumor resection.

Reconstruction Methods

Since a periacetabular tumor excision always destroys the hip joint, the most important task for reconstruction is to realize iliofemoral stability. There are several types of reconstruction: arthrodesis, resection arthroplasty, and tumor

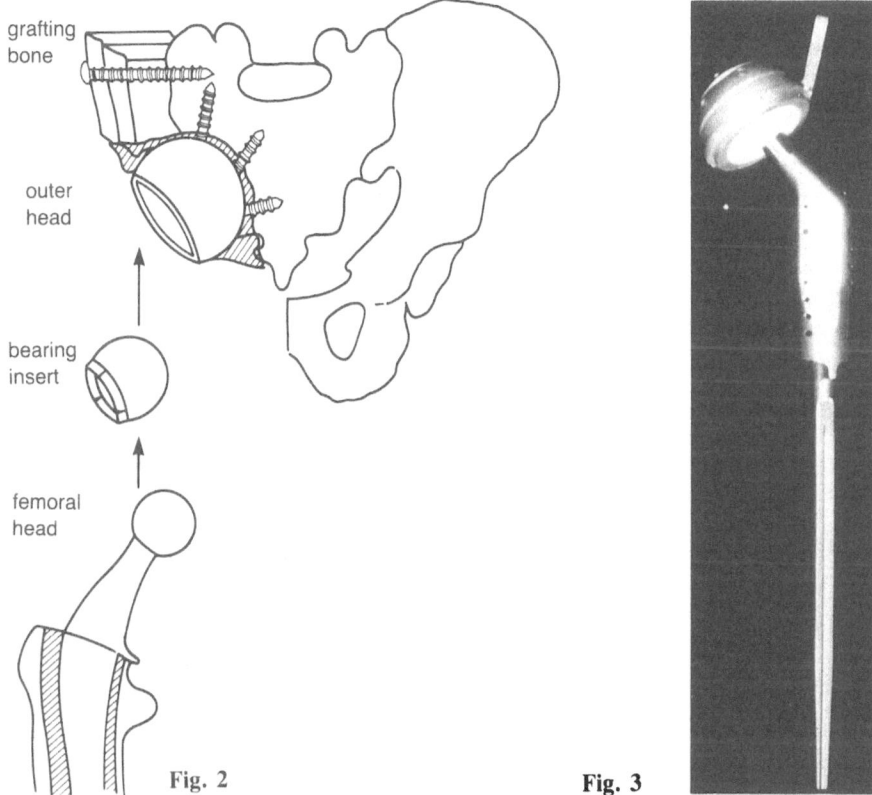

grafting
bone

outer
head

bearing
insert

femoral
head

Fig. 2   Fig. 3

Fig. 2. Illustration of an iliofemoral prosthesis following surgery for a pelvic tumor. The outer head, fixed in the ilium or sacrum, and the inner head with a long intramedullary stem cemented to the femur were connected with the bearing insert

Fig. 3. Newly designed tumor prosthesis. The socket with blade was devised in order to obtain more rigid fixation

prosthesis with or without pelvic continuity. In this series, of the 16 patients in whom the hip joint was sacrificed, 12 underwent reconstruction with a constrained-type total hip tumor prosthesis without restoration of pelvic continuity. This type of tumor prosthesis consists of 3 components. The metallic outer head is fixed with screws and bone cement in the remaining ilium and sacrum. The inner head with its long neck and long intramedullary stem, which is cemented to the femur, is firmly connected with the ultra-high-density polyethylene (HDP)-bearing insert, resulting in a constrained joint mechanism of the femoroilium (Fig. 2). In order to obtain rigid fixation of the outer head, bone grafting in the anterior and lateral portions of the remaining ilium and sacrum is needed.

A new socket design was devised for securing fixation to the bone (Fig. 3). Two patients who were treated in the early stage of this study received a non-constraining tumor hip prosthesis.

Two patients underwent resection arthroplasty at the first operation, but, 1 year later, reconstruction of the iliofemoral joint with a constrained hip tumor prosthesis was performed because of poor functional results of the flail hip. Arthrodesis with autogenous and allogeneic bone was performed in 1 case. An artificial pelvis manufactured out of alumina ceramic was tried in 1 case of malignant fibrous histiocytoma.

Of the five patients who had iliac tumors away from the acetabulum, three suffered disruption of pelvic continuity in the sacroiliac joint. In two of these patients, the pelvic ring continuity was reconstructed by bone grafting and approximation of the remaining part of the pelvic bone. The disruption in the sacroiliac joint could not be restored in one patient.

In ischiopubic tumors, we did not perform any reconstruction if the iliofemoral joint could be preserved.

Results

Control of the Disease

There were 7 local recurrences (30.4%). These seven patients, three with intralesional and four with marginal excisions, were judged to have an inadequate margin. Of the patients with marginal excisions, two with low-grade chondrosarcomas and one with parosteal osteosarcoma did not have local recurrence or distant metastasis at more than 5 years after the operation. All the six patients who were judged to have had a wide margin did not show any local recurrence at the time of follow-up, and all but one who had lung metastasis are still alive and disease-free.

The overall 5-year survival rate for pelvic tumors was 33% (Kaplan-Meiyer method). Ewing's sarcomas showed the worst prognosis, while the prognosis for osteosarcomas and chondrosarcomas was somewhat better. In terms of tumor location, prognosis for periacetabular tumors was the worst. The efficacy of chemotherapy remains unclear, but histological assessment of Ewing's sarcoma showed the highest necrotic rate. There was no correlation between prognosis of the disease and chemotherapeutic histological assessment.

Functional Results

Functional results depended on the location of the tumors and the reconstruction method. When a hip prosthesis was used for periacetabular tumors, almost all patients obtained relief from pain. The range of active motion at the trunk-limb junction was small because of massive resection of the muscles around the hip. The range of motion of the prosthesis itself was insufficient, but sitting on a chair was easily accomplished. Stability correlated with the quantity and quality of the remaining muscle around the hip. Shortening of the involved

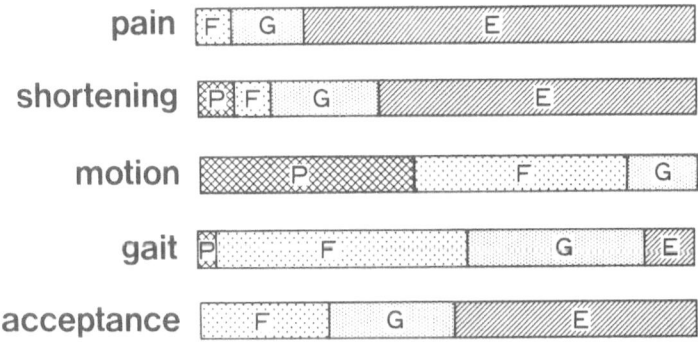

Fig. 4. Functional results of hip prosthesis following tumor surgery. Pain, shortening, motion, gait, and emotional acceptance were assessed with four grades, excellent (*E*), good (*G*), fair (*F*), and poor (P). Criteria for assessment were modified by Ennecking's method

limb was minimal. Gait was satisfactory, i.e., over 90% of the patients were able to walk with a cane or without any support. The remaining patients could walk with a crutch. In almost all cases, emotional acceptance was also satisfactory (Fig. 4).

The functional results of two flail hips were unsatisfactory because of shortening of the involved limb, instability of the iliofemoral joint, and pain. Arthrodesis and construction of an artificial pelvis did not have good functional results because of pain caused by pseudoarthrosis.

In cases of iliac tumors away from the acetabulum and of ischiopublic tumors, all patients showed excellent results if the iliofemoral joint stability could be preserved. Sacroiliac joint discontinuity did not affect the functional results.

Complications

There were 2 incidents of infection which were controlled with surgical debridement and antibiotic therapy without removal of the prosthesis. Dislocation of the prosthesis occurred in 2 unconstrained hip prostheses, while no dislocation was seen in the constrained type. There was one incident of socket loosening caused by local recurrence in the remaining ilium. Two patients had skin necrosis which was treated with a musculocutaneous pedicle flap of the abdominal rectus muscle.

Case Reports

Case 1

S.Y., a 19-year-old male, had been complaining of intermittent pain in the left iliac and buttock regions. A biopsy of the lesion in the left ilium confirmed the

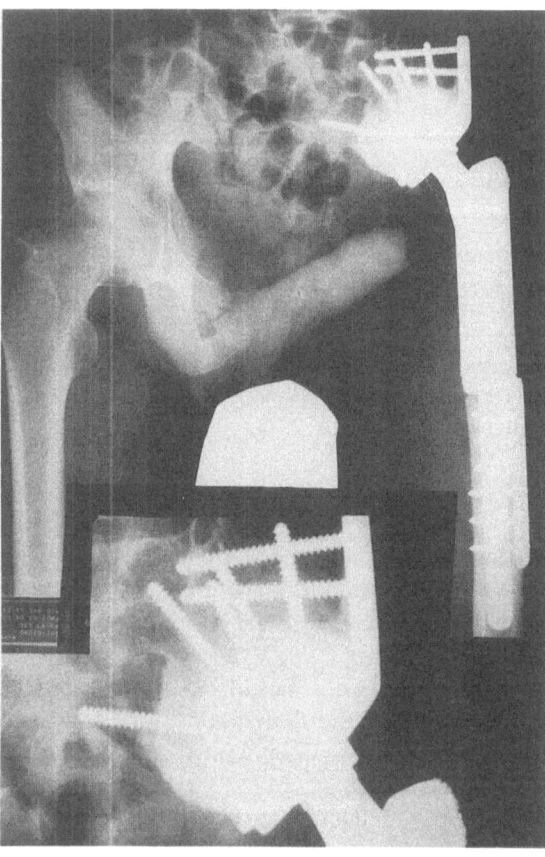

Fig. 5. Postoperative X-ray of case 1. After fixation of a constrained prosthetic socket to the grafting bone and sacrum, proximal portion of the femur was replaced with a Kotz modular prosthesis. The patient can walk without pain using a cane

diagnosis of osteosarcoma. Preoperative chemotherapy with Adriamycin and *cis*-platinum was performed resulting in regression of the tumor, followed by wide resection of the tumor with bone grafting to the sacrum without restoration of the iliofemoral joint.

Six months later, a constrained total hip replacement was performed to achieve iliofemoral stability (Fig. 5). The patient could walk with a cane 2 months after this operation.

Case 2

K.U., a 26-year-old male, noted pain in his right buttock for 6 months. Radiographs revealed an extensive osteolytic lesion with calcification, while CT and MRI findings clearly showed extension of the tumor both intra- and extrapelvically. An open biopsy showed the pathological features of a grade III chondrosarcoma. After preoperative chemotherapy with Adriamycin and *cis*-platinum, wide resection and reconstruction with a constrained total hip prosthesis were performed simultaneously (Fig. 6). Following surgery, the patient could walk without any support, but he died from lung metastasis 2 years postoperatively.

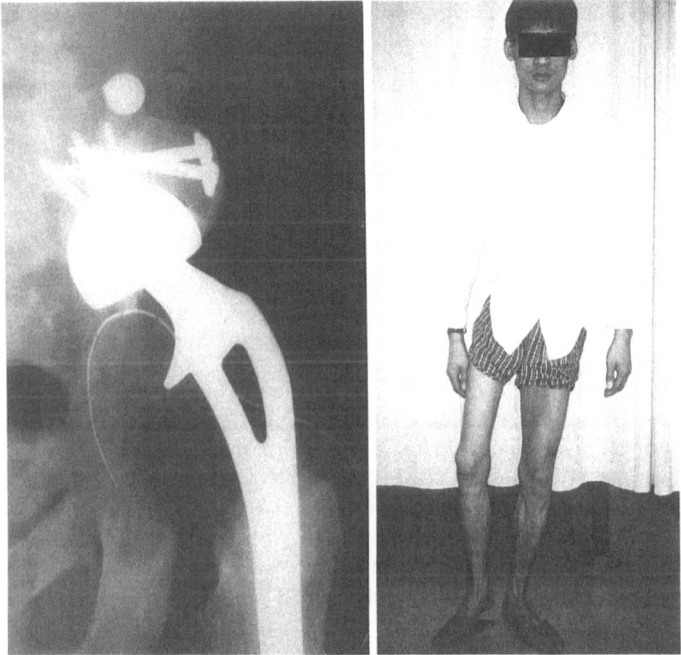

Fig. 6. Anteroposterior radiograph and functional result of the hip prosthesis in case 2. The patient was able to stand on the affected limb 1 year postoperatively

Discussion

Patients with pelvic sarcomas must be considered as having a systemic disease since many will present with metastasis or develop metastasis within 2 years from diagnosis. When treated with standard therapy, the overall prognosis for these patients is quite poor, as indicated by the 5-year survival rate of 33%. In order to improve the prognosis of patients with pelvic sarcomas, it is necessary to implement a sophisticated combined modality therapy which involves chemotherapy and radiotherapy as well as surgical resection [2].

This study shows that wide excision should be the procedure of choice for the treatment of malignant lesions involving the pelvic bone. However, it has been clearly shown by high local recurrence rates that it is very difficult to achieve the wide marginal excision planned in preoperative studies.

When selecting patients with pelvic bone tumors for a limb-saving procedure, several considerations should be emphasized. These include the precise extent and location of the tumors and the efficacy of chemotherapy and radiotherapy.

With regard to functional reconstruction after tumor resection, a constrained total hip prosthesis appears to be most useful for the restoration of iliofemoral joint stability [3]. This prosthesis can compensate for the problems caused by arthrodesis and a flail hip [4], [5]. Moreover, reconstruction with this prosthesis has good functional results even without the restoration of pelvic continuity. Although the weak point of using this prosthesis is the fixation of the socket to the remaining ilium because of poor bone stock, it is possible to overcome this disadvantage with a newly designed socket. If iliofemoral joint stability is still preserved even after tumor excision, disruption in the sacroiliac joint or pubic symphysis is negligible. These results suggest that the most important consideration for methods of reconstruction in cases of pelvic tumors is how iliofemoral joint stability can be obtained.

References

1. Enneking WF, Dunham WK (1978) Resection and reconstruction for primary neoplasms involving the innominate bone. J Bone Joint Surg [Am] 60:731–746
2. Stea B, Kinsella TJ, Triche TJ, Horvath K, Glatsein E, Miser JS (1987) Treatment of pelvic sarcomas in adolescents and young adults with intensive combined modality therapy. Int J Radiat Oncol Biol Phys 13:1797–1805
3. Uchida A, Hamada H, Yoshikawa H, Aoki Y, Ebara S, Ono K (1989) Surgical treatment of bone tumors arising from pelvic ring. In: Yamamuro T (ed) New development for limb salvage in musculoskeletal tumors. Springer, Tokyo, pp 451–458
4. Capanna R, Van Horn JR, Guernelli N, Briccoli A, Ruggieri P, Biagini R, Bettellini G, Campanacci M (1987) Complications of pelvic resections. Arch Orthop Trauma Surg 106:71–77
5. Nilsonne U, Kreicbergs A, Olsson E, Stark A (1982) Function after pelvic tumor resection involving the acetabular ring. International Orthopaedics (SICOT) 6:27–33

4.3

Limb-Salvage Procedures for Osteosarcoma Using Intraoperative Radiation Therapy

YOSHIHIKO KOTOURA, TAKAO YAMAMURO, KATSUYUKI KASAHARA,
RENPEI IWASAKI,[1] MASAJI TAKAHASHI,[2] and MITSUYUKI ABE[3]

Introduction

The survival rate of patients with osteosarcoma has been improved by advanced diagnostic techniques, the combined use of chemotherapy and radiotherapy, improved operative techniques, and integrated care systems. In the past, these patients were mainly treated by amputation combined with chemotherapy. However, in recent years, increasing advances have been made in limb salvage techniques. Since 1978, we have adopted the use of intraoperative radiation therapy (IORT) for local control of primary lesions of osteosarcoma [1] and of metastatic bone tumors. We describe the method of IORT, its antitumor effect, and clinical results.

Patients

Between 1978 and 1990, 28 patients with osteosarcoma underwent intraoperative radiation therapy in combination with chemotherapy at our clinic. The patients were 21 males and 7 females who ranged in age from 6 to 54 years at the time of IORT. Location of the lesion was the distal femur (16 cases), middle femur (1), proximal tibia (9), proximal humerus (1), and ilium (1). On admission, distant metastasis was found in one patient and pathological fracture in one.

Methods

When osteosarcoma was suspected on admission, CT, MRI, bone scintigraphy and angiography, as well as plain roentogenography were performed. In prin-

[1] Department of Orthopedic Surgery, Faculty of Medicine, Kyoto University, Kyoto, 606 Japan
[2] Chest Disease Research Institute, Kyoto University, Kyoto, 606 Japan
[3] Department of Radiology, Faculty of Medicine, Kyoto University, Kyoto, 606 Japan

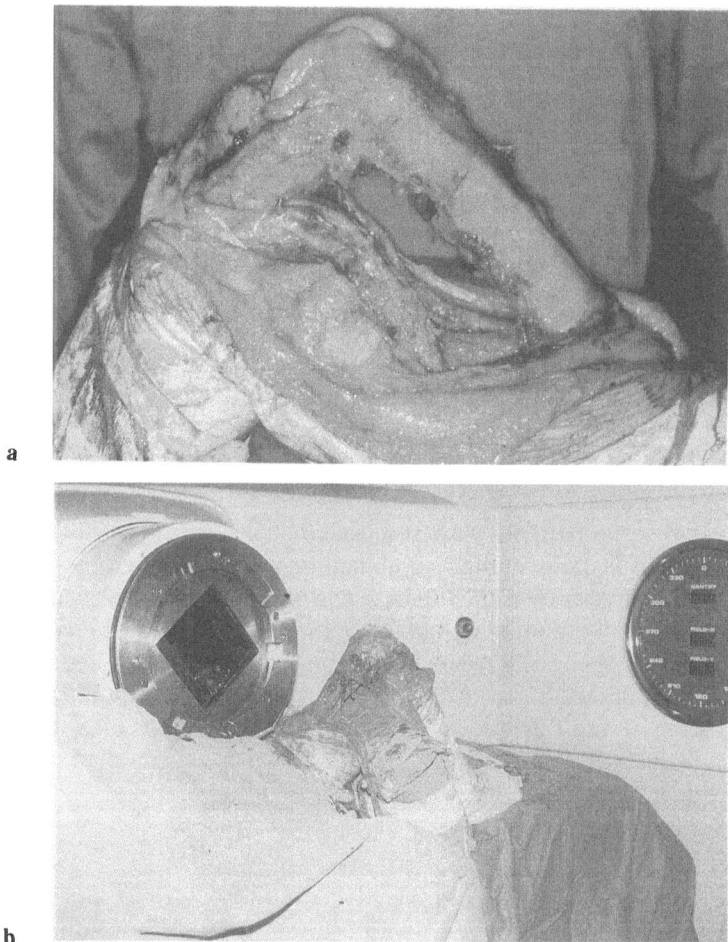

Fig. 1a–b. a Irradiation field is exposed in the operating room. **b** IORT with a betatron or Linac at a dose of 50–60 Gy

ciple, the treatment of osteosarcoma started after histological diagnosis. When osteosarcoma was diagnosed from a frozen section, Adriamycin (ADR) was immediately injected intra-arterially and intraoperative radiation therapy was performed.

When the primary lesion was located in the distal femur, a medial para-patellar skin incision was made; the vastus medialis muscle was reflected medially, and the rectus femoris and vastus lateralis muscles were reflected laterally. The joint capsule was also incised; the patellar tendon was partially dissected, and the patella was reflected. The vastus intermedius muscle was left on the femur, remaining in the irradiation field. The sciatic nerve and femoral artery and vein behind the femur were posteriorly retracted away from the irradiation field (Fig. 1.a). After adequate exposure, the surgical wound was

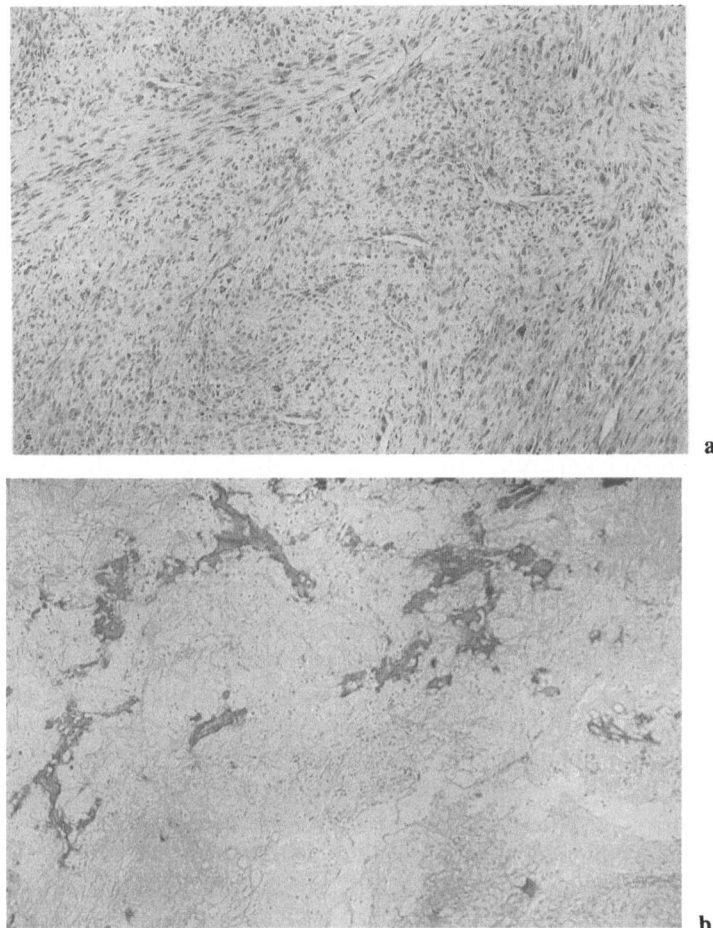

a

b

Fig. 2a–b. a Pre-IORT. **b** Post-IORT 5 months. No viable tumor cells are observed

temporarily sutured. The patient was then transferred from the operating room to the irradiation room on a stretcher equipped with an anesthetizing system and a portable ECG. The patient was placed onto the irradiation platform in the supine position; the knee joint was flexed 90°, and femoral soft tissue, nerves, and blood vessels were posteriorly retracted away from the irradiation field. Irradiation ranged from the upper 2 cm segment of the tibia to 4 cm proximal to the upper margin of the tumor, involving the entire knee joint. Parallel-opposed (internal and external) irradiation was usually given to the target area, which sometimes extended 20 cm or more in the longitudinal direction. The IORT was performed with 12–26 MeV electron beams in a dose of 50–60 Gy (Fig. 1.b). After irradiation, the incised muscles and tendons were sutured, suction drainage was inserted, and the wound was closed. After intraoperative radiation therapy, systemic chemotherapy consisting mainly of ADR and *cis*-platinum (CDDP) was continued for about 6 months.

Results

After the wound healed, spontaneous pain was relieved and swelling was reduced. At 4–5 weeks after IORT, sclerotic changes were observed in the extraosseous lesional tissue. Progression of disease in the tissue was halted, and no new periosteal reaction occurred.

Preoperatively elevated serum alkaline phosphatase values dropped sharply after IORT, subsequently returning to normal levels in all cases. The decreasing curve was nearly identical to that seen in cases of amputation.

Postoperative bone scintigrams showed a marked decrease in uptake in the irradiated area compared with those taken preoperatively. In several cases, a cold area was observed at 3 months after IORT. These effects observed on bone scintigram were long-lasting.

Histological examinations were performed in 17 patients who underwent wide resection, amputation, or autopsy after IORT for primary lesions. The 9 cases previously reported by Nagashima [2] were included among them. The duration from IORT to specimen excision was less than 6 months in 10 cases, 6–12 months in 3 cases, 12–24 months in 2 cases, and more than 24 months in 2 cases. The longest duration was 6 years.

Histological examination also revealed a marked antitumor effect of IORT. In most of the cases, previously tumor-bearing areas showed complete necrosis of sarcoma cells (Figs. 2.a,b). Most tissues with lesions showed marked fibrosis. Tumorous osteoids were only sporadically observed, and few cellular elements were seen. Although part of the cell nucleus was noted in several cases, most cell nuclei had been denatured, and were not indicative of local recurrence. In 2 cases of long-term follow-up, the histological findings showed complete necrosis 2 years and 6 years after IORT. There were no viable cells.

With regard to the antitumor effect of IORT, there were no differences among cases, while such differences are problematic when chemotherapy is used for osteosarcoma.

IORT was carried out in a total of 28 patients. None had local recurrence in the irradiated area after IORT. Three had local recurrence in non-irradiated areas: one due to tumor implantation in the vastus lateralis muscle during biopsy and the other two due to insufficiency of the area that had been irradiated.

Pathological fracture occurred in the tumor areas of ten patients 1–20 months after IORT.

Additional surgery after IORT was comprised of prosthetic replacement in 9 cases, amputation due to skin necrosis in 2 cases and due to infection in 2 cases, and internal fixation for post-irradiation pathological fracture in 3 cases. To prevent such fractures, we performed intramedullary nailing with a special titanium rod in 2 cases.

The 5-year cumulative survival rate of all patients was 44%. However, since 1984, the rate increased for 13 cases treated by IORT in combination with chemotherapy using CDDP.

Discussion

Radiotherapy for malignant bone tumors has been practiced for many years. However, it was effective only on highly radiosensitive tumors, e.g., lymphoma and Ewing's sarcoma. Osteosarcoma was also treated with a large dose of radiation, but this was virtually of no practical use, since irradiation with minimal side effects entailed insufficient antitumor effect, whereas irradiation with increased antitumor effect yielded severe side effects, such as skin and soft tissue impairments. Radiotherapy aiming at limb salvage must fulfill two conflicting requirements: providing satisfactory local control, while minimizing skin and soft tissue impairments as much as possible. Conventional irradiation procedures for osteosarcoma did not satisfy these requirements.

Abe et al. tried betatron-based IORT to prevent local recurrence of remaining minor metastasis after resection of abdominal tumors and obtained favorable results [3]. This type of radiotherapy involves effectively irradiating a surgically exposed target lesion with high-energy electron beams while minimizing radiation injury as much as possible. Therefore, IORT was considered applicable to the primary lesion of osteosarcoma. With this in mind, in 1978, we initiated IORT against primary lesions of osteosarcoma to obtain sure local-control effects with minimized side effects on the skin and soft tissue.

The purpose of IORT for osteosarcoma changed during this series. In 1978, we began IORT for osteosarcoma as an adjuvant therapy to control tumor progression until prosthetic replacement surgery. Patients underwent replacement surgery 3 months after IORT.

Since no local recurrence in the irradiated area was observed either histologically or clinically, it was presumed that IORT has a somewhat permanent antitumor effect. Recently, therefore, limb salvage with the irradiated tumor tissues preserved *in situ* has been attempted. Good range of motion and stability of the joint are often maintained.

Disadvantages of IORT include a high rate of pathological fracture in the tumor area and the difficulty of obtaining bone union at the fracture site. To prevent such fractures, we performed intramedullary nailing with a special titanium rod in 2 cases. Fractures have not been observed in these cases in the 2 years they have been monitored. The function of the affected knee joint is good and the patients can walk without support.

When an osteolytic tumor was located in the metaphysis, prosthetic replacement of the tumor including the adjacent joint was performed after IORT, enabling safe intralesional operations and maintaining good joint function.

Conclusion

IORT is an effective treatment for limb salvage in osteosarcoma because it can provide a satisfactory, long-lasting local-control effect on the lesion with fewer side effects on the skin and soft tissues.

References

1. Yamamuro T, Kotoura Y, Kasahara K, Takahashi M, Abe M (1989) Intraoperative radiotherapy and ceramic prosthesis replacement for osteosarcoma. In: Yamamuro T (ed) New developments for limb salvage in musculoskeletal tumors. Springer-Verlag, Tokyo, pp 328–333
2. Nagashima T, Yamamuro T, Kotoura Y, Takahashi M, Abe M, Nakashima Y (1983) Histological studies of the effect of intra-operative irradiation on osteosarcoma (in Japanese). J Jpn Orthop Assoc 57:1681–1697
3. Abe M, Takahashi M, Yabumoto E, Tobe T, Mori K (1974) Intraoperative radiotherapy of gastric cancer. Cancer 34:2034–2041

Replacement by Ceramic Prostheses for the Treatment of Malignant and Benign Aggressive Bone Tumors

HIDEKI HAYASHI,[1] ATSUMASA UCHIDA,[2] HIDEKI HAMADA,[3] HIDEKI YOSHIKAWA,[2] YOSHITAKA SHINTO,[2] and KEIRO ONO[2]

Introduction

Originally, the investigators of limb-salvage operations were mainly concerned with postoperative function. This objective has been realized not only by the progress of prosthetic design, but by the various efforts intended to minimize the resection area [1–5]. The next concern concentrated on two goals: to extend the yardsticks for the indication of the prosthetic replacement for the growing, younger patients and to improve the design of the prosthesis for long-term application, because most of the patients who undergo this type of operation are relatively young. In addition, the loss of bone stock around the prosthesis after long-term use would make any revision surgery more difficult. Several kinds of extending prostheses and temporary resection-arthrodesis were attempted for attaining the first goal [6–9]. Operations employing prostheses with porous-coated stems and anti-micromotion blades, prostheses with porous-coated segments for bone grafts and cement-fixed stems, long-stem prostheses with allografted segments, and ceramic prostheses were performed for achieving the second objective [10–18]. On the other hand, allograft, reimplantation of affected bone with both extracorporeal and intracorporeal irradiation were also carried out because these bones can be permanently used if they could be revascularized and reconstructed with normal bone tissue [19–22]. These methods have another advantage in that they preserve joint cartilage and the attachment of muscle or ligament because these tissues are more resistant against irradiation. However, these methods bear the problem of a high rate of complications, such as infection, fracture, or necrosis [23].

[1] Hayashi Hospital, 3-21 Mikawa, Naka-ku, Hiroshima, 730 Japan
[2] Department of Orthopaedic Surgery, Osaka University Medical School
[3] Osaka Prefecture Hospital, Osaka Japan

Among the artificial materials that are currently in use, aluminum oxide ceramic results in good tissue compatibility and minimal wear compared to the available metals [24]. Monocrystal alumina is 3 times stronger than polycrystal alumina and is also twice the strength of vitalium. Therefore, these ceramics have many features favorable to the prosthesis intended for long-term use, especially when polycrystal alumina is used for the segment and monocrystal alumina is used for the stem. Their disadvantage is that design is limited because of difficulty in their manufacture. We had adopted ceramic prostheses of this composite design since 1979. The following is a description of our experience in 71 cases.

Materials and Methods

Between September, 1979 and June, 1990, 71 patients with mostly malignant bone tumors underwent resection and reconstruction of limbs using ceramic prostheses. There were 42 males and 29 females, ranging in age from 8 to 77 years (average: 40 years). The follow-up period was from 9 to 137 months (average: 41 months).

The histological diagnoses included 20 osteosarcomas (1 = stage IIA, 16 = IIB, 3 = IIIB), 5 chondrosarcomas (1 = IA, 3 = IB, 1 = IIB), 10 of the other sarcomas (all = IIB), 12 giant cell tumors (3 = IA, 9 = IB), 20 metastatic bone tumors, 2 fractured fibrous dysplasias, 1 fractured myeloma, and 1 enchondroma surrounded with lipoma.

Eighteen patients underwent replacement for the proximal femur, 13 distal femur, 14 proximal tibia, 12 proximal humerus, 3 distal forearm, 6 midshaft, 2 pelvis, 1 scapula, 1 manubrium sterni, and 1 metacarpal bone.

The resection was of the wide type in 27 cases (for all the cases with IIA or more advanced stages), contaminated wide in 20 (for the stage I cases), and marginal in 24 cases (for all the cases with metastatic bone tumors and the 3 remaining cases).

The prostheses were all supplied by Kyocera (Kyoto, Japan). Most of them were used for the end part of long bones and consisted of polycrystal alumina segments and monocrystal alumina stems. The exceptions to these were polycrystal alumina stems in 2 early cases and titanium stems in 12 later cases. For more frequent sites of lesions, such as the proximal femur, distal femur, proximal tibia, and proximal humerus, most of the prostheses were of a semi-modular type with the segment of each 25 mm length being from 75 to 200 mm and the stem of each 1 mm diameter being from 8 to 13 mm. Prostheses for the other sites were entirely custom-made. The models with artificial joints consisted of 11 prostheses for the distal femur, 10 for the proximal tibia, and 4 for the proximal humerus. The remaining prostheses for these 3 sites and all those for the proximal femur and distal radius were the head-type models. The design of the artificial joint was a hingeless type for knee joints and a constrained type with the polycrystal-alumina scapula and high-density polyethylene

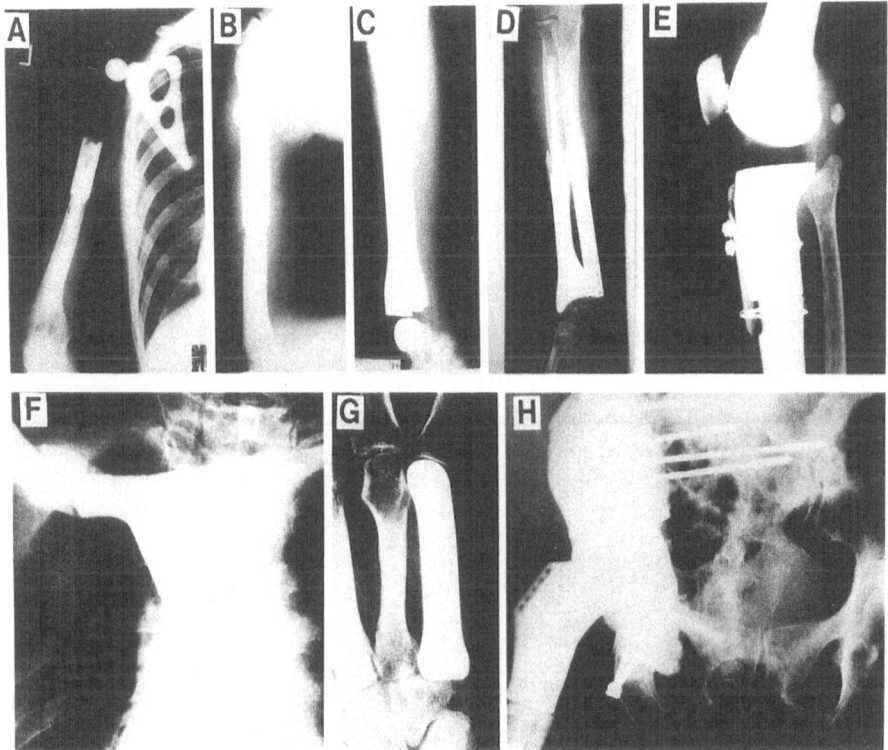

Fig. 1A–H. Postoperative radiographs of the replaced limbs using the custom-made ceramic prostheses of special design. **A** Ten years following the replacement for high-grade osteosarcoma using the constrained total shoulder prosthesis which consists of a polycrystal alumina scapula and humeral segment, high density polyethylene head, and monocrystal alumina stem. **B** Four years following the replacement for metastatic bone tumor using the segmental midshaft defect prosthesis. **C** Four years following the replacement for malignant fibrous histiocytoma with skip metastases using the total tibia prosthesis with ankle joint. **D** Eight years following the replacement for giant cell tumor of the distal radius. **E** Three months following the replacement for low-grade chondrosarcoma using the tuberositas tibia-preserving type prosthesis. **F** Six months following the replacement for high-grade chondrosarcoma in the manubrium sterni using the all-polycrystal alumina prosthesis. The *left side* is fixed with wire and bone cement. **G** Nine months following the replacement for enchondroma surrounded with lipoma. The MP joint is starting to subluxate. **H** Two months following the replacement for metastatic sarcoma on the ilium and trochanteric region using the constrained hemi-total pelvic and proximal femoral prosthesis which is fixed by bone cement, screws, and Knowles pins

head for shoulder joints (Fig. 1.A). In 4 cases in which the tumor was located on the posterior part of the proximal tibia, we used the custom-made prosthesis of the tuberositas tibia-preserving type (Fig. 1.E). With this type of prosthesis,

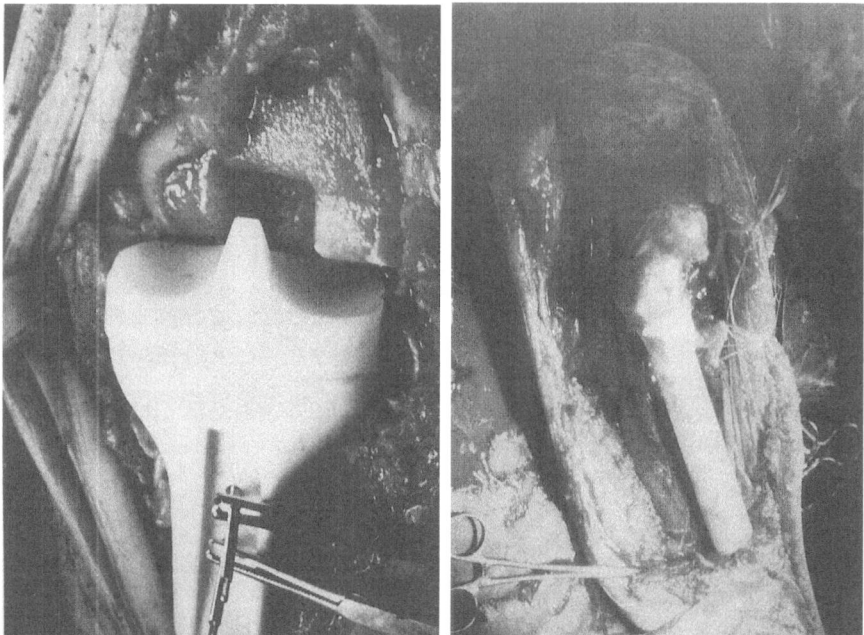

Fig. 2. Intraoperative photograph. *left* Following the resection of low-grade chondro-sarcoma in the proximal tibia and reconstruction with a custom-made prosthesis of the tuberositas tibia-preserving type. The preserved tuberositas tibia is about to be fixed into the channel of the segment using bolts and nuts. *right* Following the resection of high-grade osteosarcoma in the proximal femur and reconstruction with a custom-made head-type prosthesis. Note the joint capsule and the periost of the femoral shaft are reconstructed using a graft of tensor fascia latae and a teflon mesh

the tuberositas tibia was preserved and fixed with bolts and nuts into the channel of the segment (Fig. 2. left). The custom-made total tibial prosthesis with an ankle joint was used for the case with skip metastasis (Fig. 1.C). For the 2 pelvis, manubrium sterni, and metacarpal replacements, all prostheses were polycrystal models (Fig. 1.F,G). One of the 2 prostheses for the pelvis included the femur of a semi-modular type (Fig. 1.H). In all, the length of the prosthesis was from 50 to 360 mm, with an average length of 163 mm.

The stem was fixed without using cement in 32 cases and with cement in the rest. The latter included all the 12 cases with titanium stems.

For soft tissue reconstruction, we used a free graft from the tensor fascia latae as a joint capsule for the head-type prosthesis in the proximal humerus and proximal femur of post en bloc resection, and as collateral ligaments for the prosthesis in knee joints. We also applied teflon mesh wrapped around the segment of a prosthesis longer than 150 mm on which the origin or insertion of muscles was sutured (Fig. 2. right).

All the patients with knee joint replacements were instructed to wear a knee brace until the strength of the quadriceps muscles returned. The Functional

Evaluation Test was performed according to the new Enneking system. Radiographic analysis was done on the 15 cases with cementless fixation which were monitored for more than 3 years by the Implant Radiographic Evaluation Form of ISOLS.

Results

Oncological Results

The overall 5-year survival of 20 patients with osteosarcoma was evaluated as being 50% by the Kaplan-Meier methods. Two of the three patients, who had already developed metastases when they were initially seen, underwent thoracotomy and were both alive at 43 and 104 months after the operation. One other patient, who refused further treatment for bone metastases on the humerus and thoracic spine, died at 24 months postoperatively. Of the 17 patients who initially had no metastasis, 6 developed metastases and died at an average of 26.8 months postoperatively (range: 12–49 months), while 11 patients were disease-free at an average of 60 months postoperatively (range: 21–124 months). One patient with local recurrence seen on the distal femur at

Table 1. Functional evaluation by the new Enneking method of the results from the use of ceramic prostheses

A Replaced site	Number of cases	E	G	F	P	E and G (%)
Proximal femur	18	0	15	2	1	83
Distal femur	13	0	8	5	0	62
Proximal tibia	14	0	11	2	1	79
Proximal humerus[a]	13	2	10	1	0	92
Distal radius	3	0	2	0	1	67
Middle shaft	6	4	2	0	0	100
Pelvis[b]	2	0	0	1	1	0
Others	2	0	0	2	0	0
	71	6	48	13	4	76

[a] Includes 1 case in the scapula
[b] Includes 1 case in the pelvis with proximal femur replacement

B Resection procedure	Number of cases	E	G	F	P	E and G (%)
Wide resection	27	1	16	7	3	63
Contaminated wide resection	20	0	17	3	0	85
Marginal resection	24	5	15	3	1	83

C Stem-fixation method	Number of cases	E	G	F	P	E and G (%)
Cementless	34	2	23	7	2	74
Cemented	37	4	25	6	2	78

E, Excellent; *G*, good; *F*, fair; *P*, poor

34 months after surgery underwent amputation. He was disease-free at 59 months postoperatively.

Three out of five patients with chondrosarcoma were disease-free at an average of 57.3 months postoperatively (range: 43–82 months). One of the other two patients died from pulmonary metastases at 28 months postoperatively, and the remaining patient died from another cancer (bladder) at 14 months after surgery.

Six of the ten patients diagnosed as having the other sarcomas were disease-free at an average of 60.3 months postoperatively (range: 10–118 months) and one patient was alive with metastases at 47 months after surgery. One of the remaining three patients developed local recurrence and pulmonary metastases, and died at 10 months postoperatively. The other patient underwent replacement of hemipelvis for a huge malignant fibrous histiocytoma and died from metastases at 8 months postoperatively. The final patient was a 77-year-old female who died from heart failure at 36 months postoperatively.

All the 12 giant cell tumor cases were disease-free at an average of 59.5 months following surgery (range; 11–137 months).

Two patients with metastatic bone tumors were alive at 54 and 73 months postoperatively. The remaining 18 patients died at an average of 14.4 months postoperatively, ranging from 3 (chemotherapy-induced death) to 40 months.

Functional Results

The percentage of excellent and good was 76% in all the cases (Table 1). This percentage was better in the proximal femur, proximal tibia, proximal humurus, and midshaft than in the distal femur, distal radius, and pelvis. With regard to the results in resection procedures, this percentage was better in wide or marginal resections than in radical en bloc resections. There were no significant differences between the group with cementless fixation and the group in which cement was used.

Lower extremity. Fourteen out of 18 patients who had the lesion in the proximal femur, both of the patients with lesions in the femoral midshaft, and all of the twenty-seven patients with lesions in the knee joint could walk with or without a cane. The remaining four patients with lesions in the proximal femur needed a pair of crutches. Eight patients with lesions in the knee joint, consisting of 7 osteosarcoma and 1 huge giant cell tumor, had to wear the brace permanently. Four cases with the custom-made prostheses of the tuberositas tibia-preserving type demonstrated a better range of motion (approximately 0–90 degrees) than other cases with semi-modular types (approximately 0–60 degrees).

Upper extremity. Twelve out of thirteen patients whose lesion was in the shoulder joint could use the upper extremity satisfactory for daily life. The remaining patient had to wear the brace permanently since a head-type prosthesis was used for osteosarcoma. The range of motion of the shoulder joint was less than 90 degrees in flexion and abduction and 30 degrees in extension.

All the four patients with the humeral midshaft replacement could use the upper extremity almost normally. Two out of three patients with the replacement for the distal radius could use the hand satisfactory. In the case with replacement for the metacarpal, the prosthesis was finally removed since the joint of the proximal side dislocated.

Trunk. One of the two patients with the replacement for hemipelvis could walk with crutches. The remaining patient died before succeeding in standing.

Complications

There were 4 skin ulcers, 3 dislocations, 3 loosenings, 2 infections, 1 deformity, and 1 breakage.

All the skin ulcers, consisting of 2 cases on the proximal tibia and 2 on the proximal humerus, were successfully treated by skin flaps. All the 3 dislocated prostheses, including the foregoing 2 cases in the metacarpal and manubrium sterni, were removed. All the 3 loosenings took place in the cases with cementless fixation. Revision using a metal hinge prosthesis was done for the cases of osteosarcoma in the distal femur at 58 and 36 months after the initial replacement. Both cases with infection were successfully treated with continuous irrigation, antibiotics, cement beads, and revision using a metal prosthesis. Gradual varus deformity in the knee joint was seen in the case of a giant cell tumor, but this patient was asymptomatic except for the visible deformity at 137 months postoperatively. The breakage of the monocrystal alumina stem took place at 16 months postoperatively in the patient with osteosarcoma when he jumped on the affected limb. This patient was also given a metal hinge prosthesis.

Radiological Analysis

In each parameter of the Implant Radiographic Evaluation Form of ISOLS 1991, all the 13 patients were rated excellent or good for 1-Bone Remodelling and 2-Interface, excepting the 2 patients with clinical loosenings who were rated poor. All the 14 patients were rated excellent for 3-Anchorage, excepting the 1 patient with stem fracture. All the 15 patients were rated excellent with regard to 4-Implant body problems. In the 5-Implant Articulation Problems, all 14 patients were rated excellent except for 1 patient with valgus knee joint deformity.

Good incorporation of the prosthesis into the newly formed bone surrounding the stem and segment was observed in all the 13 patients except for the 2 patients who had complications of clinical loosenings (Fig. 3).

Discussion

The advantages of alumina ceramics as biocompatible materials were exhibited in the cases with low-grade malignant or benign aggressive tumors. However, the results in the cases with high-grade malignancies were varied,

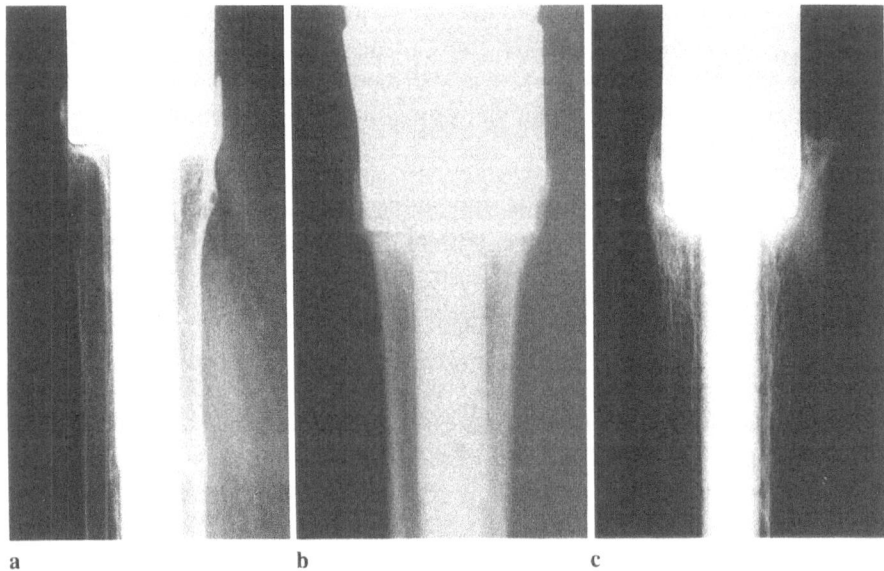

a   b   c

Fig. 3. Radiographs at the interface of the bone to the ceramic segment. Note the developing new bone along the segment and linear new bone around the stem with a thin (less than 1 mm) layer of clear zone. **a** At 4 years following the replacement for a giant cell tumor. **b** At 4 years following the replacement for a metastatic bone tumor. **c** At 7 years following the replacement for a low-grade chondrosarcoma

depending on the replaced sites. For example, in the cases of giant cell tumor, there was no complication at the 60 months' postoperative average follow-up, and functional results remained excellent or good in all the cases except for 1 case of huge tumor. Contrarily, in the cases of osteosarcoma around the knee joint, 6 out of 13 cases were rated fair or poor and four patients underwent revision. The reason for these poor results in the knee joint is that the ceramic prostheses in this series are all of the hingeless type. Wide resection and replacement with hingeless prostheses produce rather significant instability since the remaining muscle strength is not sufficient, in addition to there being defects of the sustaining ligaments. The fact that two patients who had giant cell tumor still maintain good function after 10 years suggests a favorable effect of the hingeless design for cases with minimal soft tissue resection. This may be because stress is thought to be partially absorbed by the laxity of the joint, in the same manner as in the physiological state, if the soft tissue reconstruction — especially collateral ligaments — is appropriately executed. This concept is consistent with the results of conventional total knee replacement models for osteoarthritis that have already been clarified. At present, no body has effective reconstruction methods for the soft tissues around sacrificed bone and joint [25]. Therefore, since 1987, we stopped using this ceramic prosthesis for osteosarcoma in the knee joint, although we prefer to use it for the low-grade malignant tumors.

The structure of the cup and ball mechanism in the hip and shoulder joints is also favorable for the adoption of the ceramic prosthesis which is almost a copy of the shape of the bone. Compared to these sites, the knee joint has restriction of bilateral motion. This structural difference is thought to be the explanation for the better results in the sites of the proximal femur. As to the proximal femur, a semi-modular prosthesis in this series can be indicated for any case since there was no case complicated by dislocation even in the one which included en bloc resection. However, for the case with wide resection of the proximal humerus including the deltoid muscle, we need to use the custom-made prosthesis with a scapula and constrained joint because the reconstruction of muscle insertions, which keeps the joint in physiological position, is impossible.

Any bone can be replaced with a custom-made prosthesis, but mere copy of the shape does not always work — we experienced failures in the sternum and metacarpal bones. Any functional joint structure is suitable for these sites. In any event, we need more experience in pelvis or distal radius replacements in which we have had rather satisfactory results. The reason for the good results in the midshaft of the humerus or femur is thought to be that the prosthesis is only required to supply the function of sustaining both ends of the bone without consideration of the joint function.

The strength of monocrystal or polycrystal alumina as the material for a prosthesis is considered to be satisfactory because there is only 1 case of breakage in this series. From other published reports, personal communications with other investigators, as well as from our own experience, the breakage of the prosthesis occurred during the operation, especially when the surgeon struck it with unusual force in an attempt to put the straight stem into the curved femoral shaft, or when the patient fell or jumped down on the affected limb. All these breakages occurred on the stem at a point 1–2 cm apart from the interface of the segment. These examples imply a fragile nature of the monocrystal alumina against shock, although this material is strong against gradual compression.

With regard to soft tissue reconstruction, the prosthesis of any material presently available is inferior to bone grafts, since no tissue attaches biologically to these artificial materials. To overcome this disadvantage, our methods of soft tissue reconstruction using the tensor fascia lata are useful, not only for the reconstruction of collateral ligaments in knee joints but also for that of joint capsules in other joints, such as the shoulder, hip, or wrist. Moreover, it also gives us a site on which the origins or insertions of the muscles can be attached. There were several reports that the application of artificial fabric, such as dacron or teflon, was useful for soft tissue reconstruction, and that a successful biological connection was observed [26, 27]. Our methods using the teflon mesh played a favorable role on the segment region of long prostheses.

Radiological analysis has demonstrated no problem as defined by the Implant Body and Implant Articulation. New bone formation was observed around the alunima ceramics, and the site of the interface to the host bone was stabilized spontaneously without bone graft. New bone growth was also observed on the stem. However, analysis of the cases with clinical loosening suggests the presence of a lever arm action of the prosthesis in which the stress on the joint affects the stem end, with the fulcrum at the point of the stabilized stem junction. Therefore, a very accurate fit of the stem and antirotators of the segment is required.

One more advantage of ceramic material is its minimal wear with time. The fact that there was no debris from the ceramics found around the prosthesis in autopsied subjects corroborates this finding. Debris is sometimes seen around metal prostheses in the form of metalosis.

In conclusion, alunima ceramics have clearly defined advantages over the other materials except for the restriction in constructing their design. The unfavorable results in knee joints are due to its hingeless construction, not to the fault of the material itself. It is impossible, at this time, to devise an all-ceramic hinged knee prosthesis since the axle of the hinge will break by impacting stress. We expect that the metal-ceramic composite prosthesis with a ceramic segment and a metal joint will eventually be available in order to enable long-term use as well as good postoperative function. Moreover, it would be advantageous if the surface of the ceramic part had a porous coat with beads and whose surface is also coated by bioactive ceramic, such as calcium hydroxyapatite.

References

1. Bos G, Sim FH, Pritchard DJ, Shives TC, Rock M, Askew L, Chao EYS (1987) Prosthetic replacement of the proximal humerus. Clin Orthop 224:178–191
2. Enneking WF (1986) A system of staging musculoskeletal neoplasms. Clin Orthop 204:9–23
3. Griend RAV, Enneking WF (1988) Radiologic imaging techniques in the diagnosis and treatment of osteogenic sarcoma. Sem Orthop 3-1:59–70
4. Heck DA, Chao EYS, Sim FH, Pritchard JD, Shives TC (1986) Titanium fibermetal segmental replacement prostheses. Clin Orthop 204:266–285
5. Kotz RI, Engel A (1983) Cement-free design of a tumor prosthesis for osteosarcoma of the distal femur and proximal tibia with a new technique for the ligamentum patellae. In: Chao EYS, Ivins JC (eds) Tumor prostheses for bone and joint reconstruction — the design and application. Thieme-Stratton, New York, pp 399–408
6. Capanna R, Biagini R, Ruggieri P, Bettelli G, Casadei R, Campanacci M (1989) Temporary resection arthrodesis of the knee using an intramedullary rod and bone cement. Int Orthop 13:253–258
7. Lewis MM (1986) The use of an expandable and adjustable prosthesis in the treatment of childhood malignant bone tumors of the extremity. Cancer 57:499–502
8. Scales JT, Sneath RS, Wright KWJ (1987) Design and clinical use of extending prostheses. In: Enneking WF (ed) Limb salvage in musculoskeletal oncology. Churchill-Livingstone, New York, pp 52–61
9. Verkerke GJ, Koops HS, Veth RPH, Kroonenberg HH, Grootenboer HJ, Nielsen HKL, Oldhoff J, Postma A (1990) An extendable modular endoprosthetic system for bone tumour management in the leg. J Biomed Eng 12:91–96

10. Capanna R, Leonessa C, Bettelli G, Borghi B, Cristofaro RD, Martelli C, Ruggieri P, Campanacci M (1987) Modular Kotz prosthesis — the Rizzoli experience. In: Yamamuro T (ed) New developments for limb salvage in muscloskeletal tumors. Springer, Tokyo, pp 37–44
11. Chao EYS, Sim FH (1987) Modular types of tumor endoprostheses for limb salvage. In: Enneking WF (ed) Limb salvage in musculoskeletal oncology. Churchill Livingstone, New York, pp 198–206
12. Chao EYS, Sim FH (1987) Biological and biomechanical justification of porous-coated modular segmental bone/joint prostheses. In: Yamamuro T (ed) New Developments for limb salvage in musculoskeletal tumors. Springer, Tokyo, pp 237–245
13. Knahr K, Salzer M, Plenk H Jr, Bohler M (1987) Long-term results with ceramic tumor prostheses. In: Yamamuro T (ed) New developments for limb salvage in musculoskeletal tumors. Springer, Tokyo, pp 295–304
14. Kotz RI (1988) Tumour resection and prosthesis in the therapy of the osteosarcoma. Sem Orthop 3-1:21–39
15. Malawer MM, Canfield D, Meller I (1987) Porous-coated segmental prosthesis for large tumor defects — a prosthesis based upon immediate fixation (PMMA) and extracortical bone fixation. In: Yamamuro T (ed) New developments for limb salvage in musculoskeletal tumors. Springer, Tokyo, pp 247–255
16. Okada Y, Suka T, Sim FH, Gorski JP, Chao EYS (1988) Comparison of replacement prostheses for segmental defect of bone — different porous coating for extracortical fixation. J Bone Joint Surg [Am] 70:160–172
17. Poitout D (1987) Megaprosthesis — massive osteochondral allograft. In: Yamamuro T (ed) New developments for limb salvage in musculoskeletal tumors. Springer, Tokyo, pp 377–386
18. Hayashi H, Uchida A, Hamada H, Yoshikawa H, Shinto Y, Ono K (to be published) Ceramic prostheses for the management of malignant bone tumors. Int Orthop
19. Gebhardt MC, Roth YF, Mankin HJ (1990) Osteoarticular allografts for reconstruction in the proximal part of the humerus after excision of a musculoskeletal tumor. J Bone Joint Surg [Am] 72:334–345
20. Mankin HJ, Gebhardt MC, Tomford WW (1987) The use of frozen cadaveric allografts in the management of patients with bone tumors of the extremities. Orthop Clin North Am 18-2:275–289
21. Uyttendaele D, Schryver AD, Claessens H, Roels H, Berkvens P, Mondelaers W (1988) Limb conservation in primary bone tumors by resection, extracorporeal irradiation and re-implantation. J Bone Joint Surg [Br] 70:349–353
22. Yamamuro T, Kotoura Y, Kasahara K, Takahashi M, Abe M (1987) Intraoperative radiotherapy and ceramic prosthesis replacement for osteosarcoma. In: Yamamuro T (ed) New developments for limb salvage in musculoskeletal tumors. Springer, Tokyo, pp 327–333
23. Lord CF, Gebhardt MC, Tomford WW, Mankin HJ (1988) Infection in bone allografts- incidence, nature and treatment. J Bone Joint Surg [Am] 70:369–376
24. Yamamuro T (1985) Recent advances in orthopaedic ceramic implants. J Jpn Orthop Ass 59:339–348
25. Matsumoto S, Kawaguchi N, Ammino K, Manabe J, Furuya K, Isobe Y (1987) Results of alumina-ceramic endoprostheses used for bone tumor cases. In: Yamamuro T (ed) New developments for limb salvage in musculoskeletal tumors. Springer, Tokyo, pp 309–312

26. Shinjo K, Makiyama T, Nagaya I, Asai T, Okayama N, Saito S, Miyake N, Furusawa H, Yamaji T, Tuboi S (1986) Reconstruction of malignant bone tumor by composite graft of biomaterials (in Japanese). Orthopaedia Ceramic Implants 6:115–119
27. Yanase Y, Tanaka S, Tomihara M, Soen S, Yamasaki H (1987) New technique for providing ligamentous stability in prosthetic replacement of the knee for tumors. In: Yamamuro T (ed) New developments for limb salvage in musculoskeletal tumors. Springer, Tokyo, pp 305–308

Limb Salvage by Custom Prosthesis: Madras Experience

M.V. Natarajan, V. Shantha, and S. Krishnamurthi[1]

Introduction

Management of patients with musculo-skeletal neoplasms has always been one of the most challenging areas in oncology. Current concepts in the biological behavior of tumors, clinical staging, oncological surgery and adjuvant chemotherapy have enabled local tumor control by resection without ablation [1, 2]. Reconstruction of the skeletal defect by custom prosthesis is an accepted method of management [3–8]. Limb salvage by custom prosthesis is still in its infancy in India due to the undeveloped technology for fabrication and the prohibitive cost of the prosthesis.

The present work on limb salvage in malignant bone tumors has been done at the Musculo Skeletal Tumour Service, Cancer Institute, and Muthulakshmi College of Oncologic Sciences, Madras, India.

Criteria of Selection

Cases of malignant osteoclastomas, osteosarcomas, and chondrosarcomas which are high- or low-grade and intra- or extra-compartmental are included in the program. Cases with extensive muscle involvement, neurovascular involvement, pathological fracture, and inappropriate biopsy scar are excluded.

Examinations

The examinations done at the Institute include plain X-ray, scanogram, CT scan, angiogram, and Technitium (Tc) bone scan. A scanogram is done in all cases to evaluate the extent of the tumor and level of resection. Angiograms are done in cases of osteosarcomas to determine the relation of major vascular

[1] Musculo Skeletal Tumour Service, Cancer Institute and Muthulakshmi College of Oncological Sciences, Madras 600 020, Tamil Nadu State, India

bundles to the tumor and its vascularity. Tc scans are also done in cases of sarcomas to determine the extent of the lesion and presence of metastasis.

CT scans are done to evaluate the intra- and extraosseous extension of the tumor. CT of the chest is done in cases of sarcomas to detect early metastasis. The CT scan is used for determining the dimensions of the prosthesis to be manufactured, as will be described below.

Biopsy

Closed biopsy using a trephine with the patient under local anesthesia is done for tissue diagnosis. For cases in which an open biopsy was done elsewhere, the slides are re-evaluated in the Patholgy Department of the Institute. Frozen section studies are done during surgery to determine tumor clearance, and electron microscopic studies are done on the excised tumor.

CT-Assisted Designing of Custom Prothesis

The CT scan enables the following dimensions to be evaluated accurately for manufacturing the custom prosthesis.

Distal femur/proximal tibia
1. Level of tumor clearance
2. Level of resection (length of body of prosthesis)
3. Outer diameter of bone at resection level (diameter of body of prosthesis)
4. Inner diameter of remnant bone (intramedullary (IM) component length and diameter)
5. Dimension of adjacent bone (condyle and IM component)

Proximal humerus
1. Diameter of humeral head (prosthesis head diameter)
2. Level of resection (length of body)
3. Outer diameter of bone at resection level (diameter of body)
4. Inner diameter of remnant bone (IM componant length and diameter)

Fabrication of the Prosthesis

With the above dimensions, a blueprint drawing is made of the required custom prosthesis. This is sent to the manufacturers, and a period of 3 weeks is required to fabricate the stainless steel prosthesis. More recently, we have had the prosthesis made of titanium alloy, which is comparatively stronger and lighter. All the prosthesis have required intramedullary cement fixation.

Chemotherapy Protocol

Patients with osteosarcomas who are deemed fit for the limb salvage program undergo 3 courses of preoperative chemotherapy. Following surgery, they undergo 3 more courses of chemotherapy. The cycle is repeated every 3 weeks. The chemotherapeutic schedule is as follows:

Ifosphamide $1.3 \, mg/m^2/day$ on days 1 and 2
Epirubicin $60 \, mg/m^2/day$ on day 1
Cis-Platinum $100 \, mg/m^2$ in divided doses on days 1, 2, and 3

Clinical Material

A total of 30 patients (13 males and 17 females) have thus far been treated by custom prosthesis at our Institute. Their ages ranged from 12 to 54 years (mean: 25 years). The follow-up period ranged from 2 to 30 months (mean: 16 months).

Histopathologically, there were 15 malignant osteoclastomas, 11 osteosarcomas, and 4 chondrosarcomas. The anatomical sites of lesion were the distal femur (10), proximal tibia (9), proximal humerus (9), and proximal femur (2). The tumors were staged as IA (8), IB (8), IIA (10), and IIB (4). The surgical margins of resection were wide in 25 cases and marginal in 5 cases. The length of resection ranged from 60 to 180 mm (average: 123 mm).

Case Reports

Distal Femur

The patient was a 33-year-old female who presented with an osteolytic lesion in the distal third of the left femur, involving both the condyles (Fig. 1). The closed biopsy diagnosis was that of a giant cell tumor grade III. A CT scan was done to measure the dimensions, and a custom prosthesis was designed and fabricated. Wide excision of the tumor with custom knee replacement was carried out (Fig. 2). At follow-up 30 months postoperatively, she was walking well. Knee flexion was 100° and there was no extensor lag.

Proximal Humerus

This 13-year-old female presented with an expansile lesion in the proximal third of the left humerus (Fig. 3). Biopsy revealed it to be an osteosarcoma. Preoperative chemotherapy was given in 3 cycles. Tikhoff Linberg resection and custom humeral replacement were done (Fig. 4). The patient had 3 cycles of postoperative chemotherapy. At 18 months, there was a 30° circumduction of the shoulder with good elbow and hand function.

Proximal Tibia

This 26-year-old male presented with a painful swelling in the proximal third of the right tibia of 3 months' duration. Two years previously, he had been treated elsewhere by curettage and grafting for a osteoclastoma tibia. He developed a recurrence of the tumor for which he had radiotherapy. Closed

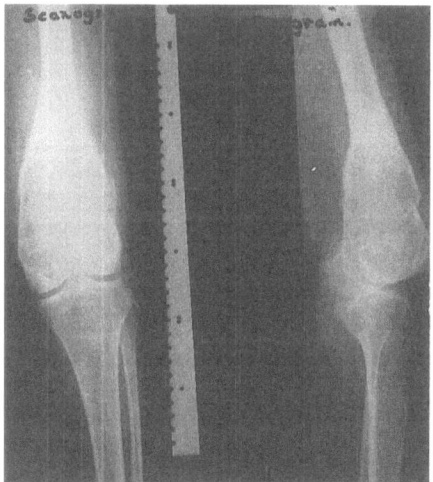
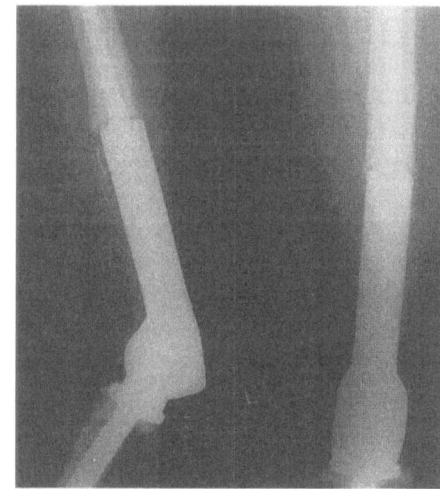

Fig. 1.   Fig.

Fig. 1. Giant cell tumor in the distal one-third of the left femur

Fig. 2. Postoperative X-ray of the custom prosthesis fitted to the left femur shown in Fig. 1

biopsy revealed the lesion to be a giant cell tumor (GCT) grade III. A wide excision was made and a custom prosthetic replacement was performed. The medial gastrocnemius with intact blood supply was transposed to cover the prosthesis. He was mobilized with an orthosis. At follow-up 21 months postoperatively there was a 100° flexion of the knee and a 20° extensor lag.

Proximal Femur

The patient, a 15-year-old female with multiple exostosis, presented with the complaint of an increasing area of swelling in the proximal third of the left femur of 7 months' duration. An open biopsy revealed the lesion to be a low-grade chondrosarcoma. The swelling was extending anteriorly, laterally, and posteriorly in the upper femur. There was no neurovascular deficit. Wide excison surgery was carried out and a custom upper femoral endoprothesis was fitted. The postoperative period was uneventful and the patient was mobilized with the use of crutches. At follow-up 12 months postoperatively, she was able to walk independently with good movements at the hip.

Functional Results

Functional results were rated according to Enneking's classification: 3% (1) had excellent results, 60% (18) had good results, 30% (9) had fair results, and 7% (2) had poor results.

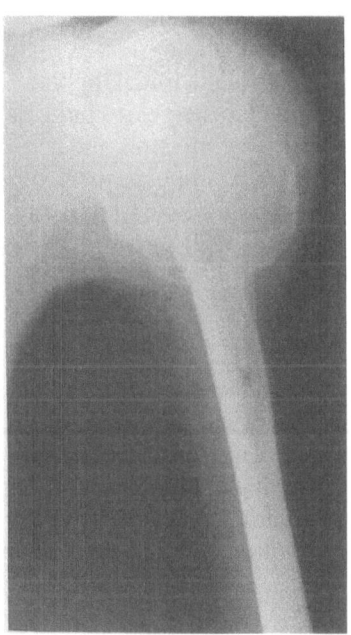

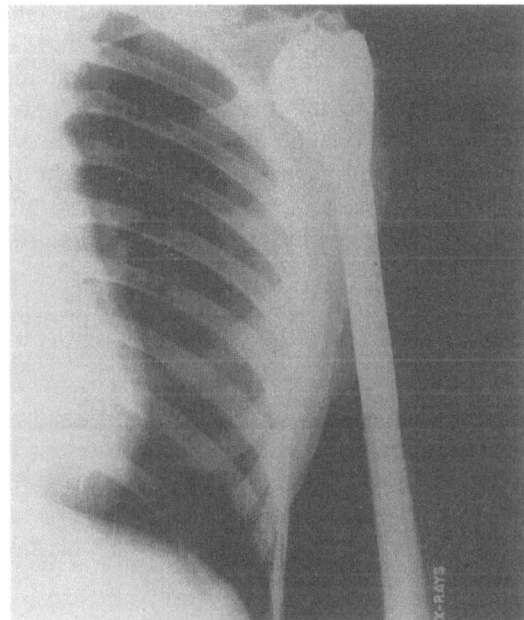

Fig. 3.   **Fig. 4.**

Fig. 3. Osteosarcoma in the proximal one-third of the left humerus

Fig. 4. Postoperative X-ray of the custom prosthesis fitted to the left humerus shown in Fig. 3

Complications

The intraoperative complications, which were later repaired, included injury to the popliteal artery in one patient and injury to the lateral popliteal nerve in another. In one patient, the intramedullary component of the tibial prosthesis had an incorrect diameter and would not enter the tibial shaft. A vertical split was made in the tibia in order to seat the prosthesis. The same patient developed superficial skin necrosis which was treated with a split skin graft. Flap necrosis, occurring in 1 case (3.3%), was excised and treated with a fascio-cutaneous flap.

Deep wound infection as the etiology for prosthesis failure occurred in 2 cases (6.6%). Ultimately, both underwent above knee amputation. The local recurrence rate in our series was 6.6% (2), and both patients had osteosarcomas. One of these patient underwent a hind quarter amputation, and both of them died of secondary metastasis to the chest.

Mechanical failure of the implant occurred in 2 cases. Three months after the first implantation, one patient with a prosthesis of the distal femur fell and bent the stainless steel hinge prosthesis at the junction between the shaft and the IM component. The implant was revised with a titanium hinge prosthesis, and the patient had excellent function for 1 year after which she fell once again. This time there was a breakage between the shaft and the IM component. The second revision was done and a Howmedica Kinematic Rotating Hinge knee was implanted. The results showed that mechanically failed initial implants can be revised with subsequent useful limb function. Flap necrosis could be avoided by obtaining adequate soft tissue coverage. Deep infection and local recurrence imply a predisposition to failure and ended in amputation in our experience. The complications which arise after limb-salvage surgery are many, but can be successfully treated in the majority of cases.

Summary

Limb-salvage surgery for malignant bone tumors has now been well established. The methods of reconstruction following resection vary. Custom prothesis is now well accepted in the treatment of tumors. The complications are many and this surgery should be performed by well-trained surgeons in selective centers for the comprehensive management of tumor patients. We at the Cancer Institute, Madras are pleased with the early results of limb preservation with custom prosthesis.

References

1. Enneking WF, Spanier SS, Goodman MA (1980) A system for the surgical staging of musculo-skeletal sarcoma. Clin Orthop 153:106–120
2. Marcove RC, Rosen G (1980) En block resection for osteogenic sarcoma. Cancer 45:3040–3044
3. Bradish CF, Kemp HBS, Scales JT (1987) Distal femoral replacement by custom-made prothesis. Clinical follow-up and survivorship analysis. J Bone Joint Surg [Br] 69(2):276–284
4. Burrows HJ, Scales JT (1975) Excision of tumour of the humerus and femur with restoration by internal prothesis. J Bone Joint Surgery [Br] 57:148–159
5. Marcove R, Lewis M, Rosen G (1977) Total femur and total knee replacement. Clin Orthop 126:147–152
6. Ross AC, Wilson JN, Scales JT (1987) Endoprosthetic replacement of the proximal humerus. J Bone Joint Surg [Br] 69(4):656–661
7. Sim FH, Chao EYS (1979) Prosthetic replacement of the knee and a large segment of tibia or femur. J Bone Joint Surg [Am] 61:887–892
8. Sim FH (1985) Limb-sparing surgery for osteosarcoma: Mayo Clinic experience. Cancer Treatment Symp 3:139–154

Vascularized Bone Grafting for Bone Defects after Removal of Bone and Soft Tissue Tumors in the Limb-Saving Procedures

Akio Minami and Kiyoshi Kaneda[1]

Introduction

Preoperative and postoperative chemotherapies and operative techniques have been developed to control malignant bone and soft tissue tumors [1, 2]. In addition, Enneking et al. reported that a surgical staging system of musculoskeletal sarcoma had a high degree of compliance and accuracy in both surgical planning and end result studies [3]. Limb-saving procedures have been attempted for malignant tumors in the extremities, and it was found that radical oncological surgery is not always incompatible with the preservation of limb functions [4–6]. On the other hand, vascularized bone graftings (VBGs) have been applied to various orthopedic diseases, of which many excellent results have been reported [7–10]. We have performed reconstructive surgery by VBGs for bone defects after wide removal of malignant bone and soft tissue tumors in the extremities. The following is a report on the operative procedures of VBGs and the limb functions regained after such surgery.

Materials and Methods

A total of twelve patients (5 males and 7 females) with bone and soft tissue tumors were involved in this study. Their ages at VBG ranged from 12 to 53 years (average: 24 years). The follow-up periods ranged from 1 year and 5 months to 13 years and 9 months (average: 5 years and 10 months). Data of all the cases are summarized in Table 1. One lesion was malignant soft tissue tumor (angiosarcoma in the flexor side of the forearm) and 11 were bone tumors. Nine of the eleven cases were malignant tumors comprised of osteosarcoma (7), chondrosarcoma (1), and angiosarcoma (1), and the remain-

[1] Department of Orthopaedic Surgery, Hokkaido University School of Medicine, Sapporo, Japan

Table 1. All data of cases with bone and soft tissue tumors

Case No.	Age (years)	Sex	Site	Diagnosis	Stage	Procedure	Chemothrapy Pre-	Chemothrapy Post-	Reconstructive surgery Primary	Reconstructive surgery Secondary	Fibula	Remarks
1	17	F	Tibia	Osteosarcoma	IIB	Wide	Yes	Yes	Total knee replacement	Knee arthrodesis	Pedicled	
2	15	M	Femur	Osteosarcoma	IIB	Marginal	Yes	Yes	Knee arthrodesis +autoclaved bone		Free	
3	17	F	Tibia	Osteosarcoma	IIB	Wide	Yes	Yes	Knee arthrodesis +autoclaved bone		Pedicled	
4	22	F	Tibia	Osteosarcoma	IIB	Wide	Yes	Yes	Total knee replacement	Knee arthrodesis	Pedicled and free	
5	17	M	Femur	Osteosarcoma	IIB	Marginal	Yes	Yes	Knee arthrodesis +autoclaved bone		Free	Metastasis
6	27	M	Tibia	Giant cell tumor	IA	Intralesional	No	No	Strut graft		Pedicled	
7	12	F	Forearm	Angiosarcoma	IIB	Wide	Yes	Yes	Strut graft		Free	
8	15	F	Ulna	Osteosarcoma	IIB	Wide	No	No	Resection	Strut graft	Free	
9	38	F	Radius	Giant cell tumor	IA	Curative	No	No	Strut graft		Free	
10	36	M	Humerus	Chondrosarcoma	IB	Curative	No	No	Shoulder arthrodesis		Free	
11	53	F	Radius	Angiosarcoma	IB	Curative	No	Yes	Strut graft		Free	
12	19	F	Humerus	Osteosarcoma	IIB	Wide	No	No	Shoulder arthrodesis		Free	Fracture

Pre., preoperative; *Post.,* postoperative

ing 2 were benign giant cell tumors. The affected sites of the 11 bone tumor cases were tibia (4), femur (2), humerus (2), radius (2), and ulna (1). A malignant soft tissue tumor (angiosarcoma) was observed in the anterior aspect of the forearm.

According to the surgical staging system of Enneking et al. [3], 8 cases were in stage IIB, 2 in IB, and the remaining 2 in IA. The surgical margin was determined according to the report of the Bone and Soft Tissue Tumor Committee of the Japanese Orthopaedic Association. At the VBG procedure, the surgical margin was curative in 3 cases, wide in 6, marginal in 2, and intralesional in 1.

In 9 cases, VBGs were primarily performed simultaneously with the wide resection of the tumor, and the graftings were secondarily performed in the remaining 3 cases. In the latter, total artificial knee replacement (2) and simple resection (1) were carried out.

The fibula was used as the donor of the vascularized bone for all cases. We performed 13 VBGs in 12 cases; the method of harvesting the fibula was described in our previous papers [7, 9, 10]. A vascularized fibula with skin was harvested in 9 out of 13 procedures. Free vascularized fibular grafting was performed in 9 cases, and pedicled grafting in 4, 1 of which was grafted with both free and pedicled fibulae.

Arthrodeses were performed following removal of the tumors surrounding the joint in 7 cases, 5 of which underwent knee arthrodesis and the remaining 2 underwent shoulder arthrodesis. Autoclaved bones including tumor tissue were applied to 3 of the 5 knee arthrodesis cases. A vascularized fibula was used as a strut graft in 4 cases and as an arthroplasty of the wrist in 1 case of a giant cell tumor at the distal end of the radius.

Preoperative and/or postoperative chemotherapies were administered in combination with surgery in 7 out of 12 cases.

Results

The vascularized bone graftings (VBGs) resulted in substantial bone unions in all cases. The time periods between the VBGs and bone unions were less than 4 months in all cases with one exception, in which the bone union occurred 6 months after the procedure. The follow-up periods averaged 5 years and 10 months. Thus far, there has been no local recurrence. However, metastasis occurred in the lung 7 months after the VBG in the case of osteosarcoma. We surgically removed the metastatic tumor in the lung and the patient is now free from the disease (1 year after removal of the metastatic tumor).

Clinical results were evaluated according to the modified system for functional evaluation of reconstruction after tumor resection described by Enneking et al. [3]. Postoperative results in all cases are summarized in Table 2. Overall clinical results in all cases were satisfactory.

Postoperative complication occurred in the case of chondrosarcoma at the proximal end of the humerus (case 10). Stress fracture occurred 1 year after

Table 2. Functional evaluation of all cases

Lower extremity lesions

Case no.	Pain	Function	Emotional acceptance	External supports	Walking ability	Gait	Total points
1	5	1	3	5	5	3	22
2	5	1	3	3	3	1	16
3	5	1	3	3	3	1	16
4	5	1	3	3	3	1	16
5	5	1	3	3	3	1	16
6	5	5	5	5	5	5	30

Upper extremity lesions

Case	Pain	Function	Emotional acceptance	Head positioning	Dexterity	Lifting ability	Total points
7	5	5	5	5	5	5	30
8	5	5	5	5	5	5	30
9	3	3	5	3	5	3	22
10	5	3	3	3	5	3	22
11	5	5	5	5	5	5	30
12	5	3	3	3	5	3	22

(by modified Enneking's functional evaluation system)

obtaining the bone union. Since the application of a body cast did not achieve bone union, the patient was successfully treated with an additional conventional bone grafting.

Case Report

Case 11

A 53-year-old housewife noticed pain in her right forearm in July, 1984. In September, excisional biopsy was performed in another hospital and, from its macroscopic appearance, the tumor was judged to be benign. Curettage and bone grafting were performed at the site of lesion. The patient was first seen in our hospital with the pathological diagnosis of the tumor being angiosarcoma (malignant hemangioendothelioma) (Fig. 1). On October 4, a wide resection of the tumor was performed. The tissues resected from the radius were 12 cm long. The muscles, including the pronator teres, flexor pollicis longus, abductor pollicis longus, and extensor carpi radialis brevis surrounding the tumor, were also removed, and the palmaris longus was transferred to the extensor pollicis longus for extension and abduction of the thumb. A free vascularized fibular grafting with skin was carried out. Postoperative circulation monitored by the peroneal flap was good. Postoperative chemotherapy started 3 weeks after surgery. Bone unions of both sides were achieved 2 months postoperatively. At 6 years after the surgery, there has been no local recurrence or distant metastasis, and almost normal functions of the hand have been achieved (Fig. 2).

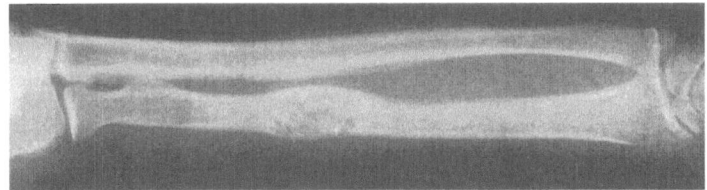

Fig. 1. A 53-year-old female with a malignant hemangioendothelioma in the right radius (case 11). Preoperative X-ray showed expansible destruction of the shaft

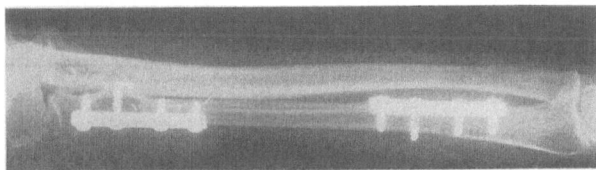

Fig. 2. X-ray 6 years after wide resection of the tumor and the vascularized bone grafting showed an excellent bone union of both ends

Discussion

Our results suggest that the VBG is effective for saving limb functions in cases of massive bone defect following wide resection of tumor in the extremities. Several reconstructive procedures for bone defects following wide resection of tumor in the extremities have been reported, including replacement by artificial joints, allogeneic bone, and conventional bone grafting [3–8]. However, various problems are inherent in these procedures: since they require the use of materials foreign to the body, the immune systems can be affected and bone union may be delayed. In VBG, the vascularized bone shows neither an immune response to the recipient nor a creeping substitution, revealing rapid incorporation of the vascularized bone into the recipient bone.

The only problem we confronted was that the fibula was too small to be loaded with more than a certain given weight. Hypertrophy of the grafted fibula can be expected in children; however, this is not anticipated our series. On the other hand, it is possibile for fatigue fracture to occur at the grafted fibula. To resolve this problem we use autoclaved bone combined with vascularized bone with the expectation that this combination would achieve bone conduction and induction. In these cases, bone union of the recipient bone with the vascularized fibula was observed within 3 months, whereas bone union of the recipient bone with the autoclaved bone was observed after about 1.5 years. This method is very easily applied to the replacement of massive bone defect and especially valuable in Japan where it is difficult to obtain allogeneic bone.

Conclusions

The VBG is a beneficial procedure for treating various orthopedic diseases; the method of the VBG with skin is particularly effective in tumor surgery, not only for monitoring but also for complementing the skin defect which frequently develops after tumor resection [7].

The question arises whether the VBG should be performed primarily or secondarily. From the technical point of view, primary reconstruction is much easier than secondary reconstruction. One of the disadvantages of the primary reconstruction is, however, that there is a possibility that local recurrence or distant metastasis of the tumor may occur. Primary reconstruction should be performed only when it is assured that the surgical margin of the tumor is sufficiently wide. Unfortunately, little is known about the countereffects of preoperative or postoperative chemotherapy on the patency of the vascular anastomosis or of the healing process of the grafted tissue [11]. This is also a disadvantage in primary reconstruction. Further basic research on this subject is recommended.

References

1. Cortes EP, Holland IF, Wang JJ, Sinks LF (1973) Chemotherapy of advanced osteosarcoma. Colston Paper No.8. Bone — Certain aspects of neoplasia. Butterworths, London, pp 265–275
2. Jaffe N, Peed D (1972) Recent advances in the chemotherapy of metastatic osteogenic sarcoma. Cancer 30:1627–1633
3. Enneking WF, Spanier SS, Goodman MA (1980) A system for the surgical staging of musculo-skeletal sarcoma. Clin Orthop 153:106–126
4. Eilber FR, Eckard J, Morton DL (1984) Advances in the treatment of sarcomas of the extremity. Current status of limb salvage. Cancer 54:2685–2693
5. Jaffe N, Watts H, Fellow K, Vawter G (1978) Local en bloc resection for limb preservation. Cancer Treat Rep 62:217–225
6. Rosen G, Murphy ML, Huvos AG, Gutierrez M, Marcov RC (1976) Chemotherapy, en bloc resection, and prosthetic bone replacement of osteogenic sarcoma. Cancer 37:1–20
7. Minami A, Ogino T, Usui M, Minami M (1986) Simultaneous reconstruction of bone and skin defects by free fibular graft with a skin flap. Microsurgery 7:38–45
8. Usui M, Ishii S, Yamamura M, Minami A, Sakuma T (1986) Microsurgical reconstructive surgery following wide resection of bone and soft tissue sarcomas in the upper extremities. J Reconstr Microsurg 2:77–84
9. Minami A, Ogino T, Sakuma T, Itoga H, Usui M (1987) Free vascularized fibular graft for the treatment of a congenital pseudoarthrosis of the tibia. Microsurgery 8:111–116
10. Minami A, Itoga H, Suzuki K (1990) Reverse-flow vascularized fibular graft: A new method. Microsurgery 11:278–281
11. Friedlaender GE, Tross RB, Doganis AC, Kirkwood JM, Baron R (1984) Effects of chemotherapeutic agents on bone. I. Short-term methotrexate and doxorubicin (Adriamycin) treatment in a rat model. J Bone Joint Surg [Am] 66:602–620

4.7

Soft Tissue Reconstruction in Limb-Sparing Tumor Surgery

Koichiro Ihara, Kazuteru Doi, Kazuhiro Sakai, Kenji Kido, Tetsuro Kishimoto, and Shinya Kawai[1]

Introduction

Limb-sparing surgery for bone and soft tissue sarcomas has become more widespread along with the development of adjuvant therapy and several kinds of imaging techniques for analyzing local tumor extension [1]. This procedure can be indicated for surgical treatment of the tumor, unless a major neurovascular structure is involved by the tumor, although vascular reconstruction may be possible in order to achieve an adequate margin [2]. However, the incision is sometimes too extensive to be closed directly after a particularly wide excision of the tumor and, furthermore, resection of muscles following tumor excision might result in a certain loss of function of the extremity. As a result, soft tissue reconstruction is regarded as the keystone of extending the indication for limb-salvage surgery and achieving favorable use of the extremities. While others have reported the use of pedicle flaps for wound coverage with satisfactory results [3, 4], the authors have been applying microsurgical tissue transfer for soft tissue reconstruction in limb-sparing tumor surgery. The selection of flaps depends on the size and content of the soft tissue defects. From our experience, the results are encouraging, and a much lower complication rate and better limb function can be expected.

Materials and Methods

Since 1985, free skin and musculocutaneous flaps have been indicated at our institution for the surgical treatment of 14 tumors, which included 11 soft tissue sarcomas and 3 locally aggressive or malignant bone tumors. The backgrounds of these patients are summarized in Table 1.

---

[1] Department of Orthopedic Surgery, Yamaguchi University School of Medicine, Ube, Yamaguchi, 755 Japan

Table 1. Clinical backgrounds of cases

Case	Age (years)	Sex	Side	Site	Diagnosis	Stage	Presentation
1	48	M	R	Post. thigh	Liposarcoma	III	1st Local recurrence
2	52	M	L	Post. thigh	Liposarcoma	IB	
3	25	F	R	Ant. thigh	Leiomyosarcoma	IIA	1st Local recurrence
4	37	F	R	Post. thigh	Liposarcoma	IB	Marginal excision
5	62	M	R	Med. thigh	Liposarcoma	IB	
6	55	M	R	Ant. thigh	MFH	IIA	Marginal excision
7	36	M	R	Lat. thigh	Liposarcoma	IB	
8	9	M	L	Popliteal	MFH	IIB	1st Local recurrence
9	75	F	R	Popliteal	Malignant schwannoma	IIB	3rd Local recurrence
10	56	F	L	Ant. thigh	Extraskeletal myxoid CS	IIA	
11	28	M	L	Femur	MFH	IIB	
12	47	M	R	Femur	Chondrosarcoma	IB	Biopsy
13	34	F	R	Dorsum of hand	Angiosarcoma	III	5th Local recurrence
14	35	F	R	Radius	GCT	3	

Post., Posterior; *Ant.*, anterior; *MFH*, malignant fibrous histiocytoma; *CS*, chondrosarcoma; *GCT*, giant cell tumor

Tumor excision was performed with the aim of preserving an adequately wide margin, although an insufficient margin (only around small areas of the tumor) was possible in 3 cases, which included 2 marginal and 1 intralesional procedure. An additional wide excision was immediately carried out for the intralesional case of angiosarcoma of the dorsum of left hand. The common peroneal nerve was resected together with the tumor in 3 cases.

In each case, a free flap was selected for wound closure and/or functional reconstruction. A groin flap was indicated for the skin coverage in 2 cases of the upper extremity (cases 13 and 14), in both of which a large area of skin needed to be excised due to skin invasion by tumor tissue and a transverse biopsy incision, respectively. The size of each flap was 17.5×13.5 cm and 12×6 cm. A latissimus dorsi musculocutaneous flap was indicated in 12 cases for the dual purpose of wound closure and functional muscle transfer. The maximum size of skin flap was 33×11 cm (average: 22×10 cm) and the maximum length of muscle was 38 cm (average: 29 cm). Both ends of the muscle were tightly sutured to a stump of excised muscle or a fascia of remaining muscles, with maintenance of an appropriate tension. The thoracodorsal nerve was anastomosed to motor nerves supplying an excised muscle at a proximal portion of the recipient site so that an activation of the transferred muscle could be accomplished following nerve regeneration. The donor site was closed by direct approximation in all cases.

Concerning the operation time required, the procedure for a tumor excision varied from 2 to 6 h, whereas the time needed for a free tissue transfer was relatively constant, taking 1 or 2 h for harvesting a flap and 1.5 h for tissue transfer and microsurgical anastomosis. A whole procedure required 5–10 h, with an average of 7 h. The volume of blood loss was 485–3,100 ml (average: 1,300 ml).

Perioperative adjuvant chemotherapy was performed in 11 cases. Preoperative administration was indicated in 10 cases, mainly by means of intra-arterial infusion of 0.8 mg/kg Adriamycin for 2 consequtive days, excepting 2 cases of systemic administration, while postoperative chemotherapy was applied in 9 cases. CYVADIC regimen, which is a combination of cyclophosphamide, vincristine, Adriamycin, and dacarbazine, was indicated for soft tissue sarcomas. In one case of malignant fibrous histiocytoma of the femur, a combination of high-dose methotrexate, Adriamycin, and *cis*-platinum was administered. Radiotherapy was not indicated in any cases.

Results

The mean follow-up period was 29 months, ranging from 8 to 58 months, and 9 cases were followed for more than 2 years.

Oncological Results

No local recurrence occurred, and a lung metastasis appeared in one case of chondrosarcoma 1.5 years after surgery. Two cases, including the latter and one of stage III, are surviving with lung metastases. The other patient with stage III of liposarcoma has died, whereas 11 patients are surviving without any evidence of disease.

Complications

In all cases, the flaps completely survived, although early surgical intervention was necessary for the salvage of vascular function in 3 cases. In 2 cases, venous thromboses were caused by a compression of adjacent arteries, whereas in the 3rd case, the area drained by the vein did not match with that of the skin flap, and another vein was anastomosed. All of these complications did not seem to be related to preoperative chemotherapy. There was no problem of wound healing, and no schedule of postoperative chemotherapy was affected in any case. Donor site morbidity was minimal in all cases.

Recovery of Transferred Muscles

Twelve transferred latissimus dorsi muscles were periodically examined by means of electromyography, and eleven recovered successfully, except in one 75-year-old patient. Motor unit potential appeared at 3.5–6 months postoperatively (average: 5 months). As the transferred muscles recovered and worked effectively as supplemental muscles, function of the involved limb gradually improved.

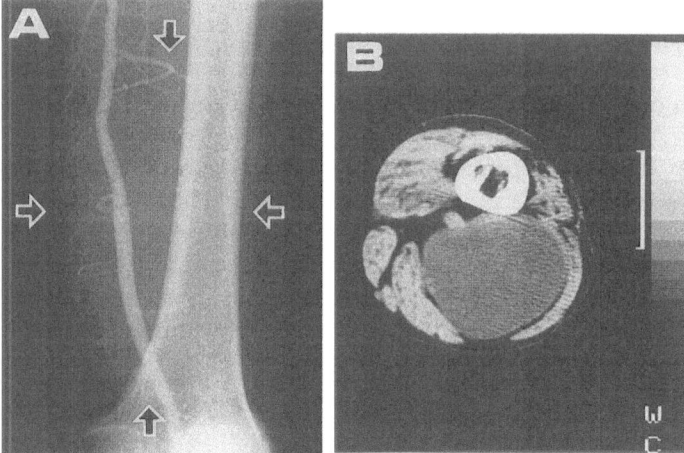

Fig. 1A,B. A The tumor is hypovascular and there is no involvement of the major vessel (*arrows*). **B** The tumor is present between hamstring muscles and is close to vessels and femur

Limb Function

Based on Enneking's system, the results in 2 cases were evaluated as excellent and in 12 as good [5]. With regard to power of knee extension or flexion for which functional muscle transfer had been indicated, the results of the evaluation of muscle manual test were good in all cases except for case 10 in Table 1.

Case Report

A 52-year-old male presented at our clinic with a large mass on the posterior aspect of the left thigh. A CT-scan revealed a large low-density tumor between the hamstring muscles (Fig. 1).

At surgery, all the posterior compartment muscles were excised with the tumor, and a common peroneal nerve was excised as well, since it was involved in a scar of the biopsy tract. A left latissimus dorsi muscle was transferred with skin flap, and thoracodorsal vessels and nerve were anastomosed at the buttock region (Fig. 2).

The patient could not flex the knee against gravity for a while after the operation. The muscle was then reinnervated (4 months postoperatively) and gradually recovered until he now obtains powerful knee flexion. The donor site healed uneventfully by direct closure (Fig. 3).

Discussion

In limb-sparing tumor surgery, a relatively high incidence of complications related to soft tissues has often been reported, especially in cases of malignant bone tumors [6, 7]. An elevation of large skin flaps and a forcible closure under

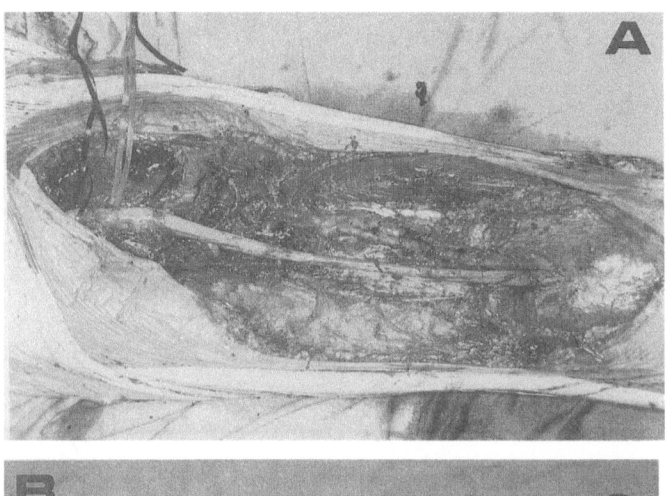

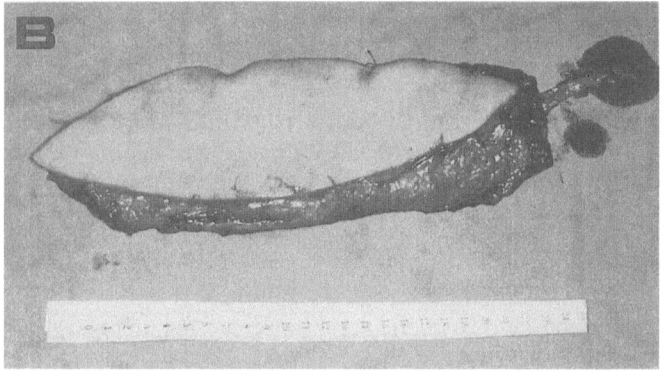

Fig. 2A,B. A Residual large soft tissue defect following wide resection of the tumor. **B** A latissimus dorsi muscle of 36 cm in length, including a skin flap of 30 × 10 cm, is harvested

tension on metal implants can give rise to massive necrosis of the skin, which might result in deep infection and failure of preserving the involved limb.

In 1984, Malawer et al. reported a gastrocunemius transposition for soft tissue coverage around the knee [4]. However, indication for this procedure is apparently limited reach of the muscle after transposition compared to the arch of rotation. Furthermore, the transposition of functioning muscles can sacrifice the remaining function of the involved limb to certain degree [8].

In 1986, Usui et al. reported the application of microsurgical tissue transfer, which includes 5 fibula grafts accompanying peroneal skin flaps and a gracilis muscle transfer [9]. Although the main portion of the series involved bone reconstruction, it clearly indicated that a microsurgical procedure was extremely useful in tumor surgery of the extremities for both skin coverage and functional reconstruction. In 1989, Hausman described a well-defined indication of microvascular surgery in limb-sparing procedures, in which not only wound coverage, but several unique problems including bone, sensibility,

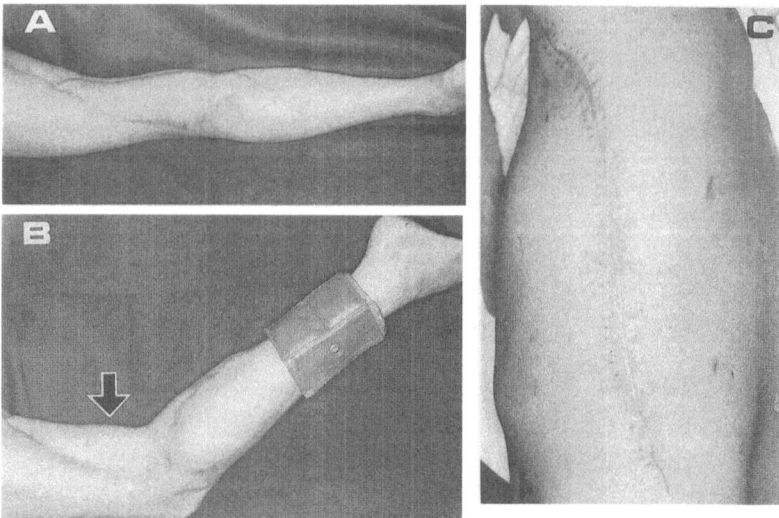

Fig. 3A–C. A The wound uneventfully healed, with a satisfactory cosmetic result of the reconstructed limb. **B** A powerful flexion of the knee is possible with a visible contraction of the transferred muscle (*arrow*). **C** A donor site is closed by direct approximation

muscle loss, infection, and cosmetic acceptance can be microsurgically salvaged [10].

How safely can a free tissue transfer be performed for malignant neoplasms of extremities, especially when regional chemotherapy is indicated? There have been reported experimental studies concerning adverse effects of chemotherapy on vascular endothelium [11], but it seems unequivocal that the procedure is reliable in combination with chemotherapy. The frequency of thrombosis was 14% in this series, which is not as high as that of microsurgery without chemotherapy [12]. Moreover, the cause of thrombosis was a compression of adjacent arteries in all cases, and no chemotherapy was employed in any of them.

Conclusions

Our results clearly showed that microsurgical tissue transfer can be a reliable strategy for soft tissue reconstruction in limb-sparing surgery of musculoskeletal tumors. In addition, recovery of functional grafted muscle can be expected despite the effects of chemotherapy, although a tendency toward delayed recovery of the muscle was noted in tumorous cases compared with traumatic cases [13]. It seems possible, therefore, to reconstruct muscle loss in cases of malignant bone tumors as well as soft tissue sarcomas. Methotrexate and *cis*-platinum, both of which are commonly used in osteosarcoma, were administered only in 1 case and their adverse effects on grafted muscles are not yet clearly understood. Lastly, a certain volume of flap can fill dead space following wide resection of tumors, thereby much more favorable cosmetic results can be obtained as a by-product of tissue transfer.

At present, microsurgical free tissue transfer is a well-established and definitive procedure with minimal complication and donor site deficit, which can reconstruct loss of muscles as well as skin defects in limb-sparing tumor surgery. These advantages may overcome the disadvantages of the time- and cost-consuming aspects in such microsurgery.

References

1. Eilber FR, Eckhardt J, Morton DL (1984) Advances in the treatment of sarcomas of the extremity — Current status of limb salvage. Cancer 54:2695–2701
2. Steed DL, Peitzman AB, Webster MW, Ramasastry SS, Goodman MA (1987) Limb-sparing operations for sarcomas of the extremities involving critical arterial circulation. Surg Gynecol Obstet 164:493–498
3. Tsuchiya K, Motegi M, Iino R, Okajima K, Maruyama Y, Kameda N, Hiruta K (1989) Reconstructive surgery after excision of malignant bone and soft tissue tumor using pedicle myocutaneous flap and fasciocutanoeus flap (in Japanese). Rinsho Seikei Geka 24:22–29
4. Malawer MM, Price WM (1984) Gastrocunemius transposition flap in conjunction with limb-sparing surgery for primary bone sarcomas around the knee. Plast Reconstr Surg 73:741–750
5. Enneking WF (1989) Modification of the system for functional evaluation of surgical management of musculoskeletal tumors. In: Enneking WF (ed) Limb salvage in musculoskeletal oncology. Churchill Livingstone, New York, pp 626–639
6. Fujinami S, Matsuoka H, Nishimura T, Sudo A, Shiokawa Y, Ogihara Y (1990) Limb salvage surgery for malignant bone tumors of the extremity (in Japanese). Orthop Surg Traumatol 33:71–76
7. Zahr KA, Sherman JE, Chaglassian T, Lane JM (1983) Prediction of skin viability following en bloc resection for osteogenic sarcoma with fluorescein. Clin Orthop 180:287–290
8. Uchida A, Yoshikawa H, Ueda T, Araki N, Aoki Y, Hamada H, Mimura K, Ono K (1989) Tumor prosthesis in malignant bone tumors of the proximal tibia (in Japanese). Orthopedic Surgery-Seikeigeka 40:1309–1316
9. Usui M, Ishii S, Yamamura M, Minami A, Sakura T (1985) Microsurgical reconstructive surgery following wide resection of bone and soft tissue sarcomas in the upper extremities. J Reconstr Microsurg 2:77–84
10. Hausman M (1989) Microvascular application in limb sparing tumor surgery. Orthop Clin North Am 20:427–437
11. Taga I, Yamamoto K, Kawai H, Kawabata H, Masada H, Tsuyuguchi Y (1987) The effects of intra-arterially injected Adriamycin on microvascular anastomosis. J Reconst Microsurg 3:153–158
12. Tsai TM, Bennett DL, Pederson WC, Matiko J (1988) Complications and vascular salvage of free-tissue transfers to the extremities. Plast Reconstr Surg 82:1022–1026
13. Doi K, Sakai K, Ihara K, Kaneko K, Kawai S (to be published) Reinnervated free muscle transfer for extremity reconstruction. J Hand Surg

Prosthetic Replacement for Malignant Bone and Soft Tissue Tumors About the Knee: Radiological Evaluation of Tumor Prosthesis

Masanobu Saito, Akira Maruoka[1], Atumasa Uchida,
and Keiro Ono[2]

Introduction

Limb salvage procedures for primary malignant bone and soft tissue tumors have become widely accepted. Recent advances in diagnostic technology, adjuvant chemotherapy, and radiotherapy have led to improvement in prognosis. Consequently, this longer life-span has increased interest in functional restoration and its durability in affected limbs. Although there are various reconstructive procedures after wide resection, such as arthrodesis, osteo-articular allograft, and prosthetic replacement, each procedure has its advantages and disadvantages, and the best among them has not yet been clearly established. Since 1981, prosthetic replacement has been the procedure of choice at Osaka University Hospital, Osaka, Japan, for limb salvage in cases of malignant bone and soft tissue tumors.

Most of the patients with primary malignant bone tumors are young, so that the long-term results of prosthetic replacement are of particular importance. For example, the results of cemented joint replacement have been reported to show a high incidence of component loosening in young patients [1]. Moreover, massive joint and segmental bone prostheses have a high risk of component failure [2], and can change the biomechanical behavior of surrounding bone which might lead to bone resorption [3]. However, there have been few clinical studies dealing with such problems [4]. We report the results of 21 cemented prosthetic replacements after resection of tumors about the knee, the most common lesions of primary malignant bone tumors.

---

[1] Division of Orthopaedic Surgery, South Osaka National Hospital, Kawachinagano-shi 586, Japan
[2] Department of Orthopaedic Surgery, Osaka University Medical School, Fukushima-ku, Osaka 553, Japan

Materials and Methods

From 1981 to 1988, 24 patients with primary malignant bone and soft tissue tumors about the knee underwent limb-salvage and prosthetic replacements at Osaka University Hospital, Osaka, Japan. Eight patients died between 4 and 30 months after surgery. Three of these, who had died within 2 years after surgery, had to be excluded from this study as such a short follow-up period does not allow exact clinical and radiographic assessments to be made. The other 5 as well as the 16 survivors were available for clinical and radiographic review for more than 2 years after surgery; the follow-up ranged from 2 to 7 years (average: 4 years). There were 13 males and 8 females with an average age at surgery of 19 years (range: 8–54 years). Of the 19 patients with malignant bone tumors, 17 had osteosarcoma, 1 fibrosarcoma, and 1 malignant fibrous histiocytoma. The distal femur was involved in 11 patients and the proximal tibia in 8. Of the two patients with malignant soft tissue tumors, one had malignant fibrous histiocytoma and the other synovial sarcoma. In terms of the surgical staging system of the Musculoskeletal Tumor Society [5], there were 19 stage IIB and 2 stage III cases.

Routine limb-salvage procedures were performed after preoperative chemotherapy with Adriamycin, high-dose methotrexate, and *cis*-platinum. None of the patients received radiotherapy. Local wide resection could be performed in all cases. In 11 patients with involvement of the distal femur, resection lengths of the femur ranged from 12 to 24 cm (average: 17 cm). The quadriceps mechanism — at least the rectus femoris — was always retained. In eight patients with involvement of the proximal tibia, resection lengths of the tibia ranged from 11 to 19 cm (average: 14 cm). The patellar tendon was always resected and reconstructed with a free tendon graft from the ilio-tibial tract or with an artificial tendon. The deep peroneal nerve had to be sacrificed in four patients. Four patients, in whom the tumor had invaded the knee joint, underwent extra-articular resection.

Three different types of prosthesis were used in this series. The one used most frequently was a hinged modified Walldius type. A non-constrained prosthesis was used in two patients, but this type was discontinued because stability of the knee joint could not be realized by reconstruction of the soft tissues alone. Since 1987, a rotating hinge prosthesis has been used for distal femoral replacements. The present study includes 14 hinged prostheses, 5 rotating hinge prostheses, and 2 non-constrained prostheses. Segmental bone defects after resection were replaced with high-density polyethylene or titanium alloy. All components were fixed with methylmethacrylate. An 8-year-old female had an extending prosthesis implanted, developed by the Stanmore group [6]. Postoperatively, a cast-type brace was applied for 2 weeks. After removal of the cast, physical therapy and partial weight-bearing exercises were begun. Full weight bearing was permitted at 6 weeks after surgery. All patients received postoperative systemic chemotherapy for approximately 1 year. From 1981 to 1983, Adriamycin and high-dose methotrexate had been administered. Since 1984, *cis*-platinum was added to that regimen. Four patients who devel-

Table 1. Functional results at the final follow-up examination

	Motion	Pain	Stability	Deformity	Strength	Functional activity	Emotional acceptance	Overall
Excellent	12[a]	18	12	14	3	7	8	5
Good	5	1	3	2	9	8	11	10
Fair	3	1	3	3	6	4	2	3
Poor	1	1	3	2	3	2	0	3

[a] Number of patients

oped pulmonary metastases underwent metastatectomy between 6 and 29 months after the limb-salvage operation.

The patients were evaluated with the Musculoskeletal Tumor Society rating system [7]. The seven factors — motion, pain, stability, deformity, strength, functional activity, and emotional acceptance — were rated excellent, good, fair, or poor. Component loosening was diagnosed when the radiographs showed either component migration or a radiolucent line more than 1 mm in width involving the entire circumference of the component. In 16 patients who showed neither postoperative infection nor component loosening, bone remodeling in relation to the insertion of a cemented tumor prosthesis was examined.

Results

Clinical Results

The overall results at the final follow-up as determined by the Musculoskeletal Tumor Society rating system were excellent in five patients, good in ten, fair in three, and poor in three (Table 1). Thus, 71% of the patients in this series obtained satisfactory (excellent or good) functional results. Most of the patients had only slight or no pain in the affected limbs. Sixteen patients (76%) could walk without support, while five used a cane. The average range of motion was 93 degrees, while 12 patients (57%) had more than 90 degrees of motion. Quadriceps muscle strength had diminished in nine patients. Diminished quadriceps muscle strength was frequently seen in the patients with proximal tibial replacement (6 out of 8 patients), because of loss of the insertion of the extensor mechanism. Two patients with non-constrained prostheses were significantly inconvenienced by instability and required a cane and a knee brace for walking.

Complications

Postoperative infection occurred in three patients (14%) within 2 months after proximal tibial replacement. Their ages ranged from 14 to 18 years. All the patients were treated successfully with debridement, irrigation, and parenteral antibiotics, and showed no signs of infection at the final follow-up. Radio-

Fig. 1a,b. a Postoperative radiograph of a 14-year-old male who received a hinged prosthesis for osteosarcoma of the proximal tibia. Two months after surgery, deep infection developed but he was treated successfully with debridement, irrigation, and parenteral antibiotics. **b** Radiograph taken 2 years after surgery shows only thickening of the cortex, but there is no evidence of component loosening

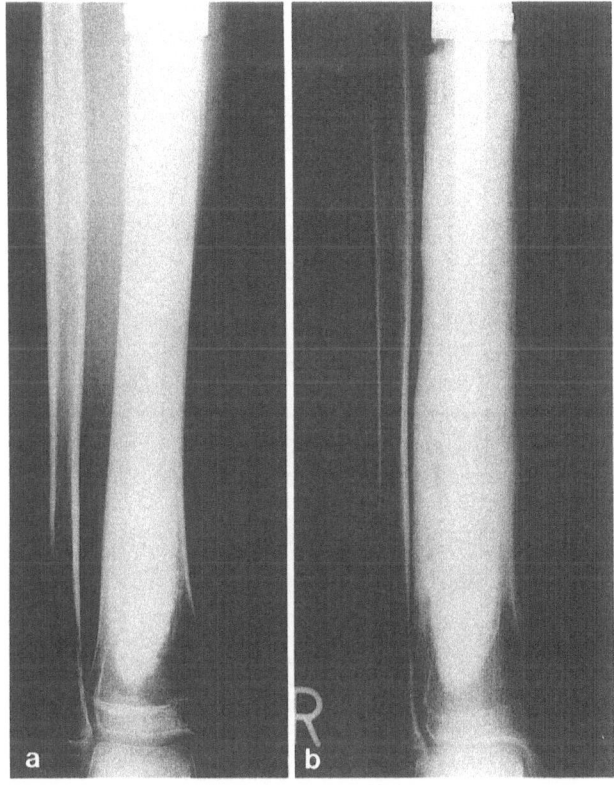

graphic findings were similar, in that they showed only thickness of the cortex surrounding the component, while neither a radiolucent line at the bone-cement interface nor any osteolytic lesions could be observed. At the time of final follow-up, thcrc was no sign of radiographic looscning (Fig. 1a,b).

Revision surgery was done on two patients. The first patient was an 18-year-old male with osteosarcoma of the proximal tibia. The postoperative radiography showed poor packing of the cement around the tibial component. Four months after surgery, a radiolucent line involving the entire circumference of the tibial component was visible, while 2 years and 7 months after surgery, subsidence of the tibial component was observed. Although the patient had no pain at that time, revision surgery of the tibial component was performed because of progressive endosteal bone loss. The second patient was a 45-year-old male who had had fibrosarcoma of the distal femur and received a rotating hinge prosthesis. However, invasion into the knee joint was detected during surgery, so that additional resection of the tibia was required. Thus, the actual resection length of the tibia was 5 cm longer than originally planned. This discrepancy made it impossible for the patient to control the rotation of the tibia. Two years after surgery, therefore, revision surgery was performed using a hinged prosthesis with a replacement segment of an adequate length, leading to a good functional result at the time of the final follow-up.

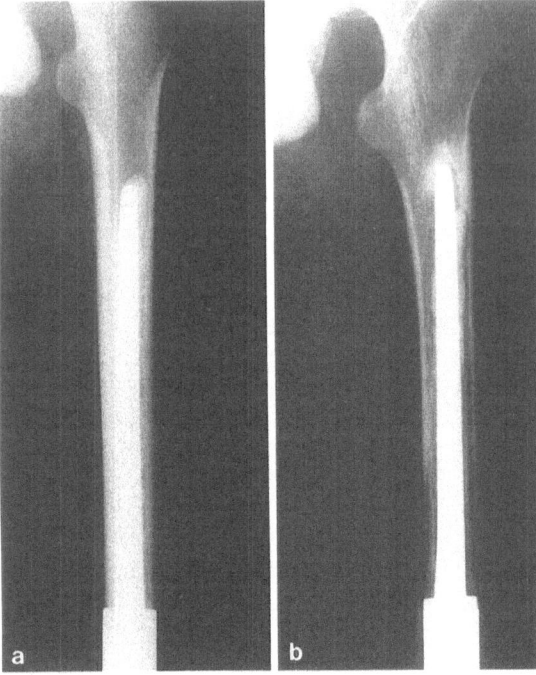

Fig. 2a,b. A 15-year-old male who had received a hinged prosthesis for osteosarcoma of the distal femur. **a** Postoperative radiograph shows poor cement packing around the femoral component. **b** Four years after surgery, there was loosening of the femoral component

Skin necrosis occurred in three patients, including two with deep infection. The limbs of these three patients could be salvaged with a local myocutaneous rotation flap. There was no fracture of the component stem. None of these patients suffered a local recurrence. Thus, although 6 of the 21 patients (29%) had at least one complication, all complications could be managed with additional therapy and no patient required amputation.

Radiographic Results

Radiographic assessment was done in 18 patients. Three patients with postoperative infection were excluded, and these patients are described in the previous section on complications.

Mechanical loosening of the component was observed in two patients (11%). The first patient underwent revision surgery because of loosening of the tibial component, as mentioned earlier. The second patient was a 15-year-old male who had had osteosarcoma of the distal femur and received a hinged prosthesis (Fig. 2.a). Six months after surgery, a radiolucent line around the entire circumference of the femoral component was visible, while 4 years after surgery, the femoral component had subsided by 20 mm (Fig. 2.b). The immediate postoperative radiographs of these two patients revealed poor packing of the cement; i.e., the cement did not extend to the tip of the stem. On the other hand, postoperative radiographs of the other 16 patients revealed adequate packing. There was a uniform mantle of cement with a width of 2–3 mm, and

Fig. 3a,b. a Postoperative radiograph shows bone at the transection site in contact with the shoulder of the prosthesis. **b** Four years after surgery, there was bone resorption in the tip of the transected bone

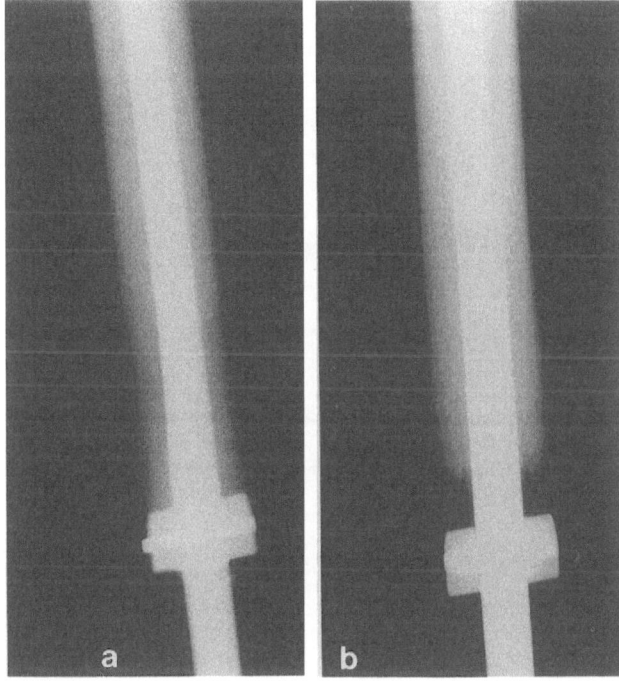

the cement was packed more than 1 cm past the tip. In these 16 patients, serial postoperative radiographs showed no evidence of component loosening, nor was there any radiolucent line visible at the cement-bone interface in 15 patients, while a non-progressive radiolucent line with a width of less than .5 mm showed only around the tip of the stem in one patient.

Bone remodeling after insertion of the tumor prosthesis was assessed in 16 patients who had neither postoperative infection nor component loosening. This analysis showed the following 2 types of bone resorption around the stem.

In five patients (31%), bone resorption in the tip of the transected bone was observed, although the radiographs taken immediately after surgery showed bone at the transection site in contact with the shoulder of the prosthesis (Fig. 3a,b.). The bone resorption was first seen on the radiographs between 2 and 8 months (average: 5 months) after surgery and was progressive at the transection site. The most severe resorption showed an extension of 15 mm over a period of 4 years. Such radiographic changes occurred in 4 out of 11 patients (36%) with distal femoral replacements, and in 1 out of 5 patients (20%) with proximal tibial replacements.

The second type of bone loss consisted of thinning of the cortex and expansion of the medullary canal not associated with component loosening (Fig. 4a,b). This radiographic change occurred in 5 patients, including 2 of the 11 patients (18%) with distal femoral replacements and 3 of the 5 patients (60%) with proximal tibial replacements. Thinning of the cortex and expansion of the medullary canal always occurred at the site of the wide resection and involved

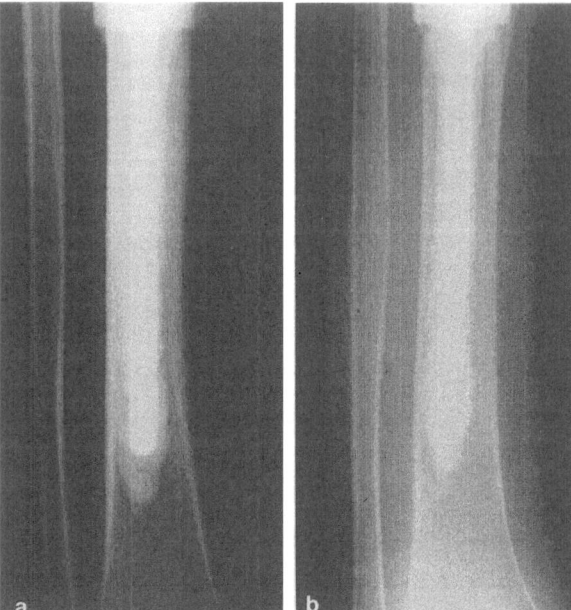

Fig. 4a,b. Serial radiographs show thinning of the cortex and expansion of the medullary canal. **a** One month after surgery. **b** Six months after surgery

the entire remaining femur or tibia. It was first seen on the radiographs between 2 and 6 months (average: 4 months) after surgery. Although such changes did not lead to component loosening, the widths of the cortex had not been restored at the time of the final follow-up.

Discussion

Prosthetic replacement is a generally accepted procedure for patients with life-threatening malignant bone or soft tissue tumors. Functional recovery and mobility of the joint can be obtained relatively soon after the operation. Furthermore, postoperative chemotherapy can be safely started immediately after surgery. Most of the patients in this series, who had received a hinged prosthesis or a rotating hinge prosthesis, did not suffer pain in their limbs and enjoyed good stability. The present study also suggests, however, that several problems will arise with regard to long-term maintenance of limb function as a result of the longer life-span realized by advances in therapeutic modalities.

Postoperative Infection

A high incidence of postoperative complications has been reported in association with limb-salvage procedures [2, 4]. Our study showed neither local recurrence nor component fracture, but three patients (14%) suffered postoperative infection. Pre- and postoperative chemotherapy, a massive prosthesis, and poor blood supply after wide resection contribute to the high risk of postoperative infection. The three patients with postoperative infection in this study were treated with debridement, irrigation, and parenteral antibiotics. At the time of the final follow-up, these three patients showed no evidence of infection. The radiographs, taken at 75 months after the onset of infection in 1 case and at 32 months in the other 2 cases, did not show any evidence of component loosening, but only thickening of the cortex around the component. Based on these results, we recommend treatment of postoperative infection with the prosthesis in place, because the removal of the prosthesis, which leads to extensive loss of bone, often means amputation.

Component Loosening

For patients with osteoarthritis or rheumatoid arthritis, the reported results of cemented total knee replacement using a hinged prosthesis have generally not been favorable, with component loosening rates of 6%–27% at 1.6–3 years postoperatively [8, 9]. For reconstruction after resection of malignant tumors about the knee, however, a hinged or a rotating hinge prosthesis should be used. There is some risk of component loosening after such operations because most of the patients requiring this operation are generally young, have a large bone defect, and do not have enough muscular stabilization after resection of the tumors.

In the present study, however, the incidence of component loosening was 11% over an average 4-year follow-up, and this result seems to be better than that for patients with osteoarthritis or rheumatoid arthritis. Decreased activity alone does not explain such results, because most of the patients studied in this series have not suffered pain in their limbs and 67% of the patients have been able to walk short distances to work or school by themselves. Recent advances in cementing techniques and stem design resulting in good canal fill are thought to be the main contributing factors for this decrease in the incidence of component loosening. In addition, the reaction of bones in young and adolescent patients in securing the cemented fixation may be different from that in older patients.

Some authors have recommended a cementless prosthesis for young patients with malignant lesions [10]. However, this procedure causes some problems with biological fixation of the prosthesis. Adjuvant chemotherapy and radiotherapy may impair bone ingrowth into the cementless prosthesis [11]. In fact, the results for cementless prosthetic replacements do not always show a lower incidence of component loosening than do those for cemented prosthetic replacement [12]. Additional studies will be necessary to establish whether a cementless or a cemented prosthesis is preferable.

Bone Resorption Around the Prosthesis

Loss of bone stock around the prosthesis also occurred in the patients who experienced neither postoperative infection nor component loosening. The mechanism of the 2 types of bone resorption — bone resorption in the tip of the transected bone, or thinning of the cortex and expansion of the medullary canal — remains unclear. Changes in the biomechanical behavior in reaction to a massive prosthesis and/or interruption of the intra-osseous blood supply may contribute to such bone resorption [3, 13]. Although neither type of bone resorption has led to component loosening within the follow-up period of this study, a better design of the prosthesis should be sought.

References

1. Dorr LD, Takei GK, Conaty JP (1983) Total hip arthroplasties in patients less than forty-five years old. J Bone Joint Surg [Am] 65:474–479
2. Quill G, Gitelis S, Morton T, Piasecki P (1990) Complications associated with limb salvage for extremity sarcomas and their management. Clin Orthop 260:242–250
3. Langlais F, Postel M, Aubriot JH, Blanquaert D (1987) The TCG prosthesis system. In: Enneking WF (ed) Limb salvage in musculoskeletal oncology. Churchill Livingstone, New York, pp 88–94
4. Sim FH, Beauchamp CP, Chao EY (1987) Reconstruction of musculoskeletal defects about the knee for tumor. Clin Orthop 221:188–201
5. Enneking WF, Spanier SS, Goodman MA (1980) A system for the surgical staging of musculoskeletal sarcoma. Clin Orthop 153:106–120
6. Scales JT, Sneath RS, Wright KW (1987) Design and clinical use of extending prostheses. In: Enneking WF (ed) Limb salvage in musculoskeletal oncology. Churchill Livingstone, New York, pp 52–61
7. Enneking WF (1987) Modification of the system for functional evaluation of surgical management of musculoskeletal tumors. In: Enneking WF (ed) Limb salvage in musculoskeletal oncology. Churchill Livingstone, New York, pp 626–639
8. Jones EC, Insall JN, Inglis AE, Ranawat CS (1979) Guepar knee arthroplasty results and late complications. Clin Orthop 140:145–152
9. leNobel J, Patterson FP (1981) Guepar total knee prosthesis: Experience at the Vancouver General Hospital. J Bone Joint Surg [Br] 63:257–260
10. Kotz R, Ritschl P, Trachtenbrodt J (1986) A modular femur-tibia reconstruction system. Orthopedics 9:1639–1652
11. Friedlaender GE, Tross RB, Doganis AC, Kirkwood JM, Baron R (1984) Effects of chemotherapeutic agents on bone: I. Short-term methotrexate and Doxorubicin (Adriamycin) treatment in rat model. J Bone Joint Surg [Am] 66:602–607
12. Salzer M, Knahr K, Kotz R, Ramach W (1987) Cementless prosthetic implants for limb salvage of malignant bone tumors of the knee joint: Clinical results of three modes of anchorage. In: Enneking WF (ed) Limb salvage in musculoskeletal oncology. Churchill Livingstone, New York, pp 26–29
13. Scales JT, Wait ME (1987) Intramedullary fixation of custom-made prostheses with bone cement. In: Coombs R, Friedlaender G (eds) Bone tumor management. Butterworths, London, pp 123–134

Surgical Reconstruction for Metastatic Malignancies of the Spine

Po-Quang Chen and Tang-Kue Liu[1]

Introduction

Patients with spinal metastasis usually have severe back pain, motor weakness, or even paraplegia due to the direct compression by the tumor mass or to spinal instability subsequent to bony destruction. Some patients must be confined to bed and require extensive care.

Although radiation to metastatic foci may relieve pain to some extent, the chance for motor recovery is rare. Since the cord was usually compressed by the tumor mass arising from the body, laminectomy alone is not only ineffective, but renders the spine more unstable. As a result of recent advances in spinal instrumentation, spinal reconstruction for this pathological condition has been emphasized. In our earlier report, surgical reconstruction of the spine after tumor excision showed encouraging results [1].

The purpose of this retrospective study was to analyze the results of surgical treatment and set guidelines for managing this challenging clinical situation.

Clinical Materials and Methods

From March, 1981 to February, 1990, 34 patients with metastatic malignancies of the spine underwent decompression and spinal reconstruction at the Department of Orthopedic Surgery, National Taiwan University Hospital. There were 18 males and 16 females whose ages ranged from 26 to 68 years (mean: 62 years). The primary cancers arose from various organs: 4 cases each from the nasopharynx and breast, 3 each from the thyroid, lung, uterine cervix, lower limbs and retroperitoneal or mediastinal region, 2 cases each from the neck, stomach, and prostate, and 1 case each from the liver and kidney. The precise

[1] Department of Orthopedic Surgery, National Taiwan University Hospital, Taipei 10016, Taiwan, Republic of China

origin could not be found in the remaining 3 cases. Histological findings included 14 cases of adenocarcinoma, 6 anaplastic carcinoma, 4 epidermoid carcinoma, and 3 cases each of sarcoma, lymphoma, and thyroid cancer. Hepatoma was found in 1 case. Metastasis spread to the cervical spine in 1 case, thoracic in 16, and lumbar in 16. One case had metastasis in both the cervical and lumbar spines.

Fourteen patients received surgery alone, because the primary tumors were thought to be resistant to other treatments. Among the remaining 20 patients, adjuvant therapy was given either before or after surgery. Eight patients received radiation to the involved spine. Chemotherapy alone was administered in 2 cases. Two patients had hormonal therapy together with either chemo- or radiotherapy to the involved spine. Six patients had combined chemo- and radiotherapy. Two patients received combined chemo-, radio-, and hormonal therapies.

All the patients were evaluated at the out-patient clinic or interviewed by telephone. The mean follow-up period was 15 months (range: 6–60 months). The severity of backache was divided into 3 grades: "marked" denoting that patients suffered from unrelenting backache inspite of strong analgesics, "moderate" denoting that pain could be relieved by analgesics, and "mild" denoting that analgesics were used occasionally to relieve back pain. The neurological status of the patients before and after surgery was also evaluated according to Frankel's scale, with ratings from A to E [2].

Surgical Considerations

The indications for surgery were: (1) intractable back pain even after local irradiation or medication, and/or (2) progressive motor weakness or impending paraplegia, or sphincter disturbance. Anterior reconstruction (AR) was preferred in most of the cases. AR included vertebral corpectomy from the anterior approach and fixation of the disrupted spines by various metallic devices, bone graft, or bone cement. Posterior reconstruction (PR) included laminectomy with decompression of the cord or cauda equina and implant fixation.

The anterior spinal devices used were the Polster-Brinckmann (P-B) prosthesis in 12 patients, Zielke's anterior implants in 11, a fracture plate in 4, and the Kaneda device in 1. Poly-methylmethacryate (PMMA) bone cement was used in 21 patients. Two patients with breast cancer received a fibular bone graft. For PR, double Harrington rodding with segmented wiring was applied (Table 1). Preoperative vascular embolization was not attempted in any patient.

Results

The present series included 13 AR, 11 PR, and 10 combined reconstructions. Of these 34 patients, 5 died within 3 months: 1 patient with hepatoma died of hepatic coma 2 days after Luque rodding, 2 died of cachexia, 1 died of massive

Table 1. Implants for spinal reconstruction

	Cases (n)
A. Anterior	
1. P-B prosthesis	12
2. Zielke's system	11
3. Kaneda device	1
4. Plate	4
B. Posterior	
1. Harrington + SW	13
2. Luque	9

P-B, Polster-Brinckmann prosthesis; *SW*, sublaminar wiring

Table 2. The neurological status of the patients before and after surgery

Frankel's scale	Pre-operative (n patients)	Post-operative (n patients)
A	4	1
B	4	0
C	14	4
D	12	10
E	0	14
	34	29 (Total)

G-I bleeding and aspiration, and 1 died of iodine anaphylaxis during the intravenous pyelography procedure. Preoperative back pain in 31 patients were rated as marked and 3 as moderate. Twenty-nine patients were available for follow-up. Postoperatively, only 2 patients still suffered from a moderate backache, 2 were mild, and the remaining 25 were pain-free.

According to Frankel's scale, the neurological status of patients before surgery was 4 each in grades A and B, 14 in C, and 12 in D. After surgery, only 1 patient remained status quo in A, while the rest were upgraded: 4 to C, 10 to D, and 14 to E (Table 2). Sphincter function was impaired in five patients before surgery, and four had normal function afterwards.

None of the patients had wound infection, implant failure, or dislodgement. Aside from the aforementioned deaths of 5 patients, 6 patients survived up to 6 months, 14 up to 12 months, 6 up to 24 months, and 3 patients lived longer than 24 months. The patient with thyroid cancer lived to 60 months. At the time of this writing, five patients were still alive.

Discussion

It is believed that the prognosis and treatment of patients with spinal metastasis depends upon the nature of the tumor, the level and extent of spinal involvement, the immune status, and the general condition of the patient [3]. We consider a predicted life expectancy of 4–6 months to be the minimal duration

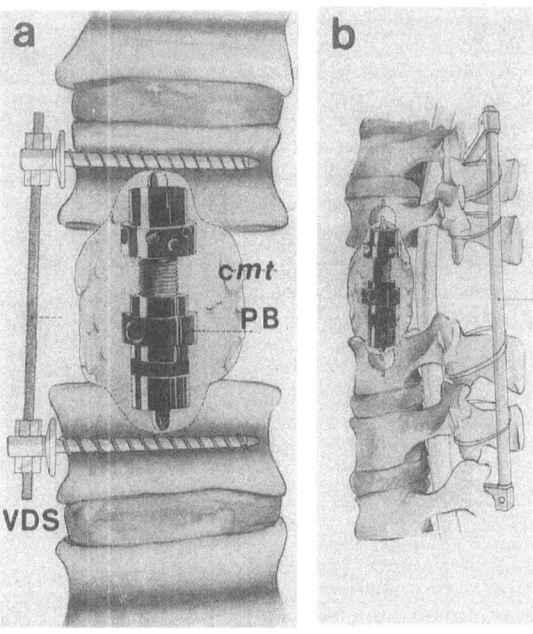

Fig. 1a,b. Schematic drawings of Polster-Brinckmann prosthesis (*P-B*) and Zielke's implant (*VDS*) fixation after corpectomy. Bone cement (*cmt*) is inserted into the defect as space filler

from which to determine surgery, because it usually takes 1 month for them to regain motor power and to become ambulatory. Surgery should be done early in order to avoid postoperative death, as was noted in four of our patients. Solini et al. [4] even proposed prophylactic surgery in order to obtain better results.

Most spinal metastases are confined to the anterior spinal column. The rapid tumor expansion eventually leads to pathological fracture or even angulation of the spine, which causes back pain and compression of the cord or cauda equina. Back pain may be relieved to a certain degree by local irradiation, but weakness of the extremities is more difficult to alleviate by conventional therapy. In the present series, 11 patients received local spinal irradiation before surgery. Their back pain persisted and motor power became decreased; some even faced impending paraplegia.

Laminectomy alone has been contraindicated, since it produces spine instability. Since compression occurs primarily because of tumors in the anterior spinal column, anterior corpectomy and reconstruction using rigid spinal implants are the logical modalities for decompression, restoration, and stabilization of the spine. Harrington [5] was the first to apply distraction rods and bone cement for reconstructions after corpectomy. Thereafter, many implants have been devised for this purpose [6–8]. AR, either single or combined with PR, was performed in 23 of our cases (67.6%). Improvement of motor power and pain relief was noted in 23 patients (91.3%). This aggressive surgical approach is justifiable in order to avoid the consequence of paraplegia.

After corpectomy, the space was filled with PMMA bone cement. Many fixation spacers have been devised in order to augment the stability and to

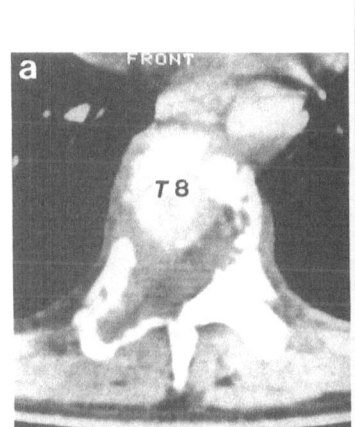
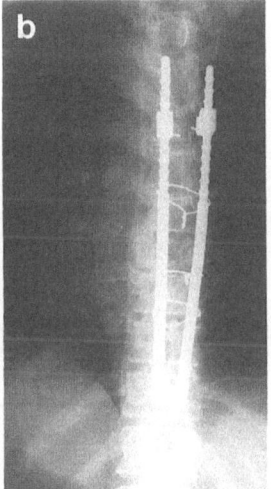
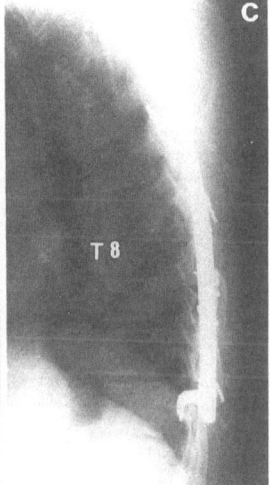

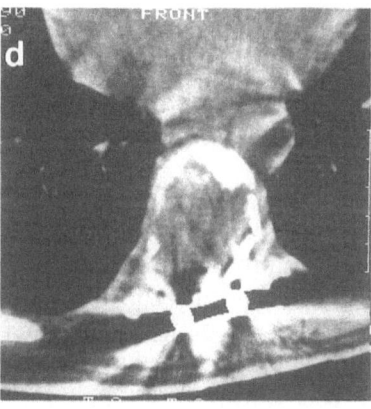

Fig. 2a–d. A 43-year-old male with a 3-year history of nasopharyngeal cancer. He had T-8 metastasis and recently was in an impending paraplegic state. **a** CT scan showed complete destruction of the T-8 body and invasion to left pedicle and posterior arch. **b, c** Anteroposterior and lateral roentgenograms showed reconstruction 5 months after laminectomy, posterior debulking, and bone grafting of the T-8 body along with Harrington rodding. **d** CT scan showed bone graft in the cavity. Two weeks after surgery, patient regained motor power. Neurological status shifted from Frankel B to D

restore the collapsed spine. Fidler [6] used stainless steel spacers along with an outer screw and rod fixator. Polster and Brinckmann [9] also devised a stainless steel implant which could be expanded into the adjacent vertebral bodies after tumor resection. Ono et al. [10] used ceramic spacers to support the bony defect. The advantage of these kinds of devices is that once inserted inside the spinal cavity, the space can be restored. They are able to resist the axial compressive loading and avoid the potential damage or encroachment to the great vessels. P-B prostheses were used in 12 patients (Fig. 1). Fibular graft was used in the two patients with breast cancer. However, they died before incorporation of the bone graft.

Curettage of the vertebral body from the posterior is known to be dangerous in the thoracic region, since the jeopardized cord might be damaged during manipulation. This procedure is less dangerous in the lumbar area [11]. Sometimes the back pain has been so severe in patients with multiple spinal

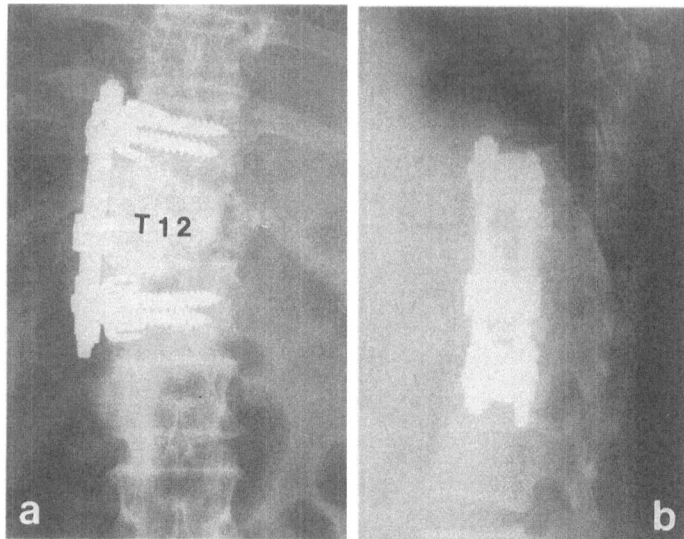

Fig. 3a,b. A 65-year-old female with breast cancer. Mastectomy was done 5 years previously. **a** Anteroposterior and **b** lateral radiographs showed that bone cement and rib grafts were inserted into the post-corpectomy space, while a Kaneda device was fixed at the adjacent bodies (T11 and L1). She survived another 2 years

metastasis that posterior fixation by spinal implants has been quite rewarding [7]. This procedure was also performed in three of our patients. When the dura was surrounded by a tumor or the tumor extended into the posterior bony structures — considered by Onimus et al. [7] to have a poor prognosis — PR or the combined procedure was helpful. These are the conditions which we considered approprite to apply posterior instrumentation (Fig. 2). Combined AR and PR was performed in 10 cases. With the improvement of anterior fixators, PR may not be necessary. The Kaneda device was used in one patient with breast cancer with satisfactory results (Fig. 3).

Conclusions

From March, 1981 to February, 1990, 34 patients with spinal metastasis were treated surgically. Their ages ranged from 26 to 68 years. Histological findings included 14 cases of adenocarcinoma, 6 anaplastic carcinoma, 4 epidermoid carcinoma, 3 thyroid cancer, 3 sarcoma, 3 lymphoma and 1 hepatoma. The involved segments were mainly in the thoracic and lumbar spines. The authors advocated anterior reconstruction of the spine whenever feasible. The procedure included: (1) vertebral corpectomy of involved segments, and (2) reconstruction and stabilization mainly by the combination of Polster-Brinckmann and Zielke's instrumentation. Bone graft or polymethylmethacrylate (PMMA) cement was chosen according to the prognosis. Posterior Harrington or Luque rodding was applied for further stabilization or for cases with involvement of posterior bony elements or multiple segments. Thirteen patients underwent anterior reconstruction, 11 posterior, and the remaining 10 a combination of the two. Postoperative pain relief was noted in all patients. At follow-up, five patients had died within 3 months of surgery. In the surviving patients, motor power improved greatly, and 14 patients were able to walk freely with only one patient remaining bedridden. In this series, anterior curettage of the involved spine with proper reconstruction gave satisfactory results with few complications.

The management of patients with malignant spinal metastasis is multidisciplinary. To improve the life of the patient, spinal reconstruction using proper implants is mandatory.

References

1. Chen PQ, Yang CY, Liu TK (1987) Surgical reconstruction as palliative treatment for metastatic malignancies of the spine. J Formosan Med Assoc 86:855–863
2. Frankel HL, Hancock DO, Hyslop G, Melzak J, Vernon JOS, Walsh JJ (1969) The value of postural reduction in the initial management of closed injuries of the spine with paraplegia and tetraplegia, part 1. Paraplegia 7:179–192
3. Tang SG, Byfield JE, Sharp TR (1981) Prognostic factors in the management of metastatic epidural cord compression. J Neurooncol 1:21–28
4. Solini A, Paschero B, Orsini G, Quercio N (1985) The surgical treatment of metastatic tumor of the lumbar spine. Ital J Orthop Traumatol 11(4):427–442
5. Harrington KD (1984) Anterior cord decompression and spinal stabilization for patients with metastatic lesion of the spine. J Neurosurg 61:107–117
6. Fidler MW (1986) Anterior decompression and stabilization of metastatic spinal fractures. J Bone Joint Surg [Br] 68:83–90
7. Onimus M, Schraub S, Bertin D, Bosset JF, Guidet M (1986) Surgical treatment of vertebral metastasis. Spine 11:883–891
8. Perrin RG, McBroom RJ (1988) Spinal fixation after anterior decompression for symptomatic spinal metastasis. Neurosurgery 22(2):324–327
9. Polster J, Brinckmann P (1977) Ein Wirbelkörperimplantat zur Verwendung bei Palliativoperationen an der Wirbelsäule. Z Orthop 115:118–122
10. Ono K, Yonenobu K, Ebara S, Fujiwara K, Yamashita K, Fuji T, Dunn E (1990) Prosthetic replacement surgery for cervical spine metastasis. Spine 13:817–822
11. Bridwell KH, Jenny AB, Saul T (1988) Posterior segmental spinal instrumentation (PSSI) with posterolateral decompression and debulking for metastatic thoracic and lumbar spine disease. Limitations of the technique. Spine 13:1383–1394

4.10

Prosthetic Replacement Surgery for Spine Metastasis

KEIRO ONO, SOHEI EBARA, KAZUO YONENOBU, NOBORU HOSONO,[1] and
EDWARD J. DUNN[2]

Introduction

In the early 1970s, we began to find an increasing number of patients with metastatic disease of the spine, primarily cervical, presenting with constant pain. Subsequently neural deficits associated with vertebral collapse occurred and there was, according to professionals in the field, "nothing to do with them" or because "they don't have long to go." When we looked more carefully at these patients, it became obvious that they had all gathered together in one group and were generally treated in one or two ways; either only supportive care was provided or they were subjected to radio-therapy and/or laminectomy. Under more careful scrutiny, it became apparent that this was not a homogenous group. There were differences in these patients based on the primary tumor, location and number of metastatic sites, their general conditions, and, considering these factors, their long-term prognoses. We began to select those patients with a reasonable remaining life span of over 6 months who have pain due to instability and/or neural compression from vertebral collapse and carried out instrument replacement supplemented by methyl-methacrylate posteriorly and, in some instances, methyl-methacrylate replacement of vertebral bodies anteriorly. We were pleased with the pain relief and return of neural function achieved in these patients. Through similar experiences in subsequent years, we developed a metal prosthesis for replacement of the metastatic tumor-affected vertebra [1] (Fig. 1).

In 1975, at the SICOT meeting in Copenhagen, the author (Ono) met Edward Dunn of the USA. It was interesting to learn that since 1972 he had been using methyl-methacrylate for the treatment of selected cases of meta-

[1] Department of Orthopaedic Surgery, Osaka University Medical School, 1-1-50 Fukushima, Fukushima-ku, Osaka, 553 Japan
[2] Department of Orthopedic Surgery, Worcester Memorial Hospital, Worcester, Massachusetts, USA

Fig. 1. A metal prosthesis for replacement of the vertebra affected by metastatic tumor. This prosthesis is anchored by bone cement

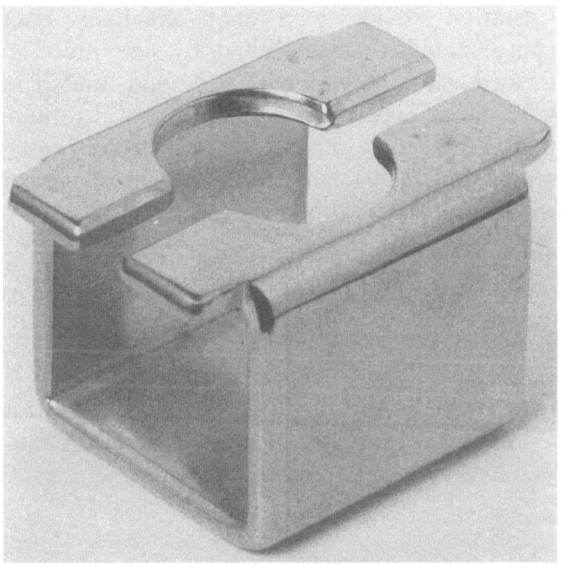

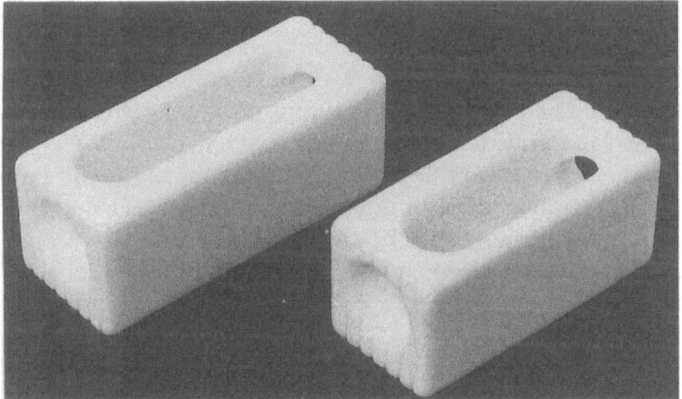

Fig. 2. A ceramic prosthesis. This prosthesis is anchored by bone cement

static tumor. The ideas incorporated in his procedure were strikingly similar to some we had entertained and his philosophy regarding indications and patient selection was in accordance with ours [2].

We began a 10-year exchange of information, ideas, and criticism, and this cooperation in the study of cervical spine problems has resulted, among other things, in the refinement of this technique as well as the critical evaluation of its results that we present below.

Since 1972, we carried out vertebral body resection and prosthetic replacement on 78 occasions in 74 patients. The first six patients received a prototype metal prosthesis [1], while a simple ceramic prosthesis was utilized for the last 68 patients [2, 3] (Fig. 2). This prosthesis is anchored by cement, and the operation provides pain relief, spinal cord decompression, and restoration of spinal stability accomplished by one procedure. When the main tumor is located within a vertebral body and limited in the number of vertebrae involved, our experience has shown that prosthetic replacement is more likely to produce a more satisfactory result than posterior decompression and instrumentation. Statistically, 60%–70% of metastatic spinal deposits are localized within the vertebral bodies, so this technique should have wide application.

Indications for Vertebral Body Prosthetic Replacement

Pain

Patients suffering from severe pain caused by an unstable spine associated with a pathological fracture of a single vertebral body are particularly benefited by this surgery.

Neural Deficit

Patients with spinal cord and/or nerve root compression secondary to collapse of the affected vertebral body and with angulation or impingement of the spinal cord or cauda equina caused by tumor mass emerging from the affected vertebral body can derive benefit from this surgery.

Patients with a more recent deterioration in neural status will do better than those with long-standing deterioration. Patients with mechanical compression secondary to tumor-induced vertebral collapse will also tend to have a better result than those who have compression to the neural structures by direct tumor invasion.

Tumor Types

Hormone-dependent tumors. Patients with hormone-dependent tumors, such as those in which the primary lesion is in the breast, prostate, or thyroid, generally have a longer survival rate and, therefore, are more liable to benefit from this surgery.

Localized metastatic lesion from well-differentiated primary tumors. These tumors are often relatively slow growing and patients can also be expected to survive longer enough after surgery (6–12 months).

Localized metastatic lesions from radio-resistant primary tumors. As long as these patients' overall physical condition is satisfactory, as reflected in their self-care activities and results from laboratory tests, this procedure may provide their only reasonable hope for pain relief and may avoid vertebral collapse and neural deficit for the rest of their lives.

Emergency. If a rapidly progressive neural deficit is found in association with a collapsed vertebra secondary to an apparent malignancy, prosthetic replacement surgery admits of biopsy, decompression, pain relief, and restoration of stability — all in one procedure.

Contraindications for Vertebral Body Prosthetic Replacement

Tumor Type

Most patients with uncontrollable or unresectable primary cancer and/or extensive lung metastases generally do not live long enough to benefit from this procedure (less than 6 months).

The presence of multiple bony metastases is usually a contraindication to the performance of this procedure. Occasionally, however, a non-debilitated patient with one of the slower-growing tumors may still benefit from this surgery.

Patient Condition

Those patients with significant debilitation and have a projected life expectancy of less than 6 months are not considered satisfactory candidates for this surgery.

Infection

The presence of active infection is a contraindication for the performance of this surgery. When a long-standing tracheostomy has been present or the need for tracheostomy is anticipated, this surgery becomes contraindicated because of the increased risk of infection.

Multiple Levels

In the laboratory, significant difficulty in anchoring the prosthesis was encountered when replacement was attempted in lesions spanning three or more vertebral levels. Therefore, we believe that patients with such vertebral body lesions should not undergo replacement surgery with this prosthesis. For these cases, radiation or an appropriate decompression with posterior instrumentation and/or fusion would be preferable.

Assessment and Examination Prior to Surgery

The patient's general status (including respiratory, cardiovascular, and renal function as well as nutritional status, and the presence of myelosuppression and an infectious condition) should be carefully evaluated before surgery. Any abnormalities (discovered) should be corrected prior to surgery. The extent of life-threatening metastases and bone metastases should be determined (by rentogenography and bone scanning).

The symptom-precipitating lesion, including not only the collapsed vertebrae but also the path and extent of intracanal tumor spread from the affected vertebrae, should be localized precisely. CT and CT myelography are indispensable for this purpose. Selective angiography can also assist in determining the extent of the lesion and its vascularity. Embolization of the feeding artery prior to surgery reduces blood loss during surgery in hypervascular cases.

Surgical Techniques and Approaches

The Antero-Lateral Approach from C_3 to T_1

An oblique incision is made in the line of the anterior border of the sternocleidomastoid muscle. After the platysma has been divided, the cervical spine is approached by blunt dissection between the great vessels and the trachea and esophagus. A wide exposure of the anterior aspects of the affected vertebra can be obtained by detaching and retracting the longus colli muscles bilaterally.

Anterior Mid-Line Approach (Sternum-Splitting Approach) to T_2 and T_3

A T-shaped incision is made with the transverse component along the lower neck crease and the vertical component along the mid-line of the sternum. The sternohyoid and sternothyroid muscles are divided and the posterior aspect of the sternum is gently dissected off the mediastinum. Once the sternum has been split, the thymus and the cardinal vessels are retracted to expose the anterior aspects of the upper thoracic vertebrae.

Thoracotomy Approach to T_4-T_{12}

The standard thoracotomy approach is used by removing one or two ribs above the affected vertebra.

Thoracoabdominal Approach to T_{12}-L_2

The tenth rib resection and detachment of the diaphragm at its periphery is preferred for creating a wide exposure.

Anterior Retroperitoneal Flank Approach to L_2-L_5

In the lumbar region, detaching the origin of the diaphragm or psoas muscle is required for creating a wide exposure of the anterolateral surface of the vertebra.

Excision of the Lesion

As a general rule, in metastatic lesions within a vertebral body, the bony fragments protruding posteriorly from the collapsed vertebra and the tumor mass impinging on the spinal cord or cauda equina should be removed. Usually, subtotal spondylectomy with excision of the two adjacent discs and curettage of the epidural space is sufficient. Meticulous hemostasis (including ligation or cauterization of the segmental vessels and application of bone wax for medullary bleeding and oxycellulose for bleeding from the vertebrae venous plexus) is mandatory before the further step of prosthetic replacement and fixation can be carried out.

The Technique of Prosthetic Replacement and Bone Cement Anchorage

After the excision of the impinging bone, tumor, and discs, we begin the procedure of prosthetic replacement and fixation of the prosthesis to the spine. A vertebral spreader is useful for providing a better view of the spinal canal and for correction of the angular spinal deformity. The adjacent two vertebrae are gently spread apart and any remaining fragments of tumor are removed, and any additional bleeding, is carefully controlled (Fig. 3).

A prosthesis 5–10 mm longer than the original space (the height of the vertebra plus the thickness of two discs) is chosen for replacement purposes. The prosthesis is usually introduced in an antero-posterior direction in the cervical spine and the uppermost 2–3 thoracic levels. In the remainder of the thoracic or lumbar spine, the prosthesis is introduced laterally.

After introduction of the prosthesis, an anchor hole is made in both the superior and inferior vertebrae (Fig. 4). These anchor holes should confirm with the intraprosthetic cavity. In order to insure this, the top and bottom surfaces of the adjacent vertebrae are excavated from inside the prosthesis by a curette or a powered apparatus. Once an appropriate hole has been made in the end plate, it can be deepened further. The prosthesis which has been used to make the initial holes can be removed during the deepening procedure. The size of the anchoring hole should not exceed the size of the aperture on either end of the prosthesis. Otherwise, bone cement may flow outside of the vertebra. When a metastatic deposit has been discovered within the adjacent vertebra during this procedure, an expansive anchoring hole within the vertebral body (that is later filled with large amount of bone cement) will generally permit firm anchorage of the prosthesis. It is also possible to use a prosthesis that will span two vertebral bodies rather than one. At any rate, the prosthesis is then introduced and its alignment carefully noted. The bone cement is then placed into the prosthesis through the anterior window and pushed with pressure into the anchor holes above and below (Fig. 5). The pressure is maintained while the cement sets. Fixation of the prosthesis can be tested by the "push — pull" method. Before closing the wound, adequate hemostasis should be assured. Figure 6a,b. shows a typical case with this spinal prosthesis.

Post-Operative Care

Immediately after surgery, the patients are allowed to change position in bed. On the first day after surgery, they can be fed in a semi-sitting position. Sitting

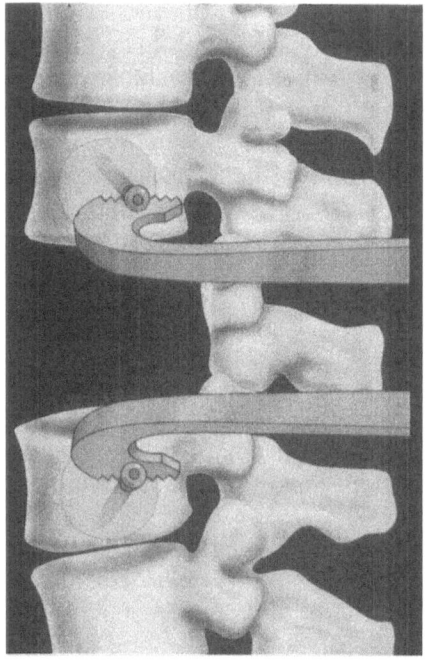

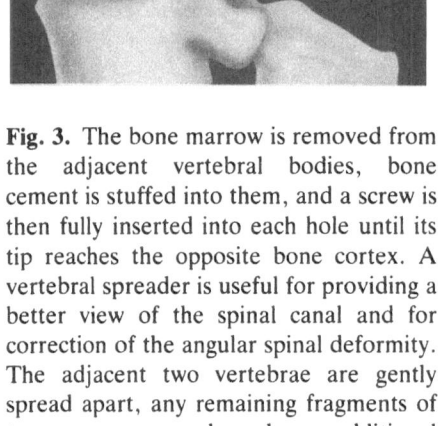

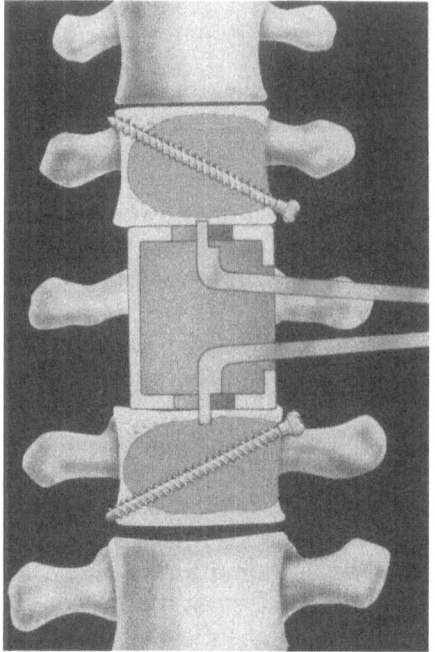

Fig. 3. The bone marrow is removed from the adjacent vertebral bodies, bone cement is stuffed into them, and a screw is then fully inserted into each hole until its tip reaches the opposite bone cortex. A vertebral spreader is useful for providing a better view of the spinal canal and for correction of the angular spinal deformity. The adjacent two vertebrae are gently spread apart, any remaining fragments of tumor are removed, and any additional bleeding is carefully controlled

Fig. 4. An anchor hole should be an extension of the intraprosthetic cavity. In order to insure this, the top and bottom surfaces of the adjacent vertebrae are excavated by a curette or a powered apparatus from inside the prosthesis. An anchor hole is then made in both the superior and inferior vertebrae. Once an appropriate hole has been made in the end plate, it can be further deepened

up in bed or standing and walking are usually permissible within the first 2–3 weeks after surgery. This progression, of course, depends on the motor recovery in the lower extremities and the patient's general condition. The rehabilitation program should start immediately after surgery. Once the wound has healed, radiotherapy, if indicated, should be instituted in the affected area. For the prevention of infection, broad spectrum antibiotics are administered routinely in a prophylactic manner, and attempts are made to maintain nutritional status.

Patient Material

There were 78 operations performed in 74 patients. The operations were carried out in the cervical area (24 cases), in the thoracic area (36), and also

Fig. 5. The prosthesis is introduced and its alignment carefully noted. The bone cement is then placed into the prosthesis through the anterior window and pushed with pressure into the anchor holes above and below. The pressure is maintained while the cement sets

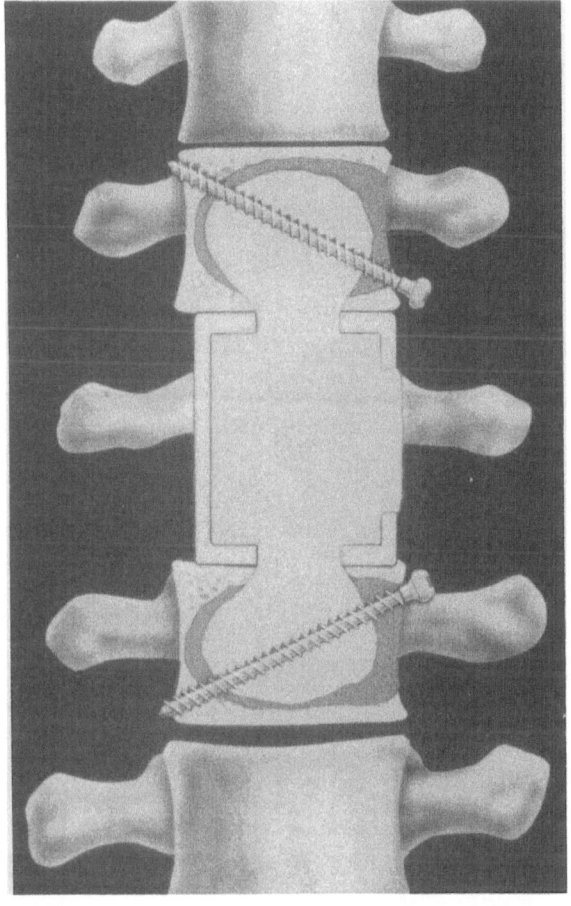

included 18 lumbar procedures. One patient had separate operations at T_4 and T_8, performed at a 3-month interval. Two patients had two level adjacent vertebral lesions resected at one operation. There were 37 males and 37 females and their ages ranged from 22 to 77 years.

Results

In summarizing the results, special note was taken with regard to pain relief and motor recovery. Of the 71 patients who complained of pain pre-operatively, 68 noted pain relief post-operatively. Of the 43 patients who had motor deficits pre-operatively, 36 noted improvement in motor function post-operatively. There were 34 non-ambulatory patients pre-operatively and 24 of these were able to ambulate post-operatively. The post-operative survival times ranged from 2 to 104 months (the longest-surviving patient is still alive). It is not particularly beneficial to discuss average survival time since it depends so much on the individual characteristics of the patient and the tumor involved. It is

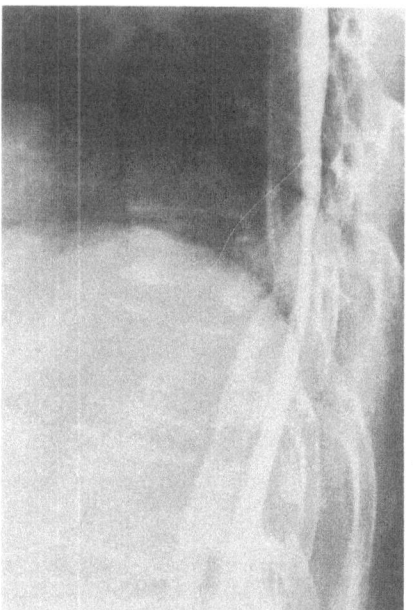

Fig. 6a,b. a The patient is a 67-year-old female whose thyroid carcinoma metastasized to the tenth thoracic vertebra and who complained of muscle weakness in both legs and very severe back pain. b Postoperative X-rays. The patient's neural symptoms and pain have been alleviated and she is now able to walk

a

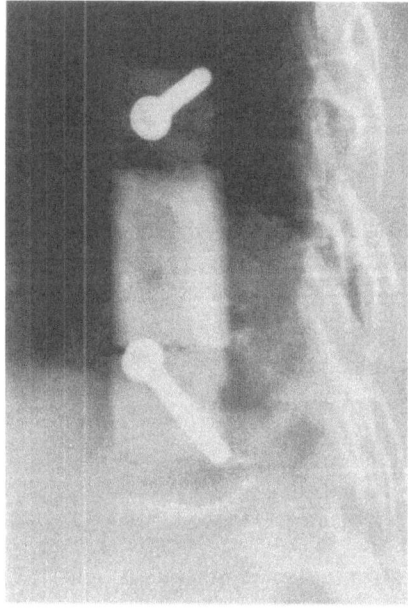
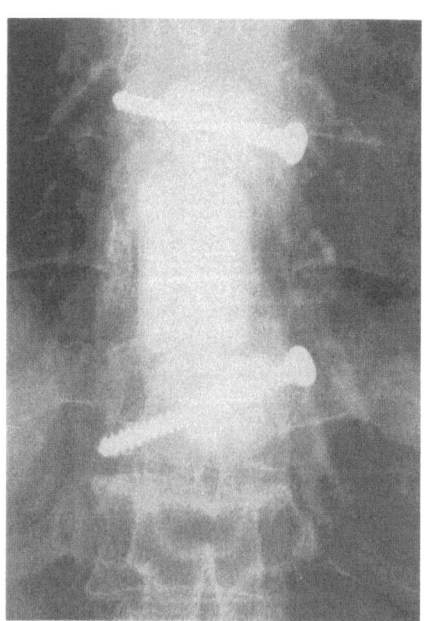

b

helpful to know, however, that 59 patients continue to maintain their surgical gain at present or maintained their surgical gain until their death. In the other 15 patients, 4 had additional metastases (femur, other spinal levels, etc.), and 11 had local recurrence, 1 having been helped by a laminectomy at a later date.

Complications

There were no intra-operative deaths, and there were no infections in the immediate post-operative period. Sixteen patients developed instability of the prosthesis of which 9 of these incidents were associated with tumor recurrence. Three patients had what was considered to be technical malplacement of the prosthesis at the time of surgery. One developed esophageal erosion and bleeding which led him to death. In one patient, the prosthesis became loose without evidence of recurrence or additional complications.

Additional Information

Six patients had posterior surgery in addition to the prosthetic replacement. Three of these procedures were carried out prior to the anterior surgery.

In four patients prosthetic replacement surgery was combined with laminectomy for the treatment of more extensive disease (two patients did surprisingly well, surviving 29 and 43 months after the first operation).

One laminectomy was carried out 11 months following the initial operation for local recurrence and the patient did well until death 40 months after the original operation.

Discussion

In a pathological study of spinal metastases, the vertebral body was proven to be the most frequent site for metastatic deposits [4]. In terms of patho-physiology, the vertebral body is the main focus precipitating the symptoms because of pain caused by pathological fracture, angulation, collapse, and tumor extension [5–8].

Despite the more frequent occurrence of metastases in the anterior aspect of the spine, until recently, the majority of surgery reported in the literature was carried out posteriorly [8, 9]. The anteriorly located tumor is rarely accessible through the posterior approach, and removal of the intact posterior elements by a laminectomy increases spinal instability.

The advent of CT scanning and improved techniques in bone scanning and myelography have allowed us to more precisely localize and delineate the extent of spinal metastases.

Because of our emphasis on patient selection (i.e., carefully delineating the indications and carefully reviewing the contraindications) in this group of patients undergoing prosthetic replacement surgery, it is not possible to compare our experience in any statistically valid way with that of previous authors, who reported on the results of laminectomy and/or radiation therapy for the treatment of spinal metastases [5, 7–9]. In general, their selections were less rigid. In our opinion, however, use of the posterior approach is partially responsible for the poorer results reported in these older series. We believe we have shown that by combining our knowledge of the location, pathophysiology, diagnostic methods, and surgical techniques for spinal metastases, we could obtain surprisingly good results in this selected group of patients upon whom we chose to operate.

Conclusions

When the indications for surgery are carefully observed and the surgery is performed in an appropriate manner, the procedure of prosthetic replacement of a vertebral body affected by metastatic tumor can contribute significantly to the avoidance of pain and neural deficit and the maintenance of the dignity and general quality of life in patients with metastatic disease.

References

1. Ono K, Tada K (1975) Metal prosthesis of the cervical vertebra. J Neurosurg 42:562–566
2. Ono K, Yonenobu K, Ebara S, Fujiwara K, Yamashita K, Fuji T, Dunn EJ (1988) Prosthetic replacement surgery for cervical spine metastasis. Spine 13:817–822
3. Ohta N, Fuji T, Fukushima F, Fujiwara K, Yamashita K, Ono K (1983) An experimental study of strength for compression force of alumina ceramic vertebral spacer. Orthopaedic Ceramic Implants 2:91–95
4. Boland PJ, Lane JM, Sundaresan N (1982) Metastatic disease of the spine. Clin Orthop 169:95–102
5. Black P (1979) Spinal metastasis: Current status and recommended guidelines for management. Neurosurgery 5:726–746
6. Constans JP, Divitiis E, Donzelli R, Spaziante R, Meder JF, Haye C (1983) Spinal metastases with neurological manifestations, Review of 600 cases. J Neurosurg 59:111–118
7. Harrington KP (1981) The use of methylmetacrylate for vertebral-body replacement and anterior stabilization of pathological fracture-dislocations of the spine due to metastatic malignant disease. J Bone Joint Surg [Am] 63:36–46
8. Onimus M, Schraub S, Bertin D, Bosset JF, Guidet M (1986) Surgical treatment of vertebral metastasis. Spine 11:883–891
9. Gilbert RW, Kim JH, Posner JB (1978) Epidural spinal cord compression from metastatic tumor: Diagnosis and treatment. Ann Neurol 3:40–51

Part 5

Prognostic Factors

5.1

Assessment of Malignancy of Bone and Soft Tissue Tumors Using DNA Cytofluorometry

Katsuyuki Kusuzaki,[1] Tsukasa Ashihara,[2] and Yasusuke Hirasawa[1]

Introduction

Many recent reports have demonstrated the usefulness of cytometric DNA ploidy analysis in assessing the nature of the malignancy of human tumors. Among the researchers who have attempted over the past 10 years to apply this technique to bone and soft tissue tumors [1–7], most believe that DNA ploidy analysis may be helpful not only for the histological diagnosis of malignancy but also in predicting prognosis. Most of these previous studies used flow cytometry, a method in which examiners are unable to determine the morphology of the studied cells, even though a large number of cells can be measured instantly. However, flow cytometry may not provide an accurate measurement of DNA content due to possible contamination with nontumorous cells, such as fibroblasts, granulocytes, and lymphocytes, and a large amount of debris from bony, cartilaginous, and collagenous matrices that commonly appear in bone and soft tissue tumors. In order to avoid these problems, we attempted to analyze the DNA ploidy of bone and soft tissue tumors using cytofluorometry. With this method, we were able to selectively measure only the tumor cells under a fluorescence microscope, although the measurable cell number was much lower than that obtained with flow cytometry and it was relatively time-consuming because we had to detect cells which had been smeared on a glass slide. The results of DNA ploidy analysis by cytofluorometry were statistically comparable with histological evaluation of malignancy performed by pathologists.

Kyoto Prefectural University of Medicine, [1] Department of Orthopaedic Surgery and [2] Pathology, Kamigyo-ku, Kyoto, 602 Japan

Materials and Methods

For a period of 8 years, we analyzed 257 patients with primary bone and soft tissue tumors who were surgically treated in our department. This study group included 141 patients with bone tumors and 116 with soft tissue tumors. Fifty-nine of the bone tumors were histologically diagnosed as benign and 49 as malignant. The other 25 cases were giant cell tumors of bone (GCT). The benign tumors included 17 enchondromas, 9 osteochondromas, 7 non-ossifying fibromas, 6 fibrous dysplasias, and 17 tumors of other types. Malignant tumors were comprised of 29 osteosarcomas, 10 chondrosarcomas, 3 lymphomas, 3 myelomas, 3 Ewing's sarcomas, and 1 chordoma. Histological diagnosis of the studied soft tissue tumors showed that 67 were benign and 49 were malignant. Twenty-one of the benign tumors were neurilemomas, 11 lipomas, 10 hemangiomas, 8 neurofibromas, and 17 were other kinds of tumors. The malignant tumors included 13 liposarcomas, 11 malignant fibrous histiocytomas (MFHs), 3 synovial sarcomas, 3 rhabdomyosarcomas, 3 leiomyosarcomas, and 16 other types of tumors. Benign tumor samples for cytofluorometry were obtained from fresh tumor tissue at resection, while malignant tumor samples were obtained at biopsy. Histological diagnosis of all patients was performed by more than one pathologist (T.A. and colleagues).

DNA Cytofluorometry

Cells were isolated from fresh tumor tissue after it was minced with scissors and filtrated through a 100-μm nylon or metal mesh. These isolated cells were smeared on a glass slide using a centrifugal smear machine (Autosmear: Sakura Seiki Co., Japan). After fixation with 70% ethanol, the smeared cells were treated with RNase (Sigma, USA) and were stained with propidium-iodide (PI: Sigma), which quantitatively intercalates between nuclear DNA strands. Since the nuclei of the PI-stained cells emitted red fluorescence under green light excitation, the DNA content of each cell was measured as fluorescence intensity by an epi-illumination-type cytofluorometer (Nikon SPM RF1-D, or OPTIPHOTO with P1: Nikon, Japan) [8]. DNA content histograms for ploidy analysis were obtained from the real-time input of the DNA content of 200 tumor cells into a personal computer connected to the cytofluorometer. By careful observation of cell morphology under a fluorescence microscope, the examiners (K.K. and colleagues), who are medical doctors with backgrounds in pathology or cytology, attempted to exclude granulocytes, lymphocytes, fibrocytes, and destructive nuclei, as well as many small fragments of bony, cartilaginous, and collagenous matrices in the smeared cell slides.

Statistical Analysis of DNA Ploidy

The DNA ploidy pattern of all tumors studied by DNA cytofluorometry was classified into 5 types: benign or malignant diploid, benign or malignant euploid-polyploid, and aneuploid. The frequency of diploid cells in all the tumors was calculated from each DNA histogram and was expressed in percentage form as the diploid index (DI). Significant differences between the average DI of benign and malignant tumors and GCTs were statistically analyzed. In soft tissue tumors, the average DI was analyzed and the frequency of DNA synthetic cells in diploid cell populations was calculated in tumors with a DI of more than 65%. The above-mentioned cells have an intermediate DNA content between that of diploid and tetraploid cells and are considered to be in the S phase of the cell cycle. This frequency was, therefore, termed the S index (SI) in our study. A statistical comparison of the SI in benign and malignant soft tissue tumors was also conducted.

Results

Except for some types of soft tissue tumors, the benign tumors analyzed in this study had DNA histograms which indicated that most of the tumor cells were diploid, while a few were tetraploid or in the S phase. This DNA ploidy pattern was the "benign diploid" type. Some of the benign soft tissue tumors, such as neurilemoma, neurofibroma, lipoma, and hemangioma, displayed the diploid-type DNA content histogram with many tetraploid and a few octaploid or double-octaploid cells. This ploidy pattern was termed the "benign euploid-polyploid-type" in which most of the cells were diploid and the frequency of tetraploid cells was usually higher than that of octaploid or double-octaploid cells. There were very few S-phase cells in the diploid or tetraploid populations in this ploidy pattern.

The DNA ploidy pattern of malignant bone and soft tissue tumors was classified into 3 types (Fig. 1). The diploid type was similar to that of benign tumors, but the frequency of S- and G_2-phase cells was increased, suggesting enhanced cell proliferation. Most cases of GCT, malignant lymphoma, Ewing's sarcoma, myxoid or round cell liposarcoma, and synovial sarcoma, and some cases of chondrosarcoma and osteosarcoma showed this type of ploidy pattern. The DNA content histogram shown in the upper panel of Fig. 1 demonstrates a typical diploid-type ploidy pattern obtained from a patient with low-grade malignant chondrosarcoma. The DNA content histogram of euploid-polyploid type tumors revealed many tetraploid cells with S- or G_2-phase cells and a few ployploid cells, although a diploid cell population was usually present. This ploidy pattern was different from the previously mentioned benign euploid-polyploid type. Some of the studied chondrosarcoma, osteosarcoma, and MFH had this kind of ploidy pattern. The representative DNA content histogram of euploid-polyploid type tumor was obtained from a patient with periosteal chondrosarcoma (Fig. 1 middle panel). The last pattern was an aneuploid type, which was characteristic of highly malignant sarcomas diagnosed by histology, such as osteosarcoma (grade III or IV), chondrosarcoma (grade III), storiform- or pleomorphic-type MFH, pleomorphic-type liposarcoma, and rhabdomyosarcoma. The DNA content histogram shown in Fig. 1 (lower panel) demonstrates the typical DNA ploidy pattern of an aneuploid tumor

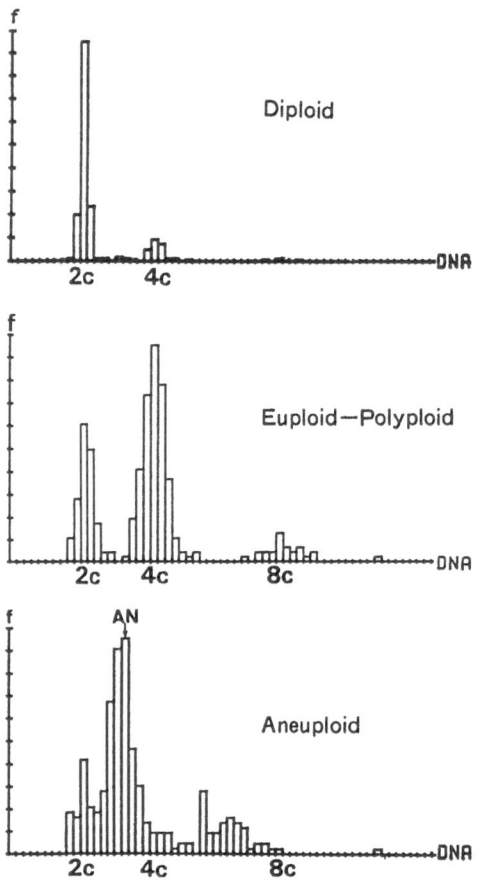

Fig. 1. Three different types of DNA ploidy patterns recognized in DNA content histograms obtained by cytofluorometry of malignant bone and soft tissue tumors. The *upper* histogram demonstrates typical diploid type obtained from a patient with low-grade malignant chondrosarcoma, and the *middle* one is a euploid-polyploid type obtained from a patient with periosteal chondrosarcoma. The *lower* histogram is of an aneuploid type obtained from a patient with osteosarcoma which consists of many hypotetraploid cells (*AN*) with their *DNA* synthetic cells. *c*, chromosome number

obtained from a patient with osteosarcoma. In all the tumors analyzed in this study, the most common DNA content of aneuploid cells was hypotetraploid.

The DI of all the studied bone tumors are shown in Fig. 2. Benign bone tumors had an average DI of 94% (SD = 0.8%), whereas malignant bone tumors had an average DI of 52.2% (SD = 25.8%). The average DI of GCT was 83% (SD = 7.8%). There were statistically significant differences with respect to DI between benign and malignant tumors ($P < 0.001$), benign tumors and GCT ($P < 0.001$), and GCT and malignant tumors ($P < 0.001$). Excluding GCT, 108 of the analyzed bone tumors (including all benign tumors) had a DI of greater than 80%; of these, only 6 were diagnosed as malignant by histological examination. Therefore, the inconsistency in determining the malignancy of bone tumors between DNA ploidy analysis and histological examination was 5.6%. In soft tissue tumors, the average DI of benign tumors was 90.3% (SD = 6.7%), while that of malignant tumors was 57.6% (SD = 29.3%). A significant difference between both kinds of tumors was also statistically confirmed ($P < 0.001$) (Fig. 3). All the benign soft tissue tumors ($n = 67$) had a DI of greater than 65%, which was much lower than that of benign

Fig. 2. The diploid index (*DI*) of all the bone tumors analyzed in this study by DNA cytofluorometry. Statistic testing revealed that the average DI is significantly different between benign tumors, giant cell tumors (*GCTs*), and malignant tumors (*). All benign tumors had a DI of greater than 80%

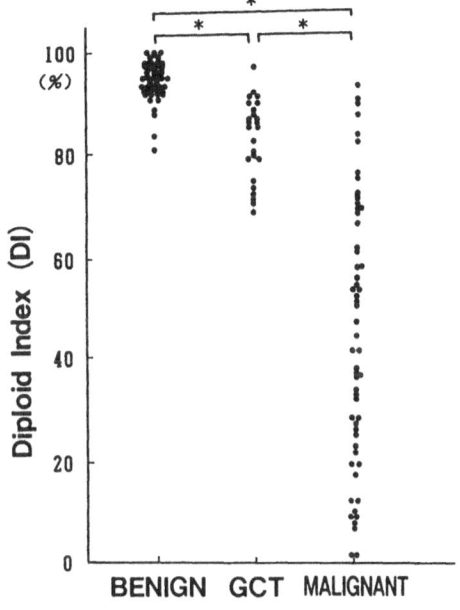

Fig. 3. The diploid index (*DI*) of all benign and malignant soft tissue tumors analyzed in this study. Although there was a statistically significant difference in the average DI between both kinds of tumors (*), many malignant tumors had a DI of greater than 65%, which was the lowest DI among the benign tumors

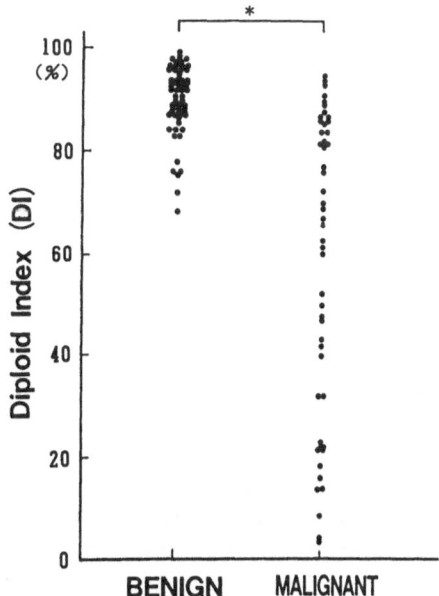

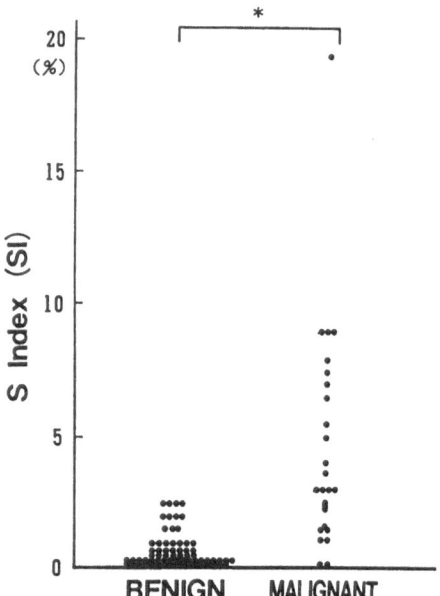

Fig. 4. The SI (frequency of DNA synthetic cells of diploid cell population: *S index*) of all the benign soft tissue tumors ($n = 67$) and malignant tumors ($n = 25$) having a DI of greater than 65%. All the benign tumors and only 9 of the 25 malignant tumors had a SI of lower than 3%

bone tumors, due to contamination of benign euploid-polyploid type tumors. However, 25 of all malignant soft tissue tumors ($n = 49$) also had a DI of greater than 65%. These tumors were classified as having the diploid type ploidy pattern; the SI of their diploid cells is, therefore, comparable to that of benign tumors having the diploid or euploid-polyploid type of the ploidy pattern. All the benign tumors displayed an SI of less than 3%, while 16 out of 25 malignant tumors had an SI of greater than 3% (Fig. 4). The average SI was significantly different between benign and malignant tumors. Consequently, in 9 out of 116 patients with soft tissue tumors, the results of assessment of malignancy by DNA ploidy analysis were inconsistent with those obtained by histological examination.

Discussion

Many DNA ploidy studies using either flow cytometry or cytofluorometry have revealed that human tumors showing an aneuploid or euploid-polyploid type ploidy pattern or having a high mean cellular DNA content are malignant [1–7]. These studies also suggested that an increased number of DNA synthetic cells in diploid cell populations may be closely related to malignancy. In bone and soft tissue tumors, the above-mentioned observations were also found to be useful for assessing malignancy in some flow-cytometric studies [1–7]. The DNA content of many tumor cells can be measured more quickly and easily with flow cytometry than with cytofluorometry. However, it is likely that DNA content histograms obtained by flow cytometry include fragments of bone, cartilage, a collagen fiber as well as non-tumorous cells. Our study was performed using cytofluorometry in order to avoid this sort of contamination and to selectively measure the DNA content of tumor cells [9, 10].

Ploidy analysis of benign bone and soft tissue tumors demonstrated that the main cell population is usually diploid with a few tetraploid cells. However, some nerve sheath tumors, hemangiomas, and lipomas have euploid-polyploid cells, such as tetraploid, octaploid, and double octaploid cells [9, 11]. Nobody using flow cytometry has reported euploid-polyploidization in soft tissue tumors, probably because flow cytometry is unable to detect such small populations among debris. Statistical analysis of the DNA ploidy shows that the average DI is significantly different between benign and malignant bone and soft tissue tumors. This finding is similar to the results of mean DNA indexing by flow cytometry [1–7]. However, statistical methods are not available to evaluate the malignancy of diploid type tumors. A diagnostic borderline between the DI of benign and malignant tumors is needed to assess malignancy in individual cases. When we made a DI of 80% as the cutoff point in this study, all analyzed benign bone tumors and only 6 malignant bone tumors had a DI of greater than 80%, whereas all other malignant tumors had a DI of less than 80%. Therefore, the inconsistency in determining malignancy between histological examination and ploidy analysis was only 5.6%. These data suggest that when DI calculated from the DNA histogram of a bone tumor is used to analyze malignancy, a value of 80% appears to distinguish between benign and malignant tumors. In GCT, as we previously reported [12, 13], some tumors showing a DI of less than 88% frequently recurred or metastasized to the lung.

All the studied benign soft tissue tumors had a DI of greater than 65%. In tumors with a DI value that was borderline between benign and malignant, the inconsistency between histological diagnosis and ploidy analytic assessment of malignancy was 27%, a discrepancy that makes ploidy analysis impractical in the clinical setting. However, we found that when SI (S index: frequency of DNA synthetic cells) was calculated from the DNA content histograms of 116 tumors with a DI of greater than 65%, all the benign tumors ($n = 67$) and only 9 of the 25 malignant tumors had an SI of less than 3%. The inconsistency between histological examination and ploidy analysis was evaluated to be 7.8%, which shows ploidy analysis to have diagnostic merit.

Conclusions

DNA ploidy analysis by cytofluorometry is useful for the quantitative assessment of malignancy of bone and soft tissue tumors. We believe that cytofluorometry is probably a better method than flow cytometry for DNA analysis of bone and soft tissue tumors.

References

1. Ashihara T, Kamachi M, Urata Y, Kusuzaki K, Takeshita H, Kagawa K (1986) Multiparametric analysis using autostage cytofluorometry. Acta Histochem Cytochem 19:51–59

2. Mankin HJ, Connor JF, Schiller AL, Perlmutter A, Alho A, McGuire M (1985) Grading of bone tumors by analysis of nuclear DNA content using flow cytometry. J Bone Joint Surg [Am] 67:404–413
3. Heilo H, Karaharju E, Nordling S (1985) Flow cytometric determination of DNA content in malignant and benign bone tumors. Cytometry 6:165–171
4. Bauer HCF, Kreicbergs A, Tribukait B (1986) DNA microspectrophotometry of bone sarcomas in tissue sections as compared to imprint and flow DNA analysis. Cytometry 7:544–550
5. Xiang J, Spanier SS, Benson NA, Braylan RC (1987) Flow cytometric analysis of DNA in bone and soft-tissue tumors using nuclear suspensions. Cancer 59: 1951–1958
6. Kreicbergs A, Tribukait B, Willems J, Bauer HCF (1987) DNA flow analysis of soft tissue tumors. Cancer 59:128–133
7. Matsuno T, Gebhardt MC, Schiller AL, Rosenberg AE, Mankin HJ (1988) The use of flow cytometry as a diagnostic aid in the management of soft tissue tumors. J Bone Joint Surg [Am] 70:751–759
8. Bauer HCF, Kreicbergs A, Silfversward C, Tribukait B (1988) DNA analysis in the differential diagnosis of osteosarcoma. Cancer 61:1430–1436
9. Kusuzaki K, Takeshita H, Kuzuhara A, Bann S, Yamashita F, Sakakida K, Kamachi M, Tsuchihashi Y, Ashihara T (1984) DNA cytofluorometry of soft tissue tumors. Jpn J Cancer Clin 30:1904–1912
10. Kusuzaki K, Takeshita H, Bann S, Kamachi M, Yamashita F, Ashihara T, Sakakida K (1985) An attempt of DNA cytofluorometry of bone tumors (abstract). Seikeigeka 36:647–653
11. Takeshita H, Kusuzaki K, Kuzuhara A, Bann S, Yamashita F, Sakakida K, Kamachi M, Ashihara T (1985) DNA cytofluorometric analysis of nerve sheath tumors. J Jpn Orthop Assoc 59:763–772
12. Kusuzaki K, Takeshita H, Kuzuhara A, Bann S, Yamashita F, Sakakida K, Kamachi M, Ashihara T (1986) The relationship between cell kinetics and histological features of giant cell tumor of bone. J Jpn Orthop Assoc 60:51–60
13. Kusuzaki K, Takeshita H, Kuzuhara A, Tsuji Y, Yamashita F, Sakakida K, Kamachi M, Ashihara T (1986) Biological malignancy of giant cell tumors of bone as analyzed by cell proliferative activity using DNA cytofluorometry (abstract). Seikeigeka: 38:559–567

5.2

The Evaluation of Clinical Prognostic Factors in Osteosarcomas

Tohru Umeda, Takeshi Ishii, Masashi Kitoh, Toshiyuki Ozawa,[1] Norihiko Takada, and Shin-ichiro Tatezaki[2]

Introduction

During the past 15 years, dramatic changes have been made in the treatment of osteosarcoma. The survival rate of patients with osteosarcoma has improved as a result of better adjuvant chemotherapeutic regimens [1–3]. There are many other factors, however, that have been shown to influence the prognosis of this disease, among them the patient's age, site and size of the lesion, chemotherapeutic regimens, and surgical procedures [4–9]. We recently reviewed all cases of conventional osteosarcoma treated at Chiba Cancer Center, and analyzed the clinical prognostic factors of this disease.

Materials

A total of 139 patients with conventional osteosarcoma were treated from 1972 to 1989. Not included in this study were cases of parosteal, periosteal, multicentric, low-grade intramedullary, and post-irradiation osteosarcoma, nor of osteosarcoma arising from Paget's disease. Adriamycin (ADR) was used as the main chemotherapeutic agent against osteosarcoma from 1975 to the present [10]. High-dose methotrexate (MTX) with citrovorum factor rescue was started in 1977 and continued to the present. The use of *cis*-platinum (CDDP) was begun in 1983 and has continued to the present [11, 12]. Starting in 1972, surgical procedures were combined with either Liniac X-ray or Co60 administered locally to tumors. Fast neutron irradiation was instituted in 1975 [10, 13]; however, the resultant poor limb function [1] led to discontinuation of radiation therapy in 1985. Although we have used intra-arterial CDDP therapy for several cases, our current chemotherapy regimen is Rosen T-12 (Fig. 1).

---

[1] Department of Orthopedic Surgery, Kashiwa National Hospital, Chiba, 277 Japan
[2] Department of Orthopedic Surgery, Chiba Cancer Center, Chiba, 277 Japan

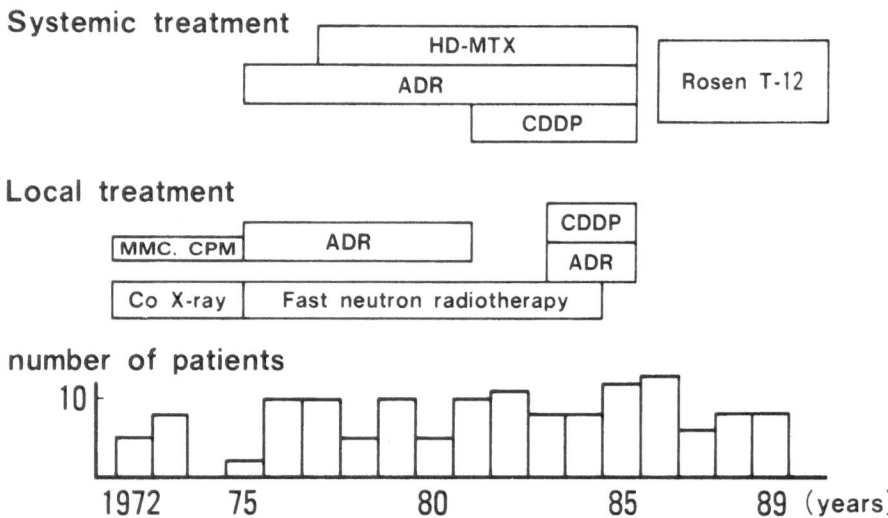

Fig. 1. The changes of the treatment modality of osteosarcoma in our institute. *MMC*, Mitomycin C; *CPM*, cychlophosphamide; *ADR*, adriamycin; *HD-MTX*, high-dose methotrexate; *CDDP*, *cis*-platinum

Seventy-four out of 139 patients were males and 65 were females. Their ages ranged from 5 to 63 years (mean: 17.6 years). Sixty-two lesions were located in the distal femur (45%), 34 proximal tibia (24%), 16 proximal humerus (12%), 11 fibula (8%), 4 pelvis (3%), 3 proximal femur (2%), 3 distal tibia (2%), and 6 in other sites (4%). Twenty-one out of 139 cases showed pulmonary metastases at the time of presentation (M1 group). Thirteen cases treated from 1972 to 1974 had not received any systemic chemotherapy (control group). Nineteen cases had inappropriate treatment histories or had refused chemotherapy (dropout group). Some cases were counted in both the M1 and dropout groups. Ninety-three cases, excluding those in the M1, control, and dropout groups, were eligible for this study of prognostic factors. The M1, control, and dropout groups were evaluated separately.

Results

Age

Patients 1–10 years of age showed a 46% 5-year cumulative survival rate (5-year SR) calculated by the Kaplan-Meier method. The 5-year SR of patients in the 11 to 20-year age group was 60% and that of the over-20 years age group was 51%. There was no significant statistical difference.

Sex

Female patients had a 62% 5-year SR and male patients had a 53% 5-year SR. Again, no statistically significant difference was detected.

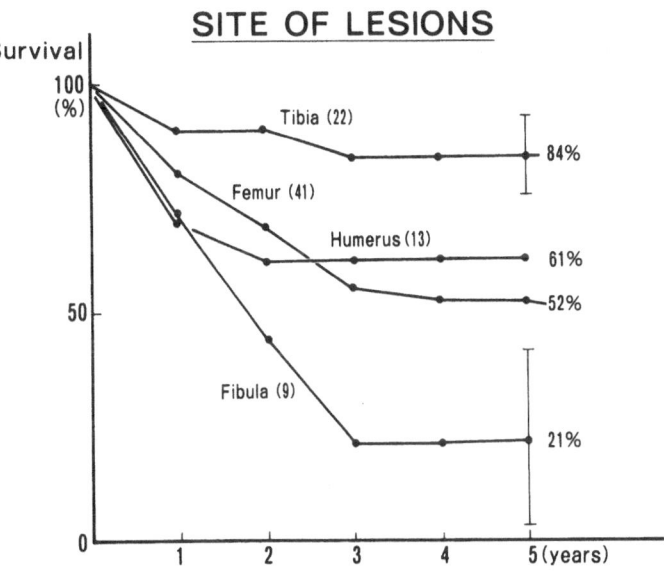

Fig. 2. The 5-year survival rates of patients with lesions of the tibia, humerus, femur, and fibula. *Longitudinal bars* indicate standard deviations

Duration of Symptoms

Twenty-eight patients experienced a 1-month duration of symptoms. Thirty-five patients experienced symptoms from 1–3 months, and 27 patients had greater than a 3-months' duration of symptoms. The 5-year SR was 58%, 58%, and 60%, respectively.

Serum Alkaline Phosphatase (ALP)

Forty patients had a normal serum ALP at presentation and 46 patients demonstrated a serum ALP of over twice the normal limit. The 5-year SR of the former group was 65% and greater than 49% in the latter group, showing no significant difference.

Tumor Site

The 5-year SR of patients with tumor originating in the proximal tibia was 84%. This was significantly better than the 52% 5-year SR of patients who had tumor originating in the femur and the 21% 5-year SR of patients with tumor originating in the fibula. Patients with tumor confined to the proximal humerus had a 61% 5-year SR (Fig. 2).

Radiological Appearance

We defined three patterns of osteosarcoma: predominantly sclerotic (31 cases), predominantly lytic (21 cases), and mixed (41 cases). The sclerotic variant demonstrated a better 5-year SR (72%) than the lytic variant (36%).

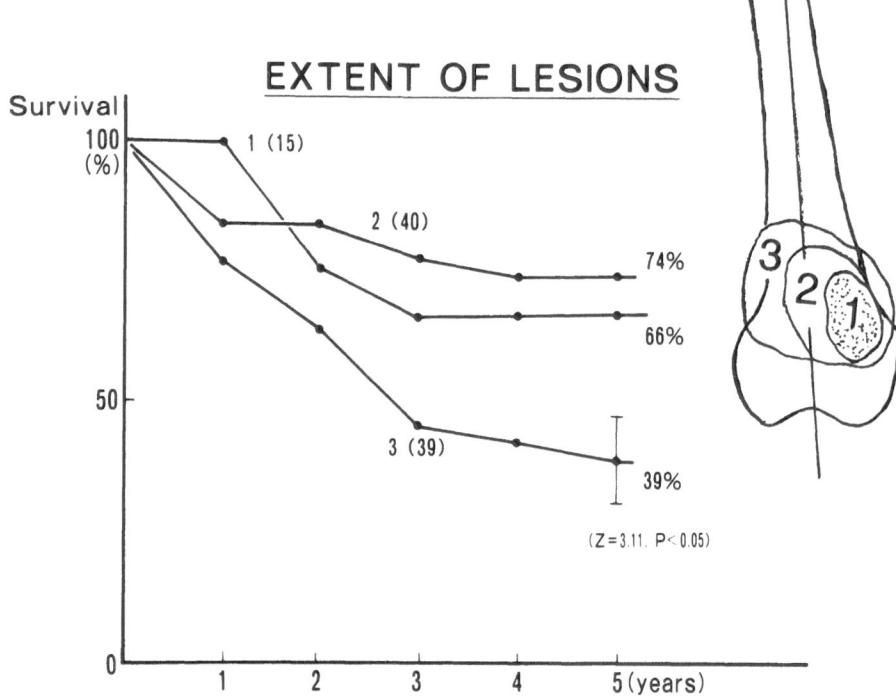

Fig. 3. The 5-year survival rates of patients with IIB-1, IIB-2, and IIB-3 lesions. The prognosis of IIB-3 was worse than either IIB-1 or IIB-2 ($P < 0.05$). Z, standard deviate; n, patient numbers

Local Extent of Tumor

According to Enneking's surgical staging system, most cases were classified as stage IIB. We further divided IIB into three subtypes, IIB-1 (15 cases), IIB-2 (40 cases), and IIB-3 (39 cases). Tumors in IIB-1 and IIB-2 are osteosarcomas with a soft tissue mass involving one side of the bone only (Fig. 3). The IIB-3 tumors have soft tissue masses involving both sides of the affected bone. The IIB-3 type showed a worse 5-year SR (39%) than either IIB-1 (66%) or IIB-2 (74%).

Histological Subtype

Of the 96 cases, 50 were classified as osteoblastic and 26 as chondroblastic. The remaining 20 cases were difficult to classify into a subtype. There were no significant 5-year SR differences between the groups.

Preoperative Chemotherapeutic Effect

We were unable to evaluate preoperative chemotherapeutic effects adequately because 93 out of 139 cases (67%) had also received preoperative radiation therapy.

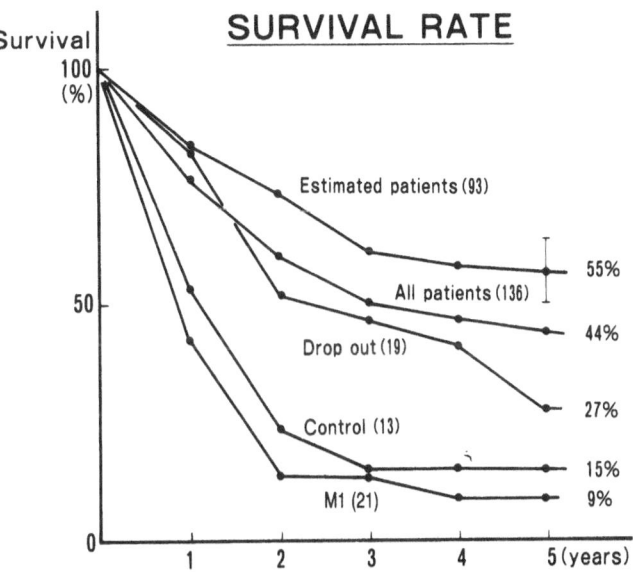

Fig. 4. The 5-year survival rates of each group. *Dropout*, Patients with inappropriate treatments; *Control*, the group which had not received any systemic chemotherapy: *M1*, patients with pulmonary metastasis at presentation, *estimated patients*, excluded dropout, control, or M1 patients

Surgical Procedure

The limb salvage group (52 cases) had a better prognosis than the amputation group (32 cases), but there was no significant statistical difference.

Pulmonary Metastasis

Out of 139 cases, 91 (65%) developed pulmonary metastases. Sixty-two of these underwent surgical excision of pulmonary nodules and exhibited a 25% 5-year SR [14].

M1 Group

Out of 21 M1 cases, 13 were initially treated at other hospitals. The following surgical procedures were carried out: 12 amputations and 8 limb salvage operations. Of the 13 patients who underwent thoracotomy for excision of pulmonary metastases, only 2 are alive [1 alive with disease (AWD), 1 no evidence of disease (NED)]. The mean survival period of patients who underwent thoracotomy was 13.6 months. This was better than that for patients without thoracotomy who had a mean survival rate of 6.0 months. The M1 group demonstrated a 9% 5-year SR (Fig. 4).

Dropout Group

Twelve cases had a history of inappropriate treatment such as intra-lesional excision or unsuitable chemotherapy. Five patients had discontinued chemotherapy after several courses and two patients had received no chemotherapy. The 1-year survival rate of this group was fairly good (84%), but the 5-year SR was only 27%.

Control Group

Thirteen patients from this group demonstrated a 15% 5-year SR.

The 5-year SR of all cases was 44% and that of the 93 cases exclusive of the M1, control, and dropout groups was 55% (Fig. 4).

Discussion

In the treatment of osteosarcoma, it is extremely important to make an accurate diagnosis and administer appropriate therapy, especially optimal chemotherapy. Our study demonstrated poor prognosis in patients who had either been misdiagnosed and treated inappropriately or who had rejected chemotherapy.

Bentzen et al. studied 184 patients with osteosarcoma and demonstrated that tumors localized to the trunk, pelvis, or femur, with a duration of symptoms of less than 6 months were poor prognostic signs [5]. They also showed that tumors dominated by fibroblastic cells in patients of approximately 25–30 years of age were good prognostic indicators. Neither sex nor radiological appearance had prognostic implications. Delepine et al. analyzed 87 patients with osteosarcoma and showed the worst prognostic factor to be in the young age group (<5 yr) among the patients treated from 1978 to 1982. However, the young patients treated from 1984 to 1987 demonstrated a better prognosis because the dose of MTX was adapted to age. They concluded that the most important prognostic factor was the amount of MTX [6]. Taylor analyzed 543 osteosarcomas in 13 institutions and presented the following prognostic factors: histological classification, site of lesion, size of lesion, histological grade, duration of symptoms, weight loss, local swelling, and radiological appearance [4]. Takeyama demonstrated that the local condition of the tumor had no significant prognostic effect other than on local recurrence and that tumors located in the tibia and tumors with a low mitotic ratio in the biopsy specimen have a better prognosis [8]. It has been shown that tumors associated with pathological fracture or skip metastasis have a poor prognosis [15, 16]. Our study demonstrated significantly better prognosis in tumors which were located in the tibia, had osteoblastic histology, or were small in size and had no pulmonary metastasis at presentation. Various papers report different prognostic factors. This is probably due to the difference of treatment methods and the relatively small series of cases. Recently, the most important prognostic factor has been thought to be chemotherapy. Our study showed a far better prognosis if patients received systemic chemotherapy compared to those who did not (control). The telangiectatic osteosarcoma which was thought to be associated with a worse prognosis than the usual osteosarcoma has now been shown to be extremely responsive to chemotherapy [17]. Rosen et al. reported that patients with good response to preoperative chemotherapy showed good prognosis [2]. Raymond et al. reported that the continuous disease-free survival rate was 91% in patients with >90% tumor necrosis by preoperative chemotherapy, while it was 14% in <90% tumor necrosis [7]. Kawano et al. indicated the most important prognostic factor to be the preoperative chemotherapy effect [18]. Thus, the effect of preoperative chemotherapy has been shown to be a more important prognostic factor than histological appearance, age of the patient, and tumor size. Therefore, we must increase the numbers of good responders to chemotherapy and improve the survival rate of poor responders in order to improve the overall survival rate of patients with osteosarcoma.

Summary

1. We evaluated the prognostic factors of 139 osteosarcomas.
2. Tumors of a sclerotic type, small in size and tibial in location showed significantly better prognosis.
3. Tumors in the 10 to 19-year age group, limb salvage procedure group, normal ALP, and osteoblastic type groups had a better prognosis, although the difference was not statistically significant.
4. The dropout and control groups showed the worse prognosis.
5. The 5-year SR of all cases was 44% and that of the 93 cases evaluated in this study was 55%.

References

1. Umeda T, Takada N (1985) The functional evaluation of osteosarcoma patients with limb salvage treatment (in Japanese). Rinsho Seikei Geka 20:216–226
2. Rosen G, Caparros B, Huvos AG, et al. (1982) Preoperative chemotherapy for osteogenic sarcoma: Selection of postoperative adjuvant chemotherapy based on the response of the primary tumor to preoperative chemotherapy. Cancer 49:1221–1230
3. Winkler K, Beron G, Kotz R, et al. (1984) Neoadjuvant chemotherapy for osteogenic sarcoma: Results of a cooperative German/Austrian study. J Clin Oncol 12:617–624
4. Taylor WF, Ivins JC, Unni KK, et al. (1989) Prognostic variables in osteosarcoma: A multi-institutional study. J Natl Cancer Inst 81:21–30
5. Bentzen SM, Poulsen HS, Kaae S, et al. (1988) Prognostic factors in osteosarcomas. Cancer 62:194–202
6. Delepine N, Delepine G, Jasmin C, et al. (1988) Importance of age and methotrexate dosage: Prognosis in children and young adults with high-grade osteosarcomas. Biomed Pharmacother 42:257–262

7. Raymond AK, Chawla SP, Carrasco CH, et al. (1987) Osteosarcoma chemotherapy effects: A prognostic factor. Semin Diagn Pathol 4:212–236

8. Takeyama S, Tateishi A (1989) Analysis for treatment of osteosarcoma — Good prognostic factors. J Jpn Orthop Assoc 63:S455

9. Scranton PE, DeCicco FA, Totten RS, et al. (1975) Prognostic factors in osteosarcoma: A review of 20 years' experience at the University of Pittsburgh Health Center. Cancer 36:2179–2191

10. Takada N, Hodaka E (1979) The treatment of osteosarcoma (in Japanese). Rinsho Seikei Geka 14:756–764

11. Umeda T, Takada N, Hodaka E, et al. (1984) Evaluation of severe side effects of high-dose methotrexate in osteosarcoma (in Japanese). Gan to Kagaku Ryoho 11:285–294

12. Umeda T, Takada N, Hodaka E, et al. (1986) Toxic effects of cisplatin in the treatment of malignant bone and soft tissue tumors (in Japanese). Gan To Kagaku Ryoho 13:1857–1861

13. Takada N, Hodaka E (1979) Radiation therapy of osteosarcomas (in Japanese). Orthop Surg Traumatol 22:681–691

14. Umeda T, Takada N, Seki Y (1983) The treatment of osteosarcoma patients developed pulmonary metastases (in Japanese). Rinsyo Seikei Geka 20:917–927

15. Jaffe N, Spears R, Eftekhari F, et al. (1987) Pathological fracture in osteosarcoma. Cancer 59:701–709

16. Wuisman P, Enneking WF (1990) Prognosis for patients who have osteosarcoma with skip metastasis. J Bone Joint Surg [Am] 72:60–68

17. Rosen G, Huvos AG, Marcove R, et al. (1986) Telangiectatic osteosarcoma: Improved survival with combination chemotherapy. Clin Orthop 207:164–173

18. Kawano H (1989) Neoadjuvant chemotherapy for osteosarcoma — The value in survival. J Jpn Orthop Assoc 63:S457

Histological Typing and Grading of Adult Soft Tissue Sarcomas: Eastern Cooperative Oncology Group (ECOG) Experience and Review of the Literature

MASANORI SHIRAKI,[1] and JOHN J.S. BROOKS[2]

Introduction

Accurate histological typing of soft tissue sarcomas (STS) is a challenging task for pathologists [1–3]. Because of the significant diagnostic discordance among pathologists, the importance of histopathology peer review in the analysis of therapeutic trials has been emphasized [1, 4, 5]. Although the histological grade of malignancy (HGM) is considered to be the most important prognostic indicator, the grading system is highly complex and is not entirely reproducible [1, 6]. This report presents (1) the experience of the ECOG Pathology Review Committee with histological typing and grading of STS, including comparison of the ECOG experience with the other sarcoma study groups, (2) prognostic significance of HGM and various grading systems used by major group studies, and (3) influence of histological type and tumor grade on chemosensitivity of advanced adult STS in the ECOG trial EST 3377 [5].

Histological Typing of Soft Tissue Sarcomas

Soft tissue sarcomas represent a diverse group of rare neoplasms with considerable variations in histological patterns and biological behavior. While some cell types show little variation in behavior from case to case, others present a wide range of behavior within each cell type [3, 7]. The difficulty in making a precise diagnosis of STS is reflected by the significant number of disagreements in diagnosis between institutional pathologists and reviewers [1, 4, 5] (Table 1). It is impossible to compare the reported incidence of STS cell types or to analyze the therapeutic response of particular cell types in the literature since the criteria for diagnosis are not uniformly applied.

[1] Baystate Medical Center, Western Campus of Tufts University School of Medicine, Springfield, MA 01199, USA
[2] University of Pennsylvania School of Medicine, PA 19104, USA

Table 1. Comparison of reviewer agreement in diagnosis of sarcomas

Study group[a]	Year	Agreement				Disagreement				Total cases (n)
		Diagnosis	(%)	Grade	(%)	Other sarcoma[b]	(%)	Non-sarcoma[c]	(%)	
SWOG [4]	1978	79	(61)			41	(31.7)	10	(7.3)	130
SEG [1]	1986	137	(66)	G1	(83)	58	(28)	12	(6)	207
				G2	(77)					
				G3	(72)					
FNCLCC [6]	1986	16	(61)							25
ECOG	1987	780	(73)		(75)	160	(15)	131	(12)[d]	1,071
Swedish Cancer Registry [9]									(10)	800[e]

[a] SWOG, Southwestern Oncology Group, USA; SEG, Southeastern Cancer Study Group, USA; FNCLCC, French Federation of Cancer Centers Sarcoma Study Group; ECOG, Eastern Cooperative Oncology Group, USA
[b] Disagreement on type of sarcoma
[c] Disagreement on presence of sarcoma
[d] Cases of non-sarcoma or ineligible cell type or cases in which diagnosis of sarcoma cannot be confirmed on review
[e] Cases in the Swedish Cancer Registry between 1958 and 1963

To minimize misinterpretation of treatment results from improper histological diagnosis, all the pathology material in the ECOG trials were reviewed
by a panel of eight experienced pathologists from various ECOG member
institutions. The review panel evaluated the eligibility of each case histopathologically by confirming or reclassifying the submitting diagnosis or reject-
ing patients with non-sarcomatous malignancies or benign neoplasms. If there
were a failure to reach a consensus on a case, or if there were uncertainty
among committee members, the case was referred to our consultant, Dr. Franz
M. Enzinger of the Armed Forces Institute of Pathology, for his opinion and
diagnosis. The histological typing of all the tumors followed the World Health
Organization (WHO) Histological Classification of Soft Tissue Tumors [8]. As
of May 1987, a total of 1,071 cases were reviewed by the panel. The overall
agreement rate between the eligible submitting diagnosis and the pathology
review panel's interpretation was 73% (780/1,071). However, disagreement
with respect to sarcoma cell type occurred in 15% (160/1,071). Diagnosis of
sarcoma was not confirmed in 12% of the cases (131/1,071). In comparison, the
Southeastern Cancer Study Group (SEG) experienced a slightly lower overall
agreement rate (66%) between the primary pathologists and the reviewer [1].
Lower agreement rates also were reported by the French Federation of Cancer
Centers (FNCLCC) Sarcoma Study Group (61%) and by the Southwestern
Oncology Group (SWOG) (61%) [4, 6]. It has been shown that the incidence
of non-sarcoma, or cases in which diagnosis of sarcoma cannot be confirmed on
peer review, varied from 6%–12% [1, 4, 9] (Table 1).

Although the overall agreement rate between the review panel and the
submitting diagnosis was 74% in the recent ECOG trial (EST 3377), the
agreement rate varied from 17% to 100% when divided into different cell types
[5]. The agreement rate was lowest for those submitted as rhabdomyosarcoma
(17%) and highest for Ewing's sarcoma (100%) and alveolar soft part sarcoma (100%). While the agreement rates for malignant fibrous histiocytoma
(MFH) and malignant schwannoma were relatively high, a significant number
of cases were submitted as other types of sarcoma (Table 2). The most commonly mislabeled submitting diagnoses for MFH were rhabdomyosarcoma or
fibrosarcoma and those for malignant schwannoma were sarcoma not otherwise
specified (NOS) or fibrosarcoma. Sarcomas with lower agreement rate included
rhabdomyosarcoma, fibrosarcoma, sarcoma NOS, and angiosarcoma (Table 3).

Grading of Soft Tissue Sarcomas and Its Prognostic Significance

Although the histologic grade of malignancy (HGM) is considered to be the
single most important prognostic indicator of soft tissue sarcomas, uniform
criteria for grading has not been well established. In most studies, HGM is
based on histological type and/or a composite of morphological features,
including cellular differentiation, pleomorphism, cellularity, mitotic count, and
necrosis. There are a number of reports indicating the prognostic significance
of various histopathological and clinical parameters. However, significant

Table 2. Sarcomas with high agreement but often unrecognized

Cell types	A. Submitting diagnosis (*n*)	B. Panel agreed (%)	C. Submitted as other sarcomas		D. Confirmed cases (B and C)
MFH	51	41 (80)	Rhabdomyosarcoma	6	63 (41 and 22)
			Fibrosarcoma	5	
			Leiomyosarcoma	2	
			Liposarcoma	1	
			Mesothelioma	1	
			No diagnosis	7	
			Total	22	
Malignant schwannoma	16	13 (81)	Fibrosarcoma	2	23 (13 and 10)
			Leiomyosarcoma	1	
			Sarcoma NOS	5	
			No diagnosis	2	
			Total	10	

MFH, Malignant fibrous histiocytoma; *NOS*, not otherwise specified

Table 3. Sarcomas with low agreement rate

Cell types	Submitting diagnosis (*n*)	Panel agreed (%)	Other sarcomas by panel	
Rhabdomyosarcoma	12	2 (17)	MFH	6
			Others	4
			Total	10
Fibrosarcoma	27	13 (48)	MFH	5
			Malignant schwannoma	2
			Leiomyosarcoma	2
			Hemangiopericytoma-	2
			Nonsarcoma	3
			Total	14
Sarcoma NOS	30	8 (27)	Malignant schwannoma	5
			Leiomyosarcoma	4
			Others	13
			Total	22
Angiosarcoma	9	3 (33)	Sarcoma NOS	2
			Synovial Sarcoma	1
			Nonsarcoma	3
			Total	6

MFH, Malignant fibrous histiocytoma; *NOS*, not otherwise specified

proportions of sarcomas in virtually all studies have been graded solely on histological cell types rather than morphological features. This might be referred to as "automatic grading" (Table 4).

Suit et al. were able to show a correlation between HGM with survival in patients with primary and recurrent STS who were treated with radical dose

Table 4. Comparison of grading system for sarcomas

Authors	Year	Cases (n)	Histologic parameters	Cell type	Other Considerations and Results
Suit et al. [10]	1975	100	Yes	Yes	(a) Major emphasis on mitoses (b) Correlation of grade with survival
Russell et al. [11]	1977	1,215	Yes	Yes	(a) Prognostic significance of staging system combined with HGM
Markhede et al. [13]	1982	97	Yes	Yes	(a) Multivariate analysis of prognostic factors (b) Correlation of survival with grade and adequacy of surgical procedure
Costa et al. (NCI, USA)	1984	163	Yes	Yes	(a) Major emphasis on necrosis (b) Correlation of necrosis with time to recurrence and survival
Trojani et al. [14] (FNCLCC)	1984	155	Yes	No	(a) Multivariate analysis of prognostic factors (b) Grading system based on tumor differentiation, mitotic score, and tumor necrosis (c) Correlation of histological grade with survival and disease-free intervals
van Unnik et al. [15] (EORTC)	1988	169	Yes	No	(a) Multivariate analysis of prognostic factors (b) Grading system based on mitotic score and tumor necrosis (c) Correlation of mitotic score and necrosis with survival and metastatic potential
Tsujimoto et al. [16]	1988	236	Yes	Yes	(a) Multivariate analysis of prognostic factors (b) Correlation of survival with tumor necrosis or tumor depth

NCI, National Cancer Institute, USA; *FNCLCC*, French Federation of Cancer Centers; *EORTC*, European Organization for Research and Treatment of Cancer; *HGM*, histological grade of malignancy

radiation therapy either alone or combined with limited surgery [10]. The prognostic significance of the TNM staging system combined with HGM was established by Russell et al. [11]. In the study by Costa et al., necrosis was the best single histopathological parameter in predicting time to recurrence and overall survival, and the following grading system, based on histological type and extent of necrosis, was proposed: grade 1, low grade sarcomas with no necrosis; grade 2, sarcoma not grade 1 with minimal necrosis; grade 3, sarcoma with moderate to marked necrosis [12]. Automatic grading was part of their study; in other words, grading based upon degree of necrosis applied to certain types of sarcoma. Prognostic significance of various clinical and pathological

parameters in STS was also evaluated by multivariate analysis [13–16].
According to the study by Markhede et al., the likelihood of survival was
related to the adequacy of the surgical procedure and the HGM [13]. In a study
by the FNCLCC, the histological grade based on tumor differentiation, mitotic
score, and tumor necrosis was found to be the most important single prognostic
factor [14]. When reproducibility of this grading system among a review panel
was tested, the crude agreement rate for tumor grade was significantly higher
(75%) than for the histological type (61%) [6]. Although the agreement rate
between institutional pathologists and the review panel in the SEG study was
also higher for tumor grades (72%–83%) than for histological types (66%),
28% of the cases originally considered grade 3 by institutional pathologists
were downgraded in review [1] (Table 1). Van Unnik et al. of the European
Organization for Research and Treatment of Cancer (EORTC) Soft Tissue and
Bone Sarcoma Group found that tumor differentiation, presence of myxoid
areas and of necrosis, and mitotic rate were all related to length survival.
When multivariate analysis was applied, the mitotic score and the presence of
necrosis retained prognostic significance, with the mitotic score being the most
important factor. Based upon these two parameters, the proposed grading
system of van Unnik et al. showed a good correlation with prognosis in terms
of survival and metastatic potential [15]. In the study by Tsujimoto et al.,
sex, tumor depth, location, histological grade, cellularity, mitotic count, and
necrosis were significant prognostic factors by monofactorial analysis, but only
the mitotic count and tumor depths were of prognostic significance after
multivariate analysis [16].

Although statistical significance of various histopathological and clinical
prognostic indicators was shown in these studies, the distribution in respect to
cell type was not uniform: the large proportion of their diagnostic groups
of STS were MFH, liposarcoma, synovial sarcoma, or undifferentiated sarcoma [13–16]. For example, 63% of Markhede's series, 61% of van Unnik's
series, 44% of Trojani's series, and 54% of Tsujimoto's series were MFH,
liposarcoma, or synovial sarcoma; only a few special sarcomas with an unusual
natural history (i.e., epithelioid or clear cell sarcoma, alveolar soft part sarcoma, angiosarcoma, or Kaposi's sarcoma) were included [13–16]. Since the
predictive significance of histological parameters is different in various types of
sarcomas, it is still extremely important to establish accurate histological diagnosis before grading malignancy [3, 17, 18]. In the ECOG studies of STS, we
have used a combined grading system with three grades — low (grade 1),
intermediate (grade 2), and high (grade 3) — based on the histological type for
some sarcomas (i.e., automatic grading) and a composite of histological parameters for the remainder of the sarcomas. After establishing the diagnoses,
tumors are divided into three groups for grading purposes, as follows:

1. For the first group of tumors (i.e., leiomyosarcoma, hemangioperiocytoma,
   chondrosarcoma, and malignant schwannoma), grading malignancy based
   on a composite of histological criteria is considered to be most valuable
   because of their wide variation in behavior (Table 5).

Table 5. Grading of soft tissue sarcomas

Grade	Description
1	Well-differentiated, non-necrotic tumors with a lower mitotic rate (less than 2/10 HPF)
3	Highly cellular, poorly differentiated tumors usually with necrosis and a high mitotic rate (greater than 6/10 HPF)
2	Tumors falling between grades 1 and 3

HPF, High power field

2. In the second group of sarcomas, the grade of malignancy can be determined by the histological type or subtype alone, since they show little variation in behavior within each cell type.
   a) Well-differentiated or myxoid liposarcoma or dermatofibrosarcoma protuberans are classified as grade 1.
   b) Myxoid malignant fibrous histiocytoma is classified as grade 2.
   c) Rhabdomyosarcoma, malignant triton tumor, extraskeletal osteosarcoma, Ewing's sarcoma, alveolar soft part sarcoma, mesenchymal chondosarcoma, pleomorphic or round cell liposarcoma, and the vast majority of MFH are classified as grade 3.
3. The third group of sarcomas that show moderate variation in behavior can be graded as follows.
   a) Malignant granular cell tumor, fibrosarcoma, malignant giant cell tumor, epithelioid sarcoma, clear cell sarcoma, epithelioid malignant schwannoma, Kaposi's sarcoma, or synovial sarcoma are classified as grade 2 or 3.
   b) Myxoid chondrosarcomas are classified as grade 1 or 2 based on a composite of histological parameters.

Influence of Histological Type and Grade of Malignancy on Chemosensitivity of Advanced Adult Soft Tissue Sarcomas

Possible effects of the histological type and grade of malignancy on treatment response of metastatic STS were investigated in patients who entered the ECOG randomized trial EST 3377 (phase III comparison of three adriamycin regimens for metastatic soft tissue sarcomas) [5, 19]. Of the 361 patients entered on this trial, a clinicopathological analysis was performed on 274 patients. There were 98 leiomyosarcomas, 58 malignant fibrous histiocytomas (MFH), 22 sarcomas not otherwise specified (NOS), 21 malignant schwannomas, 20 liposarcomas, 14 fibrosarcomas, 12 synovial sarcomas, 12 hemangiopericytomas (HPC), 3 angiosarcomas, 2 rhabdomyosarcomas, and 12 other sarcomas. After establishing the histological diagnosis, the grade of malignancy was determined by the composite morphological features (Table 5). There were 170 grade 3 (62%), 77 grade 2 (28%), and 16 grade 1 (6%) lesions. While a therapeutic response was noted in 22% of the patients (60/274), including 14 complete (5%) and 46 partial responders (17%) [5], the other patients showed

Table 6. Complete or partial response[a] by grade and cell type[b]

Type of sarcoma	Grade 1 or 2	Grade 3	Grade unknown	P-Value
MFH	1/12 (8%)	9/41 (22%)	2/5	0.42[c]
Fibrosarcoma	0/4 (0%)	1/9 (11%)	0/1	1.00[d]
Malignant schwannoma	2/6 (33%)	1/14 (7%)	1/1	0.20
Leiomyosarcoma	13/48 (27%)	12/47 (25%)	0/3	1.00
All others	5/23 (22%)	12/59 (20%)	1/1	1.00
Total	21/93 (23%)	35/170 (21%)	4/11	0.75

MFH, Malignant fibrous histiocytoma
[a] Determined by the response criteria for cooperative group sarcoma study
[b] Grade unknown in 11 patients
[c] The *P*-value for combining MFH and fibrosarcoma is 0.27
[d] The *P*-value adjusting for type of sarcoma is 1.00
(From [5] with permission)

either no change (9%, 26/274) or progression (69%, 188/274). There was a slightly higher overall response rate noted among lower grade sarcomas: 25% for grade 1 (4/16), 22% for grade 2 (17/77), and 21% for grade 3 (35/170) lesions. However, when adjusted for cell type, there was no significant difference in response rate between grades 1 and 2 versus grade 3 [5] (Table 6).

When treatment response was compared to the histological type, a slightly higher overall response rate was shown for leiomyosarcomas (26%, 25/98) than for non-leiomyosarcomas (20%, 35/176) [19]. The median survival time for patients with leiomyosarcoma was higher than for those with MFH or other sarcomas, but the difference was marginal [5] (Table 7). A higher complete response rate was observed in patients with Ewing's sarcoma, hemangiopericytoma, sarcoma NOS, and synovial sarcoma (12.2%, 6/49) than in those with all other types of sarcomas (3.5%, 8/225) [5] (Table 8).

Application of New Technologies

Recently, electron microscopy, immunohistochemistry, and flow cytometry have become valuable adjuncts in determining histogenesis, grade of malignancy, and prognosis of STS [20–25]. The application of recent molecular biological techniques for the evaluation of genetic DNA and RNA sequences, oncogenes, and nuclear chromosomes has shown promise in the analysis of biological behavior and cell origin of the tumors [26, 27].

Immunoperoxidase stains have played an important role in the diagnosis of STS in ECOG studies. The most commonly used specific phenotypic markers were desmin (skeletal and smooth muscle), factor VIII (endothelium), neurofilament (neural, neuronal), S-100 (neural, cartilagineous, and fatty), cytokeratin (synovial and epithelial), and alpha 1 chymotrypsin (fibrohistiocytic). During the period from 1984 through 1987, a total of 123 sarcomas were examined by immunoperoxidase stains (34%, 123/360). In 17% (21/123) of these, the stains were used to confirm the cell type. The stains were helpful in

Table 7. Survival for patients with advanced soft tissue sarcoma

Type	Survival rates (months)			Median (months)	P-Value
	6	12	18		
Leiomyosarcoma	66%	35%	31%	9.6	
MFH	55%	29%	12%	7.3	0.19
Others	62%	35%	21%	7.7	

MFH, Malignant fibrous histiocytoma

Table 8. Analysis of complete responders (CR) by histological type and grade (G)

Histological type	CR Total (%)		G1	G2	G3	
A. Ewing's sarcoma	1/3	(33)	0	0	1	
Hemangiopericytoma	2/12	(17)	0	0	2	
Synovial sarcoma	1/12	(8)	0	0	1	
Sarcoma NOS	2/22	(9)	0	0	2	
B. MFH	4/58	(7)	0	1	3	
Liposarcoma	1/20	(5)	0	0	1	
Leiomyosarcoma	3/98	(3)	0	2	1	
Other sarcomas	0/49	(0)	0	0	0	
Total CR/all	14/274	(5)	0/16	3/77	11/170	($P = 0.57$)

Group A tumors (12.2%, 6/49) vs group B tumors (3.5%, 8/225) ($P = 0.02$)
NOS, Not otherwise specified; *MFH*, Malignant fibrous histiocytoma

establishing accurate diagnosis in 51% (63/123) by excluding other possibilities existing morphologically. Major changes in diagnosis (from sarcoma to non-sarcomatous malignancy, one cell type to another with therapeutic implications, sarcoma to benign reactive lesion) occurred in 12% of all cases examined by immunohistochemical stains [25]. Immunoperoxidase stains may also be applied to the analysis of cell surface markers for immunotherapy, or proliferation markers for grading of sarcomas and biological markers (growth factors, receptors, or antioncogenes) for better understanding of the biological behavior of tumors [25, 28].

Summary

1. Since there is significant diagnostic discordance among pathologists, a histopathological peer review is essential for proper interpretation of the results in the therapeutic trials of STS.
2. The prognostic importance of HGM has been shown repeatedly. However, since predictive significance of histological parameters may differ in different types of sarcomas, the histological diagnosis should be established before grading of the malignancy.
3. Although the ECOG randomized trial of three adriamycin regimens was unable to confirm the predictive value of HGM on chemosensitivity of

metastatic adult STS, it demonstrated a slightly higher overall response rate for leiomyosarcomas (26%, 25/98) than for non-leiomyosarcomas (20%, 35/176) [19], and, although the number was small, identified a subgroup of sarcomas with a higher complete response rate [5].

Acknowledgments. The authors are indebted to other members of the ECOG Committee, including Drs. H.T. Enterline, formerly of the Hospital of the University of Pennsylvania, J.A. Roth, Overlook Hospital, Summit, N.J., S. Hirschl, St. Charles Hospital, Port Jefferson, N.Y., U.N. Rao, Roswell Park Memorial Institute, Buffalo, N.Y., N.S. Cooper, New York University VA Medical Center, New York, N.Y., F.M. Enzinger, (consultant), Armed Forces Institute of Pathology, Washington, D.C., D.A. Amato, Department of Biostatistics, University of Michigan, Ann Arbor, Mich., and E.C. Borden, Chairman of the ECOG Melanoma Sarcoma Committee and University of Wisconsin, Wis., who participated in the ECOG trials and the histopathology peer review.

References

1. Presant CA, Russell WO, Alexander RW, Fu YS (1986) Soft tissue and bone sarcoma histopathology peer review: The frequency of disagreement in diagnosis and the need for second pathology opinions. The Southeastern Cancer Study Group Experience. J Clin Oncol 4:1658–1661
2. Enterline HT (1981) Histopathology of sarcomas. Semin Oncol 8:133–155
3. Enzinger FM, Weiss SW (1988) Soft tissue tumors. C.V. Mosby, St. Louis, pp 10–11
4. Baker LH, Benjamin RS (1978) Histologic frequency of disseminated soft tissue sarcomas in adults (abstract). Proc Am Soc Clin Oncol 19:324
5. Shiraki M, Enterline HT, Brooks JJ, Cooper NS, Hirschl S, Roth JA, Rao UN, Enzinger FM, Amato DA, Borden EC (1989) Pathologic analysis of advanced adult soft tissue sarcomas, bone sarcomas and mesotheliomas: The ECOG experience. Cancer 64:484–490
6. Coindre JM, Trojani M, Contesso G, David M, Rouesse J, Bui NB, Bodaert A, DeMascarel I, DeMascarel A, Goussot JF (1986) Reproducibility of a histopathologic grading system for adult soft tissue sarcomas. Cancer 58:306–309
7. Dahlin DC (1989) Grading of soft tissue sarcomas. In: Ryan JR, Baker LO (eds) Recent concepts in sarcoma treatment. Kluwer, Dordrecht, pp 1–6
8. Enzinger FM, Lattes R, Torloni R (1969) Histologic typing of soft tissue tumors: International histological classification of tumors No 3. World Health Organization, Geneva
9. Angervall L, Kindblom LG (1988) The diagnosis of soft tissue tumors. The Goteborg experience. In: Ryan JR, Baker LO (eds) Recent concepts in sarcoma treatment. Kluwer, pp 22–26
10. Suit HD, Russell WO, Martin RG (1975) Sarcoma of soft tissue: Clinical and histopathological parameters and response to treatment. Cancer 35:1478–1483
11. Russell WO, Cohen J, Enzinger F, Hajdu SI, Heise H, Martin RG, Meissner W, Miller WT, Schnitz RL, Suit HD (1977) A clinical and pathological staging system for soft tissue sarcomas. Cancer 40:1562–1570

12. Costa J, Wesley RA, Glatstein E, Rosenberg SA (1984) The grading of soft tissue sarcomas. Results of a clinico-pathologic correlation in a series of 163 cases. Cancer 53:530–541
13. Markhede G, Angervall L, Stener B (1982) A multivariate analysis of the prognosis after surgical treatment of malignant soft tissue tumors. Cancer 49:1721–1733
14. Trojani M, Contesso G, Coindre JM, Rouesse J, Bui NB, DeMascarel A, Goussot JF, David M, Bonichon F, Lagarde C (1984) Soft tissue sarcomas in adults: Study of pathological prognostic variables and definition of a histopathological grading system. Int J Cancer 33:37–42
15. Unnik JAM van, Coindre JM, Contesso G, Albus-Lutter CE, Schiodt T, Miralles TG, Sylvester R, Thomas D, Bramwell V (1988) Grading of soft tissue sarcomas. Experience of the EORTC soft tissue and bone sarcoma group. In: Ryan JR, Baker LO (eds) Recent concepts in sarcoma treatment. Kluwer, Dordrecht, pp 7–13
16. Tsujimoto M, Aozasa K, Ueda T, Morimura Y, Komatsubara Y, Doi T (1988) Multivariate analysis for histologic prognostic factors in soft tissue sarcomas. Cancer 62:994–998
17. Angervall L, Kindblom LG, Rydholm A, Stener B (1986) The diagnosis and prognosis of soft tissue tumors. Semin Diagn Pathol 3:240–258
18. Hajdu SI (1986) Differential diagnosis of soft tissue and bone tumors. Lea and Febiger, Philadelphia, p 104
19. Borden EC, Amato DA, Rosenbaum C, Enterline HT, Shiraki M, Creech RH, Lerner HJ, Carbone PP (1987) Randomized comparison of three Adriamycin regimens for metastic soft tissue sarcomas. J Clin Oncol 5:840–850
20. Brooks JJ (1982) Immunohistochemistry of soft tissue tumors: Progress and prospectives. Hum Pathol 13:969–974
21. Brooks JJ (1986) The significance of double phenotypic patterns and markers in human mesenchymal differentiation: A new model of mesenchymal differentiation. Am J Pathol 125:113–123
22. Kreicbergs A, Tribukait B, Willems J, Bauer HCF (1987) DNA flow analysis of soft tissue tumors. Cancer 59:128–133
23. Xiang JH, Spanier SS, Benson NA, Braylan RC (1987) Flow cytometric analysis of DNA in bone and soft tissue tumors using nuclear suspensions. Cancer 59:1951–1958
24. Kroese MCS, Rutgers DH, Wils IS, Unnik JAM van, Roholl PJM (1990) The relevance of the DNA index and proliferation rate in the grading of benign and malignant soft tisse tumors. Cancer 65:1782–1788
25. Brooks, JJ (1988) Immunohistochemistry in sarcomas. In: Ryan JR, Baker LO (eds) Recent concepts in sarcoma treatment. Kluwer, Dordrecht, pp 48–58
26. Eilber FR, Huth JF, Mirra J, Rosen G (1990) Progress in the recognition and treatment of soft tissue sarcomas. Cancer 65:660–666
27. Druker BJ, Mamon HG, Roberts TM (1989) Oncogenes, growth factors and signal transduction. N Engl J Med 321:1383–1390
28. Cance WG, Brennan MF, Dudas ME, Huang CM, Cordon-Cardo C (1990) Altered expression of the retinoblastoma gene production in human sarcomas. N Engl J Med 323:1457–1462

Multivariate Analysis for Histological Prognostic Factors in Soft Tissue Sarcoma of Extremities and Trunk

Takafumi Ueda,[1] Katsuyuki Aozasa,[2] Masahiko Tsujimoto,[3] Akira Myoui, Shigeyuki Kuratsu,[4] Atsumasa Uchida, and Keiro Ono[5]

Introduction

Soft tissue sarcoma (STS) is a heterogeneous group of malignant mesenchymal tumors of which a histological grade based on the histological type could be one of the most important prognostic factors [1]. The clinicopathological staging system for STS proposed by the American Joint Committee (AJC) in 1977 utilized the histological grade as well as tumor size and extent of the tumor for staging factors [2]. However, a lack of concrete criteria for histological grading seemed to limit the value of this staging system. This might be due to discrepancies in the diagnosis and classification even among experienced pathologists because of its relative rarity and complex histology. To establish a useful grading system for STS, the prognostic significance of various histological factors were evaluated by nonparametric univariate and multivariate analysis in 169 patients with localized STS in extremities and trunk.

Materials and Methods

From a histological and clinical review of 420 cases of STS, excluding those arising from bone and visceral organs treated between 1962 and 1985 at 14 hospitals (Osaka University Hospital, Osaka, Japan and affiliated hospitals), we accepted 290 cases as STS [3]. Among these, 62 cases of STS located in the head and neck (33) or retroperitoneum (29) were excluded. Another 59 cases were also excluded because of the presence of distant metastasis at first admission (29) and/or inadequate clinical information (32). Finally, 169 consecu-

[1] Department of Orthopaedic Surgery. The Center for Adult Diseases, Osaka, Japan
[2] Department of Pathology, Nara Medical College, Nara, Japan
[3] Department of Pathology, Osaka Police Hospital, Osaka, Japan
Departments of [4] Pathology and [5] Orthopaedic Surgery, Osaka University Medical School, Osaka, Japan

tive patients with localized STS in extremities and trunk were selected for the current study.

Without knowledge of the patients' survival, the hematoxylin and eosin-stained sections were reviewed independently by three pathologists (T.U., K.A., and M.T.); the number of mitotic figures (per 10 high-power fields [HPF]), cellularity, cellular pleomorphism, and degree of tumor necrosis were evaluated. For evaluation of the mitotic counts, we selected the area with the highest mitotic figures for counting, and then took the average of the mitotic counts submitted by the three pathologists. The cases were divided into 2 groups: low score group (average count $\leqslant$5/10 HPF) and high score group (>5/10 HPF). In terms of tumor necrosis, the cases were classified into 3 categories by each pathologist: absent and minimal (score 1), moderate (score 2), and marked (score 3). The scores given by the pathologists were totaled and all cases were divided into 2 groups: low score (scores of 3 and 4) and high score (scores from 5–9). Cellularity and cellular pleomorphism were estimated in a similar manner: low score group (scores from 3–5) and high score group (scores from 6–9). Histological diagnosis and grade were decided on the basis of the criteria of Enzinger and Weiss [1].

Precise clinical data including follow-up information were available in all cases. The follow-up period calculated from the date of initial definitive surgical treatment ranged from 1 to 176 months (median, 35 months). Actuarial survival curves were calculated by the method of Kaplan and Meier, and the log-rank test was used to evaluate the prognostic significance of individual factors. Subsequently, a multivariate analysis of these prognostic factors was made using the Cox's proportional hazards model.

Table 1. Histological type and grade in 169 Patients

Histological type	Number of patients (%)	Histological grade		
		G1	G2	G3
Malignant fibrous histiocytoma	59 (35)	5	14	40
Synovial sarcoma	24 (14)	0	14	10
Liposarcoma	19 (11)	17	1	1
Rhabdomyosarcoma	13 (8)	0	0	13
Malignant schwannoma	11 (7)	1	4	6
Fibrosarcoma[a]	9 (5)	1	7	1
Leiomyosarcoma	5 (3)	1	3	1
Dermatofibrosarcoma protuberans	4	4	0	0
Clear cell sarcoma	3	0	2	1
Alveolar soft part sarcoma	2	0	2	0
Extraskeletal Ewing's sarcoma	2	0	0	2
Extraskeletal chondrosarcoma	1	0	0	1
Angiosarcoma	1	0	0	1
Malignant hemangiopericytoma	1	0	1	0
Epithelioid sarcoma	1	0	1	0
Unclassified	14 (8)	3	4	7
Total	169	32	53	84

[a] Including 4 cases of infantile fibrosarcoma

Table 2. Actuarial survival rates according to various clinical and histological factors

Factors		Patients (n)	Actuarial survival rates		
			2-Year	5-Year	P-value
Age	<50 Years	100	84.8 (%)	65.5 (%)	N.S.
	≥50 Years	69	90.5	54.8	
Sex	Male	92	87.0	54.3	P < 0.1
	Female	77	87.3	68.5	
Tumor size	≤5 cm	54	93.7	61.3	N.S.
	>5 cm	84	81.6	54.7	
Tumor depth	Superficial	16	93.3	93.3	P < 0.05
	Deep	86	84.6	44.2	
Location	Upper extremity	32	82.1	51.9	
	Lower extremity	86	88.3	59.5	N.S.
	Trunk[a]	51	88.5	69.8	
Histological grade	G1	32	100	78.9	N.S.
	G2	53	87.4	68.5	P < 0.025
	G3	84	81.8	48.5	
AJC Stage	Ia + b	28	100	76.7	N.S.
	IIa + b	34	90.2	71.0	P < 0.01
	IIIa + b	52	83.9	48.2	N.S.
	IIIc	5	40.0	20.0	N.S.
	IVa	24	77.9	36.5	
Cellularity	Low score	39	100	89.1	P < 0.001
	High score	130	83.5	52.9	
Cellular pleomorphism					
	Low score	118	87.5	59.7	N.S.
	High score	51	86.3	63.4	
Mitosis	≤5/10 HPF	86	94.6	72.3	P < 0.005
	>5/10 HPF	83	79.4	49.8	
Tumor necrosis					
	Low score	132	91.5	67.0	P < 0.001
	High score	37	71.8	37.7	

N.S., Not significant; *AJC*, American Joint Committee; *HPF*, high-power fields
[a] including limb-girdles

Results

The present series included 92 males and 77 females with an age range from 0 to 84 years (median, 43 years). The primary tumors were located in the upper extremity in 32 cases, lower extremity in 86, and trunk (including limb-girdles) in 51. The distribution of histological diagnosis and grade is shown in Table 1. The actuarial 5-year survival rate in all patients was 60.8%.

The comparison of survival rates for all variables of clinical and histological factors is shown in Table 2. Among the clinical factors, tumor depth (superficial vs deep, $P < 0.05$) was the only significant prognostic factor. Age, tumor size, and location of the primary tumors did not significantly affect survival. With respect to histological factors, histological grade (G2 vs G3, $P < 0.025$), cellularity ($P < 0.001$), mitosis ($P < 0.005$), and degree of tumor necrosis ($P <$

Table 3. Multivariate analysis for prognostic factors in 91 patients with soft tissue sarcoma

Factors	Category	P-value
Age	0: <50 Years , 1: ≥50 Years	0.2605
Sex	0: Female , 1: Male	0.1848
Tumor size	0: ≤5 cm , 1: >5 cm	0.2866
Tumor depth	0: Superficial , 1: Deep	0.0001
Histological grade	0: G1 and G2 , 1: G3	0.1184
Cellularity	0: Low score , 1: High score	0.0304
Cellular pleomorphism	0: Low score , 1: High score	0.3610
Mitosis	0: ≤5/10 HPF, 1: >5/10 HPF	0.1574
Tumor necrosis	0: Low score , 1: High score	0.2005

HPF, High-power fields

Table 4. Histological prognostic factors of soft tissue sarcomas in previous studies

	Markhede et al. [4]	Myhre-Jensen et al. [5]	Trojani et al. [6]	Costa et al. [7]
Histological type	(+)	+	−	+
Cellularity	+	+	−	+
Differentiation	−	−	+	−
Cellular pleomorphism	+	+	−	+
Mitotic activity	+	+	+	+
Tumor necrosis	−	−	+	+

0.001) were prognostically significant. Cellular pleomorphism was not correlated with survival.

Subsequently, the factors proven to be significant by the univariate analysis were selected for the Cox's multivariate analysis to define independent prognostic factors in STS. For this purpose, 91 representative patients on whom full information was available were selected. The results showed that tumor depth ($P = 0.0001$) and cellularity ($P = 0.0304$) proved to be the most significant prognostic factors (Table 3). Among the histological factors, histological grade ($P = 0.1184$), mitosis ($P = 0.1574$), and tumor necrosis ($P = 0.2005$) subsequently influenced the prognosis.

Discussion

The present univariate analysis revealed that cellularity, mitosis, and degree of tumor necrosis were histological prognostic factors in patients with STS. The use of all these factors has been proposed for grading STS in several recent studies [4–7] (Table 4). However, cellular pleomorphism was not prognostically significant in the present study, confirming the findings reported by Trojani et al. [6].

Cellularity proved to be the most important histological prognostic factor in STS by the present multivariate analysis, whereas mitosis [4–6, 8] and tumor necrosis [6, 7] had been found to be the most important ones in several previous studies on STS. The major reason for this might be due to the difference in distribution of the primary tumors: the present series included only cases located in the extremities and trunk, whereas the other series also included those located in the head and neck and in the retroperitoneum. Indeed, our previous study, which included head and neck and retroperitoneal cases of STS, showed mitosis to be the most important histological prognostic factor in STS [8]. These combined findings show that histological parameters for STS grading must be modified according to the location of the primary tumors.

Histological grading in STS was determined primarily on the basis of the histological subtype of the tumor, and secondarily on histological variables such as mitotic count, cellularity, cellular pleomorphism, amount of stroma, infiltrative or expansive growth, and tumor necrosis [1]. Even when we could not make a precise histological diagnosis or when we obtained conflicting results, such as high cellularity and low mitotic count in the same tumor, accurate grading of the STS in the extremity and trunk could be made based on cellularity together with mitosis and necrosis of the tumors.

Conclusions

The present multivariate analysis showed that cellularity and tumor depth were the most important prognostic factors in the patients with STS located in the extremities and trunk. The prognostic significance of cellularity and mitosis suggests that further evaluation of cell proliferative activity, using for example the Ki-67 monoclonal antibody [9, 10] and the silver-staining nucleolar organizer region (AgNOR) [11] as markers, would make prediction of the prognosis of STS more accurate.

References

1. Enzinger FM, Weiss SW (1983) Soft tissue tumors. CV Mosby, St. Louis
2. Russell WO, Cohen J, Enzinger FM, Hajdu S, Heise H, Martin RG, Meissner W, Miller WT, Schmitz RL, Suit HD (1977) A clinical and pathological staging system for soft tissue sarcomas. Cancer 40:1562–1570
3. Tsujimoto M, Aozasa K, Ueda T, Sakurai M, Ishiguro S, Kurata A, Ono K, Matsumoto K (1988) Soft tissue sarcomas in Osaka, Japan (1962–1985): Review of 290 cases. Jpn J Clin Oncol 18:231–234
4. Markhede G, Angervall L, Stener B (1982) A multivariate analysis of the prognosis after surgical treatment of malignant soft tissue tumors. Cancer 49:1721–1733
5. Myhre-Jensen O, Kaae S, Madsen EH, Sneppen O (1983) Histopathological grading in soft-tissue tumors. Relation to survival in 261 surgically treated patients. Acta Pathol Microbiol Immunol Scand [A] 91:145–150
6. Trojani M, Contesso G, Coindre JM, Rouesse J, Bui NB, Mascarel A, Goussot JF, David M, Bonichon F, Lagarde C (1984) Soft-tissue sarcomas of adults: Study of pathological prognostic variables and definition of a histopathological grading system. Int J Cancer 33:37–42

7. Costa J, Wesley RA, Glatstein E, Rosenberg SA (1984) The grading of soft tissue sarcomas. Results of a clinicohistopathologic correlation in a series of 163 cases. Cancer 53:530–541
8. Tsujimoto M, Aozasa K, Ueda T, Morimura Y, Komatsubara Y, Doi T (1988) Multivariate analysis for histologic prognostic factors in soft tissue sarcomas. Cancer 62:994–998
9. Ueda T, Aozasa K, Tsujimoto M, Ohsawa M, Uchida A, Aoki Y, Ono K, Matsumoto K (1989) Prognostic significance of Ki-67 reactivity in soft tissue sarcomas. Cancer 63:1607–1611
10. Zehr RJ, Bauer TW, Marks KE, Weltevreden A (1990) Ki-67 and grading of malignant fibrous histiocytomas. Cancer 66:1984–1990
11. Kuratsu S, Aozasa K, Myoui A, Tsujimoto M, Ueda T, Uchida A, Hamada H, Ono K, Matsumoto K (1991) Prognostic significance of AgNOR reactivity in soft tissue sarcomas. Int J Cancer 48:211–214

A Classification of Bone Metastases from Breast Cancer

Kazuo Yamashita, Takafumi Ueda, Yoshio Komatsubara,[1]
Hiroki Koyama,[2] Hideo Inaji,[3] Kazuo Yonenobu, and Keiro Ono[4]

Introduction

A classification of disseminated cancer with bone metastases is urgently needed. This classification would facilitate the evaluation of therapeutic results and provide guidelines for the treatment of individual patients. We verified the clinical value of a classification exclusive to patients with disseminated breast cancer with bone metastases, according to the distribution of the metastases in terms of visceral metastases-free rate and survival rate after diagnosis of the bone metastases.

Patients and Methods

Breast cancer patients undergoing bone scan for detection of metastatic bone lesions and for monitoring of their distribution in the skeleton were eligible for this study. The medical records of 112 females who had histologically diagnosed breast cancer and had relapsed with bone metastases ($n = 101$), and those who had stage IV breast cancer with bone metastases ($n = 11$) were reviewed. These patients had been treated between 1975 and 1988 at the Center for Adult Diseases, Osaka, Japan or Osaka University Medical School. Skeletal images were obtained 2–3 h after intravenous injection of Tc-99m-labeled methyldiphosphonate and recorded using a gamma camera. By means of multiple overlapping views, the skull, cervical spine, thoracic spine, lumbar spine, pelvis (including sacrum), rib cage, proximal humeri, femora, and proximal tibiae were examined. The radiologists' reports on bone scans were reviewed and the diagnosis of bone metastases was ultimately made by one of us (K. Yamashita), taking into account the radiographic findings. Hot or cold

[1] Departments of Orthopaedic Surgery and [2] Surgery, The Center for Adult Diseases, Osaka, Japan
[3] Departments of Surgery and [4] Orthopaedic Surgery, Osaka University Medical School, Osaka, Japan

lesions on bone scan were interpreted as "not significant" if there were a benign radiographic explanation and "metastatic" if there were a radiographic confirmation of metastasis or if no benign radiographic explanation could be found.

Concerning the detection of extraosseous metastases, aspiration of pleural effusion, lymph nodes or skin biopsy, radiography or computed tomographic (CT) scan of the lung, CT or ultrasonic scan of the liver, and CT scan of the brain were performed. Interdisciplinary collaboration was needed for these investigations, involving specialists of general surgery, pathology, radiology, and orthopedic surgery.

According to the distribution of bone metastases at the time of their first manifestation, patients were classified into 3 groups as follows: group I, including patients who had bone-only metastases; group II, including patients who had extraosseous soft tissue lesions in lymph nodes, skin, and contralateral breast; group III, including patients who had extraosseous lesions in viscera with or without soft tissue lesions. Patients in group I were further classified into 2 subgroups as follows: group I_A, including patients who had metastases in bones cranial to the lumbosacral junction, which was selected arbitrarily as a cut-off point to separate cranial bone metastases from caudal bone metastases, and group I_B, including patients who had caudal bone metastases or both cranial and caudal bone metastases. Survival rates after the diagnosis of bone metastases were compared among the 3 groups. Visceral (lung, pleural, liver, or brain) metastases-free rates after the diagnosis of bone metastases were also compared between groups I and II and between groups I_A and I_B.

Survival and visceral metastases-free rates were calculated by the method of Kaplan and Meier [1]. Differences in these rates among the various patient groups were tested using the log-rank test.

Results

The median age of the 112 patients was 52 years (range: 26–80 years). Forty-two patients (38%) were premenopausal and the other 70 (63%) were post-menopausal. After the diagnosis of bone metastases, 95 patients received chemotherapy (single agent, $n = 72$; combination chemotherapy, $n = 23$) and 102 received endocrinic treatment.

When bone metastases were first documented, 82 patients had bone-only metastases (group I), 12 had extraosseous lesions in soft tissue (group II), and 18 had extraosseous lesions in viscera or in both viscera and soft tissue (group III). At the time of this analysis, 85 patients had died and the other 27 were alive or lost to follow-up. The survival rate in group I was significantly higher than in groups II and III ($P < 0.001$) and the survival rate in group II was significantly higher than in group III ($P < 0.05$) (Fig. 1). The 50% survival time in groups I, II, and III were 35, 14, and 5 months, respectively. When patients who had distant metastases at the initial diagnosis of breast cancer ($n = 11$) were excluded, the survival rate in group I ($n = 71$) was also significantly higher than in groups II ($n = 12$) and III ($n = 18$) ($P < 0.001$).

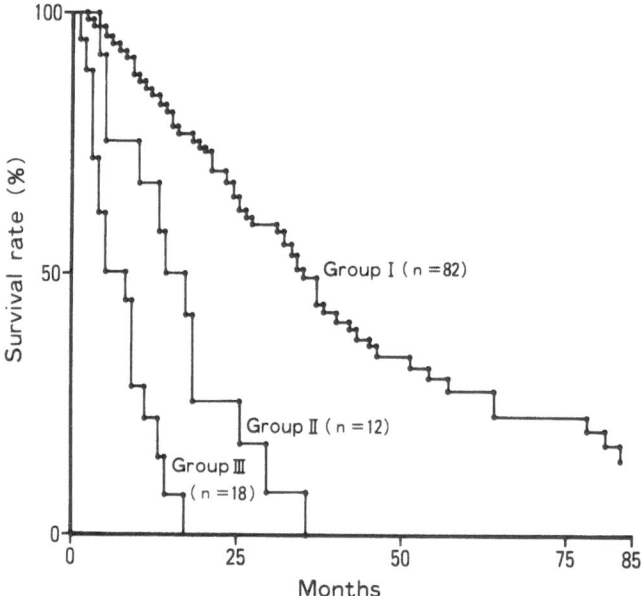

Fig. 1. Survival rate after the diagnosis of bone metastases according to their distribution: groups I (bone only, $n = 82$), II (bone and soft tissue, $n = 12$), and III (bone and visceral organs, $n = 18$). The differences between groups I and II, between groups I and III, and between groups II and III were significant at P levels of <0.001, 0.001, and 0.05, respectively

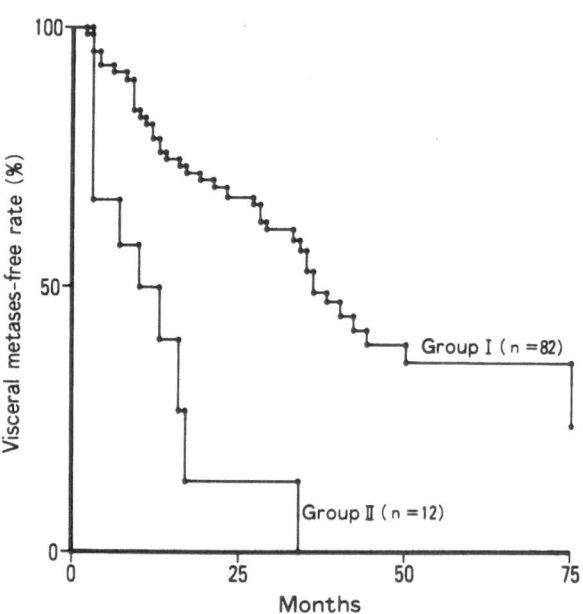

Fig. 2. Visceral metastases-free rate after the diagnosis of bone metastases according to their distribution: groups I (bone only, $n = 82$) and II (bone and soft tissue, $n = 12$). The difference was significant at a P level of <0.001

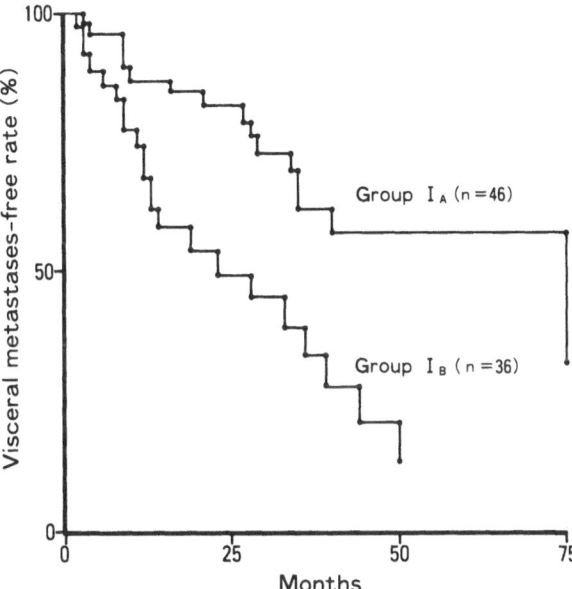

Fig. 3. Visceral metastases-free rate after the diagnosis of bone metastases in group I according to the distribution of the metastatic bone lesions: groups I_A (affecting cranial bones only, $n = 46$) and I_B (affecting caudal bones, $n = 36$). The difference was significant at a P level of <0.005

Among the patients in group I ($n = 82$), 42 died of visceral complications, 14 died without visceral metastases, 2 were still alive with visceral metastases, and the other 24 were still alive with bone metastases or lost to follow-up. Among the patients in group II ($n = 12$), 10 patients died of visceral complications and the other two died without visceral metastases. The visceral metastases-free rate in group I was significantly higher than in group II ($P < 0.001$) (Fig. 2). The 1-year, 2-year, 3-year, 4-year, and 5-year visceral metastases-free rates in group I were 79%, 68%, 49%, 40%, and 36%, respectively. Survival after the appearance of visceral metastases was short (range: 1–26 months and 1–22 months, median, 6 and 2 months in groups I and II, respectively).

When bone metastases were first documented, 42 patients in group I had cranial bone metastases (group I_A), 6 had caudal bone metastases, and the other 30 had both cranial and caudal bone metastases (group I_B). The visceral metastases-free rate in group I_A was significantly higher than in group I_B ($P < 0.005$) (Fig. 3).

Discussion

A bone-only metastatic pattern has been identified as one of the reasonably well-defined metastatic patterns from breast cancer [2, 3]. As reported in the literature [4, 5], metastases often remain localized in the bone for an extended time in patients with breast cancer with this pattern. In this review of our patients with breast cancer with bone metastases, 3 well-defined metastatic patterns were identified as follows: pattern I, metastases in bone only; pattern II, metastases in bone and soft tissue; and pattern III, metastases in bone and visceral organs. The differences in survival rates after the diagnosis of bone metastases were significant among the respective groups of patients. Inclusion or exclusion of patients with distant metastases at the initial diagnosis of breast cancer did not greatly affect the differences in survival rates among the 3 groups of patients; however, patients with distant metastases at the initial diagnosis of breast cancer should be analyzed separately from patients in whom the disease was disseminated subsequent to treatment of the primary cancer. The prolonged survival rates in patients with pattern I might be related to the confinement of the disease to a less extensive area. In addition, the high visceral metastases-free rate in patients with pattern I showed that their bone metastases remained localized in the bone for a relatively long time. This peculiar selectivity and chronicity might be explained by a bone-seeking and less aggressive biological behavior of the tumor in pattern I metastases.

Among patients with pattern I bone metastases, the visceral metastases-free rate in patients with bone metastases cranial to the lumbosacral junction (I_A) was higher than in patients with caudal bone metastases only or with both cranial and caudal bone metastases (I_B). The prolonged visceral metastases-free interval in patients with cranial bone metastases might only be related to a direct route to the cranial bones by retrograde venous seeding [6]. Moreover, the appearance of visceral metastases is a poor prognostic sign in patients with pattern I bone metastases, because survival after the appearance of visceral metastases was short (median, 6 months) compared with the whole course of the disease.

We propose the following classification based on the distribution of the metastatic lesions of bone metastases from breast cancer:

1. Pattern I, metastases are found in bone only
   a) I_A, involving only bones cranial to the lumbosacral junction
   b) I_B, involving bones caudal to the lumbosacral junction
2. Pattern II, metastases are found in bone and soft tissue including lymph nodes, skin, and contralateral breast
3. Pattern III, metastases are found in bone and visceral organs

Although this classification of disseminated breast cancer is not fundamentally different from the traditional classification [2, 3, 7], this classification provides new information regarding treatment of bone metastases from breast cancer. Specifically, this distinguishes that (1) patients with bone-only metastases form a distinctive group with a favorable prognosis and with a long visceral metastases-free interval, (2) the visceral metastases-free interval in patients with metastases at bone and soft tissue is shorter than in patients with bone-only metastases, and (3) the presence of visceral metastases is a poor prognostic sign in patients with breast cancer and bone metastases. This classification will provide useful guidelines for the treatment of individual patients with breast cancer and bone metastases. Aggressive surgical treatment of pathological fractures or spinal cord compression is indicated for patients with pattern I bone metastases because of their favorable prognosis. On the other hand, less aggressive treatment is indicated for patients with pattern III bone metastases. To classify bone metastases more precisely, clinical signs related to the biological markers of the metastatic tumors should be taken into account in addition to their distribution or the extent of dissemination. Such a classification could produce meaningful results in comparing different treatments.

Summary

The medical records of 112 patients with bone metastases from breast cancer were reviewed. According to the distribution of bone metastases at the time of their first manifestation, three well-defined metastatic patterns were identified as follows: pattern I, metastases in bone only; pattern II, metastases in bone and soft tissue; pattern III, metastases in bone and visceral organs. Metastases remained localized in the bone for an extended time in patients with pattern I bone metastases, especially in metastases involving only bones cranial to the lumbosacral junction. The visceral metastases-free interval in patients with pattern I bone metastases was longer than in those with pattern II. Patients with pattern I bone metastases survived longer than those with either patterns II or III. Aggressive surgical treatment of pathological fractures or spinal cord compression is indicated for patients with pattern I bone metastases because of their favorable prognosis.

References

1. Kaplan EL, Meier P (1958) Nonparametric estimation from incomplete observations. J Am Stat Assoc 53:457–481
2. Cutler SJ, Asire AJ, Taylor SG (1969) Classification of patients with disseminated cancer of the breast. Cancer 24:861–869
3. Smalley RW (1976) Five clinical patterns of recurrence of cancer of the breast. Proc Am Assoc Cancer Res 17:172
4. Sherry MM, Greco FA, Johnson DH, Hainsworth JD (1986) Metastatic breast cancer confined to the skeletal system: An indolent disease. Am J Med 81:381–386
5. Perez JE, Machiavelli M, Leone BA, Romero A, Rabinovich MG, Vallejo CT, Bianco A, Rodriguez R, Cuevas MA, Alvarez LA (1990) Bone-only versus visceral-only metastatic pattern in breast cancer: Analysis of 150 patients: A GOCS study. Am J Clin Oncol 13:294–298
6. Yamashita K, Ueda T, Komatsubara Y, Koyama H, Inaji H, Yonenobu K, Ono K (1991) Breast cancer with bone-only metastases: Visceral metastases-free rate in relation to anatomic distribution of bone metastases. Cancer 68:634–637
7. Valagussa P, Bonadonna G, Veronesi U (1978) Patterns of relapse and survival following radical mastectomy: Analysis of 716 consecutive patients. Cancer 41:1170–1178

5.6

Alteration of the Metastatic Pattern of Osteosarcoma Associated with Adjuvant Chemotherapy: An Analysis of 38 Autopsy Cases

Atsumasa Uchida, Yoshitaka Shinto, Nobuhito Araki,
Hideki Yoshikawa, Tsugio Kato, and Keiro Ono[1]

Introduction

Osteosarcoma is the most frequent primary malignant bone tumor, and mostly affects adults in their 20s. The lung is the major site of metastasis in more than 90% of cases, and this is the cause of death in most patients with osteosarcoma [1–3].

Extrapulmonary metastases, such as in the bone, brain or liver, are usually found in the terminal stage of the disease or at autopsy. After adjuvant chemotherapy was widely introduced for treatment of patients with osteosarcoma in the early 1970s, the prognosis has been markedly improved due to the decrease of pulmonary metastases [4]. However, even though the total incidence of metastasis has decreased following adjuvant chemotherapy, cases of extrapulmonary metastases have shown an increase in number.

Several investigators have recently reported an alteration of the pattern of metastases in osteosarcoma patients treated with adjuvant chemotherapy [5, 6], but there have been no detailed papers investigating alteration of the metastatic pattern in autopsied osteosarcoma patients. To clarify more precisely whether adjuvant chemotherapy has altered the metastatic pattern of osteosarcoma, we analyzed the metastatic sites of 38 autopsy cases of osteosarcoma.

Materials and Methods

Thirty-eight patients with high grade conventional osteosarcoma of the extremities were treated and autopsied at Osaka University Hospital from 1960–1990. Osteosarcoma arising from Paget's disease of the bone and postradiation osteosarcoma, as well as low grade parosteal osteosarcoma were excluded.

---

[1] Department of Orthopaedic Surgery, Osaka University Medical School, Fukushima-ku, Osaka, 553 Japan

There were 27 males and 11 females, and the mean age was 16.5 years (range, 9–27 years). The patients were divided into chemotherapy and nonchemo-therapy groups. The chemotherapy group included 22 patients treated with surgical resection of the tumor and adjuvant chemotherapy from 1975–1990. The nonchemotherapy group included 16 patients treated only with amputation and without chemotherapy before 1975, and were evaluated as a control group. There were no significant differences between age, primary site, and histo-logical subtype among the two groups. Clinical follow-up for local recurrence and metastasis was carried out for both groups through physical examinations and chest and local bone X-rays every month for the 1st year and every 2–3 months after the 2nd year. Laboratory examinations on serum and urine were routinely performed for the early detection of metastasis in other organs. In the chemotherapy group, technetium-99 m (Tc 99 m) and gallium (Ga) scintigrams were performed every 6 months for 2 years after operation, and after that they were performed when the patients symptoms were suggestive of local recurrence and metastasis. Twenty-two patients in the chemotherapy group were treated with $50 \, mg/m^2$ Adriamycin (ADR), $300 \, mg/kg$ high-dose methotrexate (HD-MTX), and $100 \, mg/m^2$ cis-platinum (CDDP) for about 1 year. After preoperative chemotherapy with these drugs, wide excision (12 patients) or amputation (10 patients) of the primary lesion was done, and 2–3 weeks after surgery, postoperative chemotherapy was started according to the Rosen T-10 B protocol using ADR and HD-MTX [7]. CDDP was also used with them. In some patients with lung metastasis, thoracotomy was performed [3].

Pulmonary metastases were not clinically apparent but always found by chest radiography or whole lung tomography. However, extrapulmonary metastases, especially bone and central nervous system (CNS) metastases were clinically apparent; almost all the bone and CNS metastases were not initially detected by specific imaging methods, such as scintigrams or computer tomography, but by clinical symptoms, such as pain, swelling, or neurological abnormality. Symptoms of convulsion, palsy, and loss of sight suggested brain metastasis, and paraplegia was caused by spinal metastasis. However, most metastases to unusual sites, such as the peritoneum, diaphragm, or adrenal gland, were found at autopsy. Autopsy was performed by a certified pathologist according to established methods.

Results

Autopsy on 38 patients showed 116 metastatic sites; 37 metastatic sites (31.8%) were detected before autopsy and 79 sites (68.2%) at autopsy. Pulmonary metastasis alone without evidence of disease in other organs was observed in 17 out of 38 cases (44.7%), pulmonary and extrapulmonary metastasis were observed in 20 out of 38 cases (52.6%), and extrapulmonary metastasis alone was observed in only 1 case (2.7%) in this study.

The cases were divided into the two groups: 16 cases in the nonchemo-therapy group treated with amputation only and 22 cases in the chemotherapy

Table 1. Metastatic pattern of osteosarcoma in 38 autopsy cases

	Chemotherapy group (n = 22)	Nonchemotherapy group (n = 16)
Extrapulmonary metastasis and pulmonary metastasis	16 (73%)	4 (25%)
Pulmonary metastasis only	5 (23%)	12 (75%)
Extrapulmonary metastasis only	1 (4%)	0 (0%)

Table 2. Metastatic sites of osteosarcoma in 38 autopsy cases

Metastatic site	Chemotherapy group (n = 22)	Nonchemotherapy group (n = 16)
Lung	21	16
Bone	12	3
Lymph node	6	2
Brain	5	1
Liver	3	1
Kidney	3	1
Pancreas	1	1
Subcutaneous site	1	1
Muscle	5	0
Peritoneum	4	0
Diaphragm	3	0
Adrenal gland	3	0
Ovary	2	0
Esophagus	1	0
Uterus	1	0

group treated with radical procedures and adjuvant chemotherapy. Mean survival from diagnosis until death was 17 months (6–28 months) in the nonchemotherapy group and 27 months (14–62 months) in the chemotherapy group (Kaplan Meier, $P < 0.005$).

Twelve cases (75%) in the nonchemotherapy group and 5 (23%) cases in the chemotherapy group developed only pulmonary metastasis. In the chemotherapy group, 16 cases (73%) developed both pulmonary and extrapulmonary metastases, whereas only 4 cases (25%) in the nonchemotherapy group did (Fisher's exact test, $P = 0.028$). Only 1 case in the chemotherapy group developed extrapulmonary metastasis alone (Table 1). Details of the metastatic sites in each group are shown in Table 2. In the chemotherapy group, the rate of metastasis to bone (55%) was higher than that in the nonchemotherapy group (19%) ($P = 0.008$). Metastasis to unusual sites, such as the peritoneum and diaphragm, was also found after chemotherapy.

In the nonchemotherapy group, bone metastases developed in the terminal stage of this disease. In contrast, chemotherapy appeared to hasten clinical manifestation of bone metastasis, as well as increase the rate of metastasis to bone (Fig. 1). In 4 cases in the chemotherapy group, bone metastasis was detected before lung metastasis.

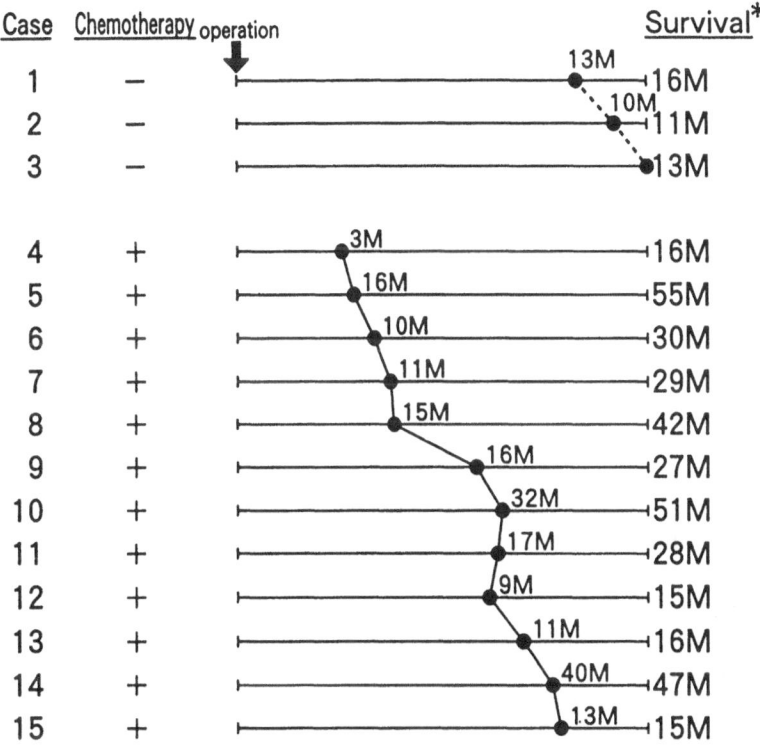

Fig. 1. Time after resection of primary tumor to bone metastasis (*solid circles*). *Survial** is the period from the first operation to death. Bone metastases in the chemotherapy group were relatively more developed in earlier stages of the disease than those in the nonchemotherapy group. The average period from the first operation to bone metastasis and survival were 12 months and 14.4 months in the nonchemotherapy group, and 16.7 months and 29.1 months in the chemotherapy group. —, months

Discussion

Before the development of adjuvant chemotherapy, the major metastatic site of osteosarcoma was the lung [1–3]. Extrapulmonary metastases were very rare in patients with osteosarcoma and were usually found in the terminal stage of disease or at autopsy. In this study, 12 out of 16 cases (75%) in the nonchemotherapy group had only pulmonary metastasis and the remaining 4 cases (25%) had both pulmonary and extrapulmonary metastasis, which were detected in the terminal stage. In contrast, 5 out of 22 cases (23%) developed only pulmonary metastases and 17 out of 22 cases (75%) developed extrapulmonary metastases in the chemotherapy group.

The prolonged period of survival caused by chemotherapy may have some effect on the increase of extrapulmonary metastasis. However, extrapulmonary metastasis in the chemotherapy group did not rapidly increase during this period, and even in earlier stages of the disease, the rate of extrapulmonary metastasis in the chemotherapy group is higher than that seen at anytime in the nonchemotherapy group. In some reports, development of better diagnostic techniques was attributed to the increased detection of extrapulmonary metastasis in osteosarcoma. However, in our study, extrapulmonary metastasis was usually diagnosed by the onset of clinical signs or symptoms in both the nonchemotherapy and the chemotherapy group. Therefore, we believe that cases with extrapulmonary metastasis can be compared between the groups.

Bone metastasis was detected in the earlier stage of the disease in the chemotherapy group, whereas in the nonchemotherapy group, it occurred in the terminal stage. Brain metastasis also tended to develop earlier in the chemotherapy group, as compared with the nonchemotherapy group. Extrapulmonary metastases were always found after pulmonary metastasis in the nonchemotherapy group, but in the chemotherapy group, 5 cases (23%) (4 cases, bone; 1 case, brain) were diagnosed as the initial indication of disease recurrence before pulmonary metastases. McNeil [8] also found bone metastasis only after pulmonary metastasis in his nonchemotherapy study, but in this study, 13% of cases treated with adjuvant chemotherapy were found to have bone metastasis before pulmonary metastasis.

The increase of extrapulmonary metastasis to unusual sites, such as the ovary, adrenal gland, uterus, colon, small intestine, and other organs, was also found in cases treated with chemotherapy. There may be a slight association between metastasis to these unusual sites and prolonged survival, because these metastases were usually found at autopsy. However, a more important reason for rapid development of metastasis to such organs seems to be an immunological dysfunction caused by chemotherapy.

The present results suggest that chemotherapeutic agents could cause alteration of the biological behavior of osteosarcoma. It is unclear whether this phenomenon is provoked by a change at the tumor cellular level or a change of the defense mechanism in the patients.

References

1. Jeffree GM, Price HG, Sissons HA (1975) The metastatic pattern of osteosarcoma. Br J Cancer 32:87–107
2. Pratt CB (1982) Outcome of patients failing adjuvant chemotherapy for osteosarcoma. Cancer Bull 34:100–103
3. William HM, Michael JS, Kuma APM, Bhaskar NR, Alexander AG, John C, Charles BP (1987) Thoracotomy for pulmonary metastasis osteosarcoma: An analysis of prognostic indicators of survival. Cancer 59:374–379
4. Sutow WW, Sullivan MP, Fernback DJ, Cangir A, George SL (1975) Adjuvant chemotherapy in primary treatment of osteosarcoma: A Southwest Oncology Group Study. Cancer 36:1598–1602
5. Armando EG, Stephen F, Friedreich RE (1984) Changing metastastatic patterns of osteosarcoma. Br J Cancer 54:2160–2164

6. Jaffe N, Smith E, Abelson HE, Frei E (1983) Osteogenic sarcoma: Alterations in the pattern of pulmonary metastasis with adjuvant chemotherapy. J Clin Oncol 1:252–254
7. Rosen G, Caparros B, Huvos AG (1982) Preoperative chemotherapy for osteogenic sarcoma: Selection of postoperative adjuvant chemotherapy based on the response of the primary tumor to preoperative chemotherapy. Cancer 49:1221–1230
8. McNeil BJ, Hanky J (1980) Analysis of several radionuclei bone images in osteosarcoma and breast carcinoma. Radiology 135:171–176

Part 6

Total Care

6.1

Gait Analysis and Its Significance in Patients with Total Knee Prosthesis after Wide Resection of Malignant Tumor

Hiroyuki Kawamura, Toshihiko Yoneda, Yoshitaka Hayashi,[1]
Atsumasa Uchida, Shigeyuki Kuratsu, Kazuo Hiroshima,
and Keiro Ono[2]

Introduction

While limb-salvage surgery, which has been commonly used for malignant tumor in recent years, has many advantages, there are several problems which need to be resolved. If, in addition to the bones, the muscles are widely resected, motor control of the affected limb can be difficult to achieve after the surgery.

Some methods of post-operative functional evaluation, such as Enneking's, focused mainly on assessment of the affected joint functions, but there are few method to precisely and accurately evaluate the supporting and locomotor functions of the extremities. In addition, there are few methods of evaluation which are useful for determining physical therapy geared to improve the locomotive ability of the patients [1, 2]. The purpose of this study was to evaluate the efficacy of reconstructive surgery and devise a physical therapy program by means of gait analysis of the patients who received total knee prosthesis after wide resection limb-salvage surgery.

Materials and Methods

Gait analysis was performed on ten patients who underwent a wide resection and total knee replacement procedure for malignant bone tumors around the knee joint. Their ages ranged from 16 to 25 years (mean age: 19.5 ± 2.8 years). The site of the bone tumor was the distal femur in seven patients and the proximal tibia in three patients. The follow-up period ranged from 3 to 46 months (mean: 16 months) (Table 1).

[1] Department of Physical Therapy, and [2] Department of Orthopedic Surgery, Osaka University Medical School, Osaka, Japan

H. Kawamura et al.

Table 1. Subjects

Case	Age	Sex	Site of tumor	Knee Extensor : Flexor (MMT grade)	Gait profile	Stairs
A	16	Male	Distal part of femur	1+ : 3+	Knee in extended position during stance phase	Step-to-step*
B	17	Male	Distal part of femur	2+ : 4	Knee in extended position during stance phase	Step-to-step*
C	17	Male	Distal part of femur	1+ : 4 −	Knee in extended position during stance phase	Step-to-step*
D	17	Male	Proximal part of tibia	3− : 4	Knee in extended position during stance phase	Step-to-step*
E	19	Male	Proximal part of tibia	1+ : 3+	Knee in extended position during stance phase	Step-to-step*
F	19	Female	Proximal part of tibia	1 : 3+	Knee in extended position during stance phase	Step-to-step*
G	20	Female	Distal part of femur	1 : 4	Knee in extended position during stance phase	Step-to-step*
H	23	Female	Distal part of femur	3 : 4	Knee in extended position during stance phase	Step-to-step*
I	20	Male	Distal part of femur	4 : 4	With double knee action	Step-by-step**
J	25	Male	Distal part of femur	4 : 4	With double knee action	Step-by-step**

* step-to-step: stepping up with the sound leg or down with the affected leg, and placing the other leg next to it.
** step-by-step: stepping up or down with one leg, and placing the other leg next through it.

Surgical Procedures

The rectus femoris muscle and the knee flexors were saved, and all the vastus muscles and part of the hip adductors were resected in the cases with the bone tumor in the distal femur. Part of the tibialis anterior muscle and part of the soleus muscle were resected, and the insertions of the patellar tendon and the knee flexors were cut in the cases with the bone tumor in the proximal tibia. In addition, the patellar tendon was reconstructed by being attached with an artificial ligament onto the stem of the prosthesis, and the knee flexors were reactivated by being sutured into the soft tissue around them. The prostheses used for reconstruction of joint function were of the hinge type in all but one patient [3].

Gait Analysis

For conducting the gait analysis, the patients were instructed to walk at a comfortable pace and speed. We measured floor reaction force by means of a force platform and activities of the muscles by means of surface electromyography. In the surface electromyography test, five muscles (the gluteus maximus, rectus femoris, biceps femoris, tibialis anterior, and gastrocnemius) were examined. Eleven healthy males (age range:20–29 years; mean: 25.2 ± 3.1 years) comprised the control group. All measurements were performed on both the affected and sound legs of the patients and on both legs of the controls. In addition to these measurements, we examined the abilities of ascending and descending stairs, the lower limb muscle strength by the manual muscle testing (MMT) technique, and the range of joint motion of the lower limbs.

Results

Two patients, who maintained a knee extension strength of MMT grade 4 or more, had a double knee action, which is a normal phenomenon in which the knee joint moves in the consecutive form of extension-flexion-extension during the stance phase. In the other eight patients whose knee extension strength was less than MMT grade 4, the knee was fixed in the fully extended position and no knee flexion was observed during the whole period of the stance phase. This finding was not related to whether or not the patient showed signs of extension lag. Additionally, we observed that the patients whose knee extension strength was MMT grade 4 or more could ascend and descend stairs using a reciprocal step-by-step form.

The patients whose knee extension strength was less than MMT grade 4 could ascend the stairs only by first raising the sound leg and then the affected leg on the same step, and could descend only by first putting down the affected leg and then the sound leg on the same step. That is to say, they could only go up and down the stairs using a step-by-step technique.

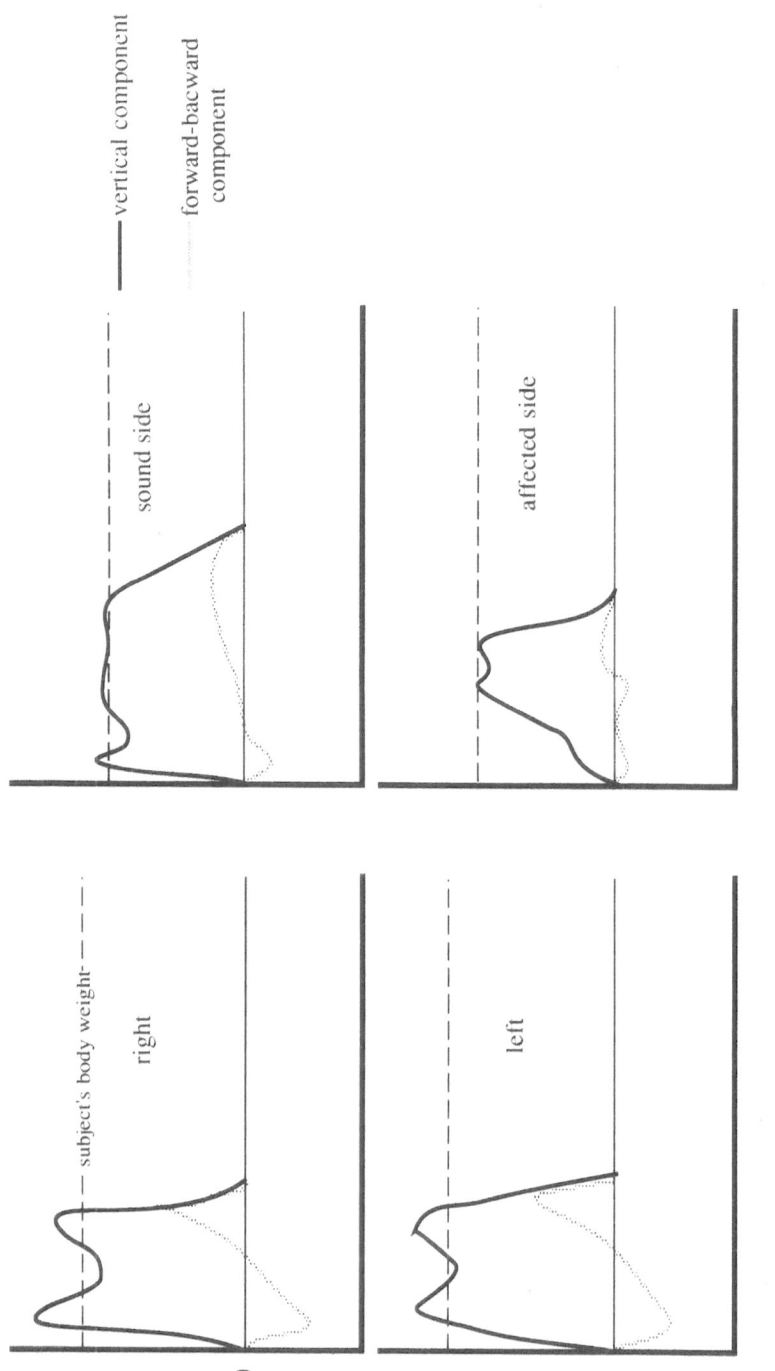

Fig. 1. Floor reaction force

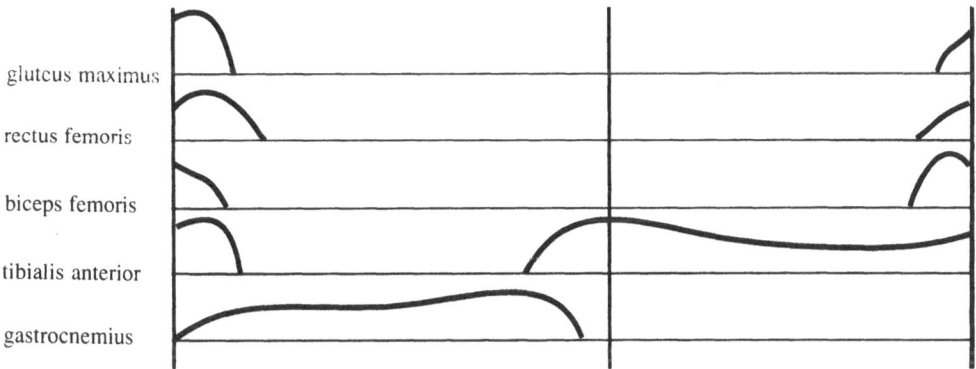

glutcus maximus

rectus femoris

biceps femoris

tibialis anterior

gastrocnemius

Fig. 2. Electromyography of the five muscles in a normal subject

Floor Reaction Force

In the control group, the stance phase time and wave pattern were almost the same for the right and left sides, while the vertical component of the floor reaction force rose rapidly to the first peak. Considering the difference in gait speeds between the patients and healthy subjects, the floor reaction force was measured in various cadences for the control subjects in whom the stance phase was prolonged if the cadence was slowed down. However, the duration up to the first peak of the vertical component of the floor reaction force was not changed even if the cadence was decreased.

In the two patients whose knee extension strength was MMT grade 4 or more, both the vertical and the forward-backward components of the floor reaction force showed a slightly smaller but almost identical pattern between the affected and the sound sides, and were similar to those of normal subjects.

In the eight patients whose knee extension strength was less than MMT grade 4, both the vertical and forward-backward components of the floor reaction force showed deformed shapes, and the forward-backward component was smaller in the sound side as well as in the affected side compared with that of the normal subjects. In addition, the stance phase and the duration up to the first peak of the sound side was prolonged (Fig. 1). In observing the course of the gait profile, the pattern of the floor reaction force was seen to be distinctly deformed from the very beginning of gait training. It tended to approach the normal pattern gradually with time after the onset of walking, but did not sufficiently reach normal levels in these patients.

Surface Electromyography

The two patients with MMT grade 4 or more in extension strength showed the same pattern of discharge as that of the normal subjects (Fig. 2). The patients whose knee extension strength was less than MMT grade 4 showed a continuous discharge pattern in the gluteus maximus, biceps femoris, and gastrocnemius muscle during the entire stance phase only in the early period of

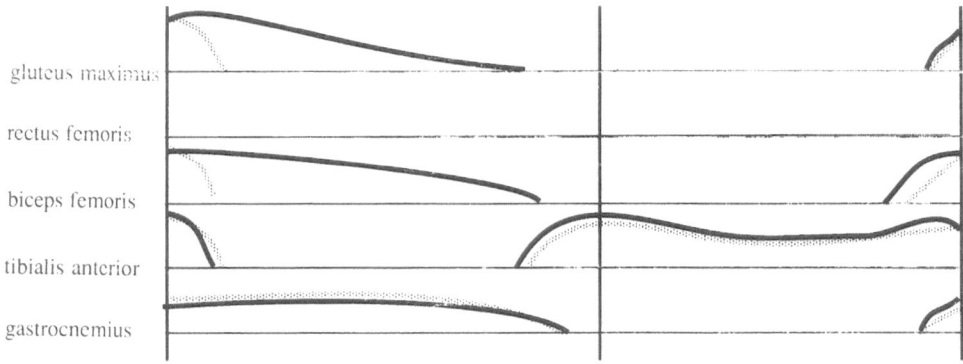

Fig. 3. Electromyography of the five muscles examined at the beginning of gait training and after acquisition of a skillful gait

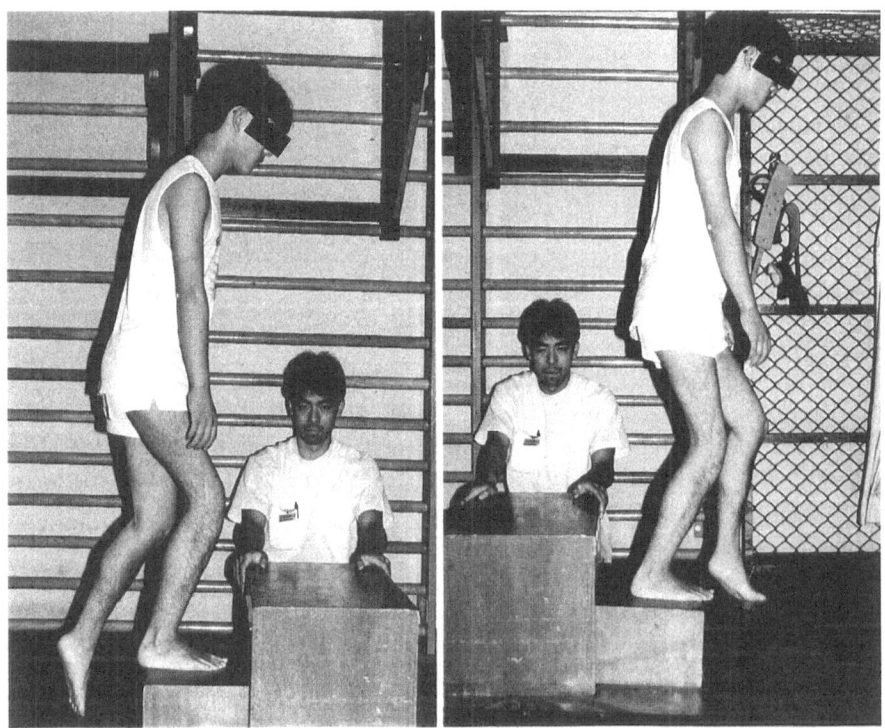

Fig. 4. Stepping up and down a footstool. Case D acquired the ability of negotiating stairs after compensatory muscle training

gait training. Then, the discharge pattern changed with time following surgery, and the discharge of the gluteus maximus and the hamstrings muscles became limited within a short early period of the stance phase. However, there were no detectable changes in the discharge pattern of the gastrocnemius muscle (Fig. 3).

Compensatory Muscle Training

Based on the results of surface electromyography, the lack of knee extensor strength during the stance phase appeared to be compensated by the gluteus maximus, biceps femoris, and gastrocnemius muscles in the patients with knee extension strength of less than MMT grade 4. Therefore, we conducted a gait exercise by compensatory muscle training in two patients (Table 1, cases D and H). The reason for selecting these cases was that it was considered to be easier to examine the compensatory function of each of their muscles since the knee extensor strength was selectively decreased while the other muscles maintained good condition.

The training was conducted by instructing the patients to stand with one leg in a flexed position or to go up and down a footstool using the affected leg while being alert to the contractions in each muscle. Without any improvement of muscle strength, they became able to walk with the double knee action in the stance phase and to ascend and descend the stairs with a step-through-step form (Fig. 4). When the double knee action was observed in a patient, examination of the floor reaction force revealed that the period for reaching the first peak was shortened and both the vertical and forward-backward components were decreased, compared with those in patients with a knee-extended gait (Fig. 5). Moreover, the discharge durations of the gluteus maximus and biceps femoris were prolonged, and the discharge amplitude of the gastrocnemius was increased (Fig. 6).

Discussion

This study demonstrated that the patients whose knee extension strength was MMT grade 4 or more had conserved a basic ability of locomotion, such as walking and going up and down the stairs, and showed a strenuous propelling force of each side, identical to that of the normal subjects. From these findings, we concluded that it was essential to reconstruct the knee extensor mechanism.

On the other hand, the patients whose knee extension strength was less than MMT grade 4 showed a distinctly deformed wave pattern of floor reaction force on the affected side. It was also observed that the two-peak pattern of the vertical component disappeared, and that both vertical and forward-backward components decreased on the sound side. From this finding, it was concluded that the propelling force decreased not only in the affected side but in the sound side as well. In addition, the stance phase of the sound side was prolonged as was the time to the first peak of the vertical component in the

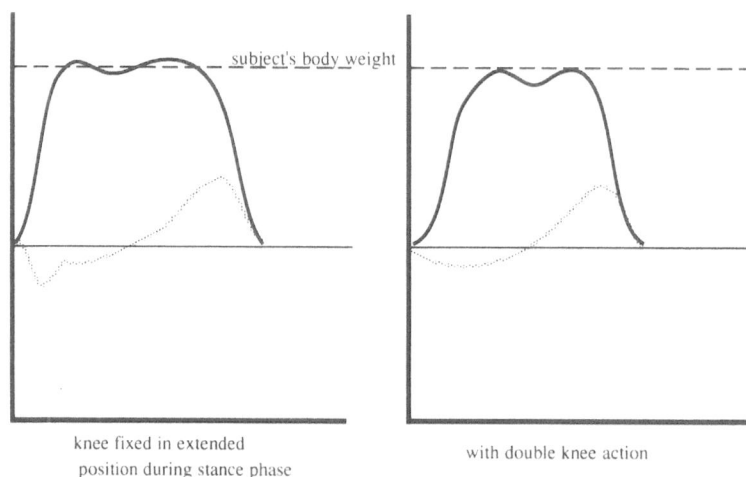

knee fixed in extended
position during stance phase

with double knee action

Fig. 5. Scheme of a floor reaction force pattern with and without double knee action. *Solid line*, vertical component of the floor reaction force; *dotted line*, forward-backward component of the floor reaction force

affected limb, expressing the difficulty of weight-shifting onto the affected limb. The decreased vertical component in the affected side showed that the affected limb did not function adequately in supporting weight.

Because the floor reaction force of a patient gradually approached the normal pattern with time, following the onset of gait training, it is useful for the assessment of motor learning in walking. This enables us to quickly judge the extent of weight-bearing ability in the affected limb by examining the vertical component and the extent of the propelling force by observing the forward-backward component. Examination of the floor reaction force is also useful in judging whether or not we achieved precise and appropriate gait profile modification in the physical therapy program.

Although the patients whose knee extension strength was less than MMT grade 4 showed continuous discharges of the gluteus maximus and hamstrings muscles during the whole stance phase in the early stage of gait training, discharges of these muscles were limited only in the early period of the stance phase and unecessary discharges decreased as the patients became more skillful in walking. We concluded that the patients could acquire the ability of using the muscles efficiently through gait training. Moreover, with the acquisition of skillful walking, the insufficiency of knee extension strength during the stance phase appears to be compensated by the hip extension force of the gluteus maximus and the hamstrings (in the early stage of the stance phase), and that collapsing was prevented by the inhibition of dorsiflexion of the ankle by the gastrocnemius muscles (after the midstance phase) [4]. This discharge pattern was very similar to that of the control subjects, except that discharge of the rectus femoris was seldom found in the patients. Even in a gait in which the knee was fixed in a fully extended position, other muscle groups excepting the rectus femoris showed the same electromyographic discharge as those of normal gaits.

The patients who received compensatory muscle training could walk with the double knee action when the biceps femoris and the gluteus maximus showed an electromygraphic pattern with a prolonged period of discharge. From these data, it was evident that those muscles together with the gastrocnemius were very essential as compensatory muscles. Thus, if it is difficult to reconstruct the knee extensors sufficiently, a method of surgery or reconstruction technique should be chosen in which the biceps femoris and the triceps surae are saved. As for a physical therapy program for these patients, it is necessary to provide them with muscle strengthening exercises and compensatory muscle training.

A gait with a double knee action, in which vertical and forward components of the floor reaction force are diminished, may enable the prevention of loosening and breakage of prostheses, since the impact to the prosthesis is mitigated. It seems highly beneficial to provide compensatory muscle training to the patients, most of whom are young.

Summarizing these findings and considerations, we conclude that gait analysis is very important in assessing the function of affected limbs and in establishing a physical therapy program for patients with bone tumors.

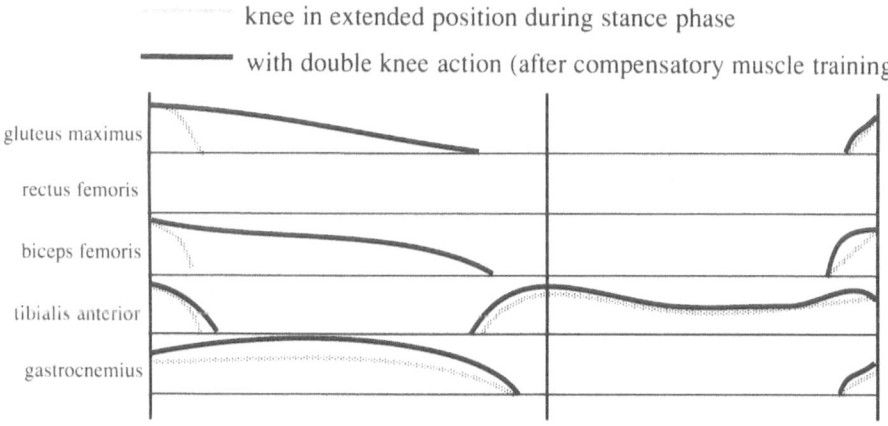

Fig. 6. Electromyography of the five muscles in gait with and without double knee action

References

1. Enneking WF (1983) Evaluation of surgical management of muscleskeletal tumors. The second international workshop on design and application of tumor prostheses for bone and joint reconstruction, Vienna
2. Nomura T, Tomita K (1986) Rehabilitation for patients with malignant bone tumor treated by tumor prosthesis. Sogo Rehabilitation. 14:605–612
3. Hamada H et al. (1986) En bloc resection for osteosarcoma. Journal of Joint Surgery. 5:101–108
4. Sutherland DH (January 1966) An electromyografic study of the plantar flexors of the ankle in normal walking on the level. JBJS vol 48.A, No 1

Nutritional Support of Children with Cancer

Masahiro Fukuzawa and Akira Okada[1]

Introduction

The association between malnutrition and poor prognosis in cancer patients is well known [1–3]. Nutritional support of children with cancer has become more sophisticated, paralleling the increasing complexities of oncological therapy. Data from several studies of children with cancer demonstrated the need to integrate nutritional staging, assessment, and support in treatment protocols [4–7]. Most notably, parenteral nutritional support effectively reversed or prevented protein energy malnutrition (PEM) [4–10] and improved tolerance to chemotherapy in children with certain tumor types, such as advanced neuroblastoma [4]. It was documented that benefits from an improved nutritional status in children with cancer improved immune competence [7, 8], decreased the incidence of *Pneumocystis carinii* [11] and other opportunistic infections [6], decreased the incidence of anthracycline-induced cardiotoxicity [12], and improved prognosis [13]. PEM frequently occurs in children with cancer and relates both to the disease and therapy. It may also affect the general well-being and quality of life of the patients and their families. It is important to adequately evaluate the nutritional status and provide proper nutritional support to patients with cancer.

Etiology of PEM

High-dose chemotherapy, radiotherapy, unpalatable drug regimens, and previous disease all contribute to anorexia, taste abnormalities, nausea, vomiting, mucositis, and diarrhea, which lead, in turn, to reduced dietary intake and greater nutritional depletion. Infection, graft-versus-host disease in bone marrow transplantation (BMT), and drug treatment may have adverse

---

[1] Department of Pediatric Surgery, Osaka University Medical School, Fukushima-ku, Osaka, Japan

catabolic effects, increasing the rate of nutritional depletion. The question of tumor-induced change in host energy expenditure remains unanswered, because it is difficult to separate the tumor from the host. It is also probable that one answer does not apply to all tumors and all patients, since individual tumor types and individual host metabolisms differ greatly. Anorexia can be a direct consequence of cancer treatment. The nausea, vomiting, and anorexia induced by chemotherapeutic agents can be severe. Indeed, in pediatric patients, cancer treatment results in a greater degree of anorexia than does the cancer itself [14]. However, in some patients, the uncontrolled continued growth of tumors places a further demand on the host for essential nutrients that causes muscle wastage and anorexia.

Evaluation of Nutritional Status

Standard Measurements

The initial measurements needed for assessing the nutritional status are age, height, weight, and, in children younger than 3 years old, head circumference. Any recent weight loss of 5% or greater, including that caused by dehydration, requires further investigation [15]. Values of height-for-age, weight-for-age, weight-for-height, and head circumference for age are plotted against the growth curves, which depict standards derived from the populations of healthy children. Any measurement below the tenth percentile should be investigated as a sign of growth impairment due to inadequate nutrition. A weight-for-height value below the fifth percentile may reflect acute malnutrition, whereas a height-for-age value lower than the fifth percentile may reflect chronic malnutrition. These simple measurements are one of the best indicators for a decision regarding the need for nutritional support [16]. Nutritional support is indicated if a patient has lost 5% of body weight.

Investigational Measurements

Serum proteins, which include total protein, albumin, transferrin, prealbumin, and retinol-binding protein, are common laboratory measures of nutritional status. The value of total lymphocyte count is also used. Albumin is probably the most common of these measures. A concentration of albumin less than 3.0 g/dl may reflect PEM. However, with a turnover of approximately 14 days, serum albumin responds slowly to change in nutritional status. Measurements of rapid turnover proteins, such as prealbumin, retinol-binding protein, and transferrin, are valid indicators for early diagnosis of PEM in children with malignancies. While the half-life of serum transferrin is only 8–10 days, values will be artificially elevated by iron deficiency anemia or chronic blood loss. Retinol-binding protein has a half-life of only 12 h, and prealbumin has a half-life of 2–3 days. Both measurements are good indicators of nutritional repletion in children. The total lymphocyte count is an unreliable indicator of nutritional status in most patients with cancer because of the effects of chemotherapy on the blood counts [17]. Anthropometry has been used to examine the body composition of patients with cancer. The results indicate that, in young patients with solid tumors, changes in major body compartments can precede changes in body weight [18]. Anthropometric tests assess protein and fat compartments by the measurement of mid-upper arm circumference (MUAC) and triceps skinfold thickness (TSFT) [19]. The TSFT measurements are taken on the nondominant arm halfway between the olecranon and the acromial process. A skinfold caliper is used to measure the thickness of the skinfold pinched at the back of the arm, taking care to include only skin and subcutaneous fat. Measurements are then compared with tables of established normal values for age and gender [19]. A percentile value of less than 5% for MUAC is indicative of muscle depletion, whereas a TSFT score of greater than 90% may reveal excess fat stores. Anthropometry can help ascertain the nature of weight gain or loss.

Recommended Intake of Calories and Protein

No standard formulas for estimating caloric needs are available for children. The Recommended Dietary Allowance of the National Academy of Science (USA) categorized by age, gender, and body weight, can serve as an initial estimation of caloric need [20] (Table 1). Nitrogen balance and actual energy balance can be measured to ensure that the desired results have been achieved. Alternatively, monitoring changes in weight or serum proteins can give an indication of the adequacy of the prescribed regimen.

Indication for Nutritional Support

An assessment of nutritional status requires physical (weight, height) and laboratory (protein, albumin) examinations as well as an accurate dietary history. Aggressive nutritional support should be considered in patients who cannot maintain food intake to meet energy demands. Any child who has sustained a weight loss of 5% during a 1-month period or less, has an albumin of 3.0 g/dl or lower, and is receiving treatment expected to inhibit adequate nutrient consumption, such as BMT, is a candidate for aggressive complete enteral or parenteral nutritional support.

Enteral Nutrition

When the voluntary intake of food is inadequate to meet caloric needs, calorically dense oral feedings in the form of special supplements should be the first step. If the child has a functional gastrointestinal tract, enteral supplementation offers many advantages over intravenous feeding, including the avoidance of deep-vein catheters and the maintenance of gut mucosal integrity. Intestinal mucosa can become significantly atrophied if the patient takes nothing enterally for an extended period of time [21]. Pharmaceutical companies are developing new products in accord with the latest nutritional re-

Table 1. Recommended intakes of calories and protein for infants and children (derived from [20])

Age (years)	kcal/kg Body weight[a]	Protein (g/kg body weight)
0–0.5	110–120	2.2
0.5–1	100–110	2.0
1–3	90–100	1.8
4–6	80–90	1.5
7–10	75–85	1.2
11–14	M 60–70	1.0
	F 50–60	
15–18	M 45–55	0.8
	F 35–45	

[a] Factors that increase caloric requirement: fever (12% for each degree over 37°C), surgery (20%–3%), sepsis (40%–50%), growth failure (50%–100%)

M, males; *F*, females

search findings. These products should be used to augment the patient's usual diet in order to provide sufficient nutrients for meeting individually estimated needs. The greatest limitation to the use of oral supplements in the pediatric cancer population is patient acceptance. The presence of mouth sores will limit tolerance for oral supplements of any kind, and diarrhea may be aggravated by hyperosmolarity or products containing lactose. If the oral intake is inadequate to meet caloric needs, a small soft tube is passed through the nasopharynx and stomach into the small intestine, and elemental feedings are provided as a constant infusion. Initially, the solution is infused at half-strength, and the volume is increased slowly until maintenance volumes are provided. Ultimately, the concentration of the solution is increased until the required caloric needs are met. If diarrhea occurs during the increase in volume or concentration, corrective measures should be taken. If adequate caloric needs cannot be provided by tube feeding because of diarrhea or vomiting, total parenteral nutrition (TPN) should be considered. Clinical conditions that contraindicate the use fo tube feeding include a nonfunctional or obstructed gastrointestinal tract, gastrointestinal bleeding, severe ulcerations that may be irritated by the tube, persistent nausea and vomiting, and severe uncontrollable diarrhea.

Parenteral Nutrition

Unfortunately, the pediatric cancer patient sometimes cannot ingest, digest, or absorb food via the gastrointestinal tract. Total parenteral nutrition serves as a reliable source of nutrition. Since TPN does not appear to improve survival or response to therapy, the main indication for it is to maintain normal body composition in the growing patient and to prevent starvation. Numerous intravenous solutions for parenteral nutrition are now available. A synthetic amino

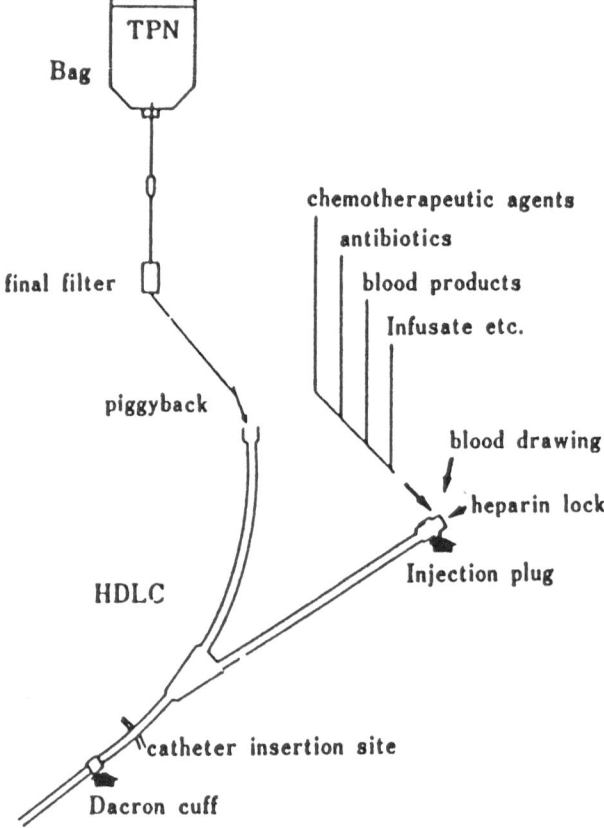

Fig. 1. Infusion system with Hickman's dual lumen catheter. *TPN*, total parental nutrition; *HDLC*, Hickmans dual lumen cather

acid source is required, and an energy source, usually glucose, is also administered. Special amino acid solutions are available for patients in hepatic or renal failure. Since vitamin deficiencies are common in young patents receiving vitamin-free TPN, vitamins should be administered daily to prevent any deficiency. Venous access is still via a repetitive venous puncture for the administration of chemotherapy and monitoring of hematologic toxicity. TPN requires a central site of infusion because of the high osmolarity of the solution, and the subclavian or external jugular route is the preferred site. We use multilumen catheters, such as Hickman's dual lumen catheter, and allow the administration of drugs and sampling of blood through the other ports [22] (Fig. 1). An incidence of subclavian vein thrombosis as high as 10% has been described in patients with cancer undergoing chemotherapy and nutritional support. Fever commonly accompanies chemotherapy, especially in patients with a white cell count of less than 1000/mm^3. The fever is not usually caused by the use of catheters, and when the white count recovers, the fever disappears [23]. However, if there is any evidence that the catheter is the source of sepsis and the infection cannot be eradicated with antibiotic therapy, the catheter should be removed without hesitation. Total caloric and protein requirements are estimated in Table 1. Thirty percent of calories are sometimes provided as fat emulsion (Intralipid). No more than 4g/kg of body weight per day of fat emulsion is given to children. Guidelines for providing adequate fluid intake must take many factors into account. In terms of body weight, adequate fluid intake is calculated as approximately 130 ml/kg per day for ages 0–12 months, 80–120 ml/kg per day for 1–8 years, and 50–75 ml/kg per day for 8–15 years. The most common abnormal finding in patients on TPN is abnormal liver function test results. The precise etiology of the liver function abnormalities observed during TPN is not known; however, several theories exist. Excessive carbohydrate administration is associated with fatty infiltration and excessive liver glycogen deposition.

One treatment involves reducing the amount of carbohydrates and replacing those calories with lipid emulsion [24]. Since the abnormalities of liver function with TPN are mild, greater abnormalities usually indicate another cause of liver toxicity.

Both enteral and parenteral nutrition have merits and demerits for nutritional support in children. It is important to adequately evaluate the nutritional status and provide proper nutritional support to patients with cancer.

References

1. DeWys WD, Begg C, Lavin PT, Band PR, Bennett JM, Bertino JR, Cohen MH, Douglass HO, Engstrom PF, Ezdinli EZ, Horton J, Johnson GJ, Moertel CG, Oken MM, Perlia C, Rosenbaum C, Silverstein MN, Skeel RT, Sponzo RW, Tormey DC (1980) Prognostic effect of weight loss prior to chemotherapy in cancer patients. Am J Med 69:491
2. Nixon DW, Lawson DH, Kutner MH (1981) Effect of total parenteral nutrition on survival in advanced colon cancer. Cancer Detect Prev 4:421
3. Clamon GH, Feld R, Evans WK, Weiner RS, Moran EM, Blum RH, Kramer BS, Makuch RW, Hoffman FA, DeWys WD (1985) Effect of adjuvant central IV hyperalimentation on the survival and response to treatment of patients with small cell lung cancer: A randomized trial. Cancer Treat Rep 69:167
4. Rickard KA, Loghmani ES, Grosfeld JL, Lingard CD, White NM, Foland BB, Jaeger B, Coates TD, Yu PL, Weetman RM, Provisor AJ, Oei TO, Baehner RL (1985) Short and long term effectiveness of enteral and parenteral nutrition in reversing or preventing in advanced neurolastoma: A prospective randomized study. Cancer 56:2881
5. Rickard KA, Kirksey A, Baehner RL, Grosfeld JL, Provisor A, Weetman RM, Boxer LA, Ballantine TVN (1980) Effectiveness of enteral and parenteral nutrition in the nutritional management of Wilms' tumor. Am J Clin Nutr 33:2622
6. van Eys J, Copeland EM, Cangir A (1980) A clinical trial of hyperalimentation in children with metastatic malignancies. Med Pediatr Oncol 8:63
7. Hays DM, Merritt RJ, Ashley J, White L, Siegel SE (1983) Effect of total parenteral nutrition on marrow recovery during induction therapy for acute non-lymphocytic leukemia in children. Med Pediatr Oncol 11:134

8. Rickard KA, Grosfeld JL, Kirksey A, Ballantine TVN, Baehner RL (1979) Reversal of protein-energy malnutrition in children during treatment of advanced neoplastic disease. Ann Surg 190:771

9. Donaldson SS, Wesley MN, Ghavimi F, Shils ME, Suskind RM, DeWys WD (1982) A prospective randomized clinical trial of total parenteral nutrition in children with cancer. Med Pediatr Oncol 10:129

10. Ghavimi R, Shils ME, Scott BF, Brown M, Tamroff M (1982) Comparison of morbidity in children requiring abdominal radiation and chemotherapy with and without total parenteral nutrition. J Pediatr 101:530

11. Hughes WT, Price RA, Sisko F, Havron WS, Kafatos AG, Schonland M, Smythe PM (1974) Protein-calorie malnutrition: A host determination for *pneumocystis carinii* infection. Am J Dis Child 128:44

12. Obama M, Cangir A, van Eys J (1983) Nutritional status and anthracycline cardiotoxicity in children. South Med J 76:577

13. Donaldson SS, Wesley MN, DeWys WD, Suskind RM, Jaffe N, van Eys J (1981) A study of the nutritional status of pediatric cancer patients. Am J Dis Child 135:1107

14. Ohnuma T, Hollad JF (1977) Nutritional consequences of cancer chemotherapy and immnunotherapy. Cancer Res 37:2395

15. Mize CE, Cunningham C, Teitell BC (1984) Undernutrition in pediatric inpatients: Repeated nutritional status evaluation. Nutr Suppl Serv 4:4

16. Merritt RJ (1981) Nutritional assessment and metabolic response to illness of the hospitalized child. In: Suskind RM (ed) Textook of pediatric nutrition. Raven, New York, p 285

17. Romirez I, van Eys J, Carr D, Coody D, George PC, Washington J, Richie E, Taylor G (1985) Immunologic evaluation in the nutritional assessment of children with cancer. Am J Clin Nutr 41:1314

18. Smith DE, Stevens MCG, Booth IW (1991) Malnutrition at diagnosis of malignancy in childhood: Common but mostly missed. Eur J Pediatr 150:318

19. Frisancho AR (1974) Triceps skinfold and upper arm muscle size norms for assessment of nutritional status. Am J Clin Nutr 27:1052

20. National Reseach Council (1980) Recommended dietary allowances (9th edn). National Academy of Sciences, Washington DC.

21. Torosian MN, Rombeau JL (1980) Feeding by tube enterostomy. Surg Gynecol Obstet 150:918

22. Lameris JS, Post PJM, Zonderland HM, Gerritsen PG, Kappers-Klunne MC, Schutte HE (1990) Percutaneous placement of Hickman catheters: Comparison of sonographically guided and blind techniques. AJR 155:1097

23. Maher MM, Henderson DK, Brennan MF (1982) Central venous catheter exchange in cancer patients undergoing TPN. J Natl Intravenous Ther Assoc 5:54

24. Wagner WH, Lowry AC, Silberman H (1983) Similar liver function abnormalities occur in patients receiving glucose-based and lipid-based parenteral nutrition. Am J Gastroenterol 78:199

Index

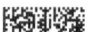